Rainforest Medicine

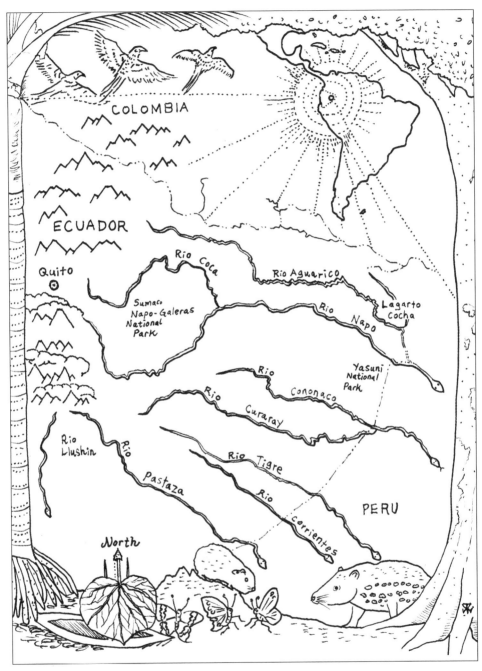

Northwestern South America, the Epicenter of Terrestrial Biodiversity

Rainforest Medicine

Preserving Indigenous Science and Biodiversity
in the Upper Amazon

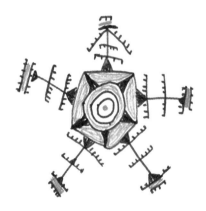

Jonathon Miller Weisberger

Foreword by Daniel Pinchbeck

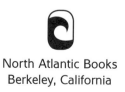

North Atlantic Books
Berkeley, California

Published by North Atlantic Books, Berkeley, California

Cover art by Pablo Amaringo
Cover and book design by Suzanne Albertson
Illustrations by Thomas Wang, Agustin Piaguaje, and the author
Artwork by Pablo Amaringo photographed by Ben Blackwell
Photo editing by Don Bright
Printed in the United States of America

Cover art: *Rondadores del Mundo* (2002) by Pablo Amaringo (1943–2009). The title of this painting means "Those Who Circulate the World," referring to spirit healers. Perhaps today we can say it's the plant-medicine tradition of the Amazon circling the world to bring understanding and healing to many. In each of his visionary paintings, Amaringo reveals multiple aspects of this traditional science. Here in the foreground we see an ayahuasca ceremony among a group of indigenous healers; radiating from beneath the vessel containing the entheogenic ayahuasca are energetic outpourings known as the *estera pinta*, the "designs mat," seen here beneath the drinkers as a rainbow-like spider-web. Ancestors as well as celestial beings of higher dimensions, and primal energies represented by jaguars, extend outward along the edges of the ceremony. Standing witness are a goddess with her scepter, and the Designs Boa. Above the drinkers is a diverse group of spirits formed from the clouds. The vision shows the human realm and the rainforest merged as one. We can see certain powerful medicinal plants and sacred trees united with realms of celestial spirits and angelic beings. Other elements include artifacts of the people's ceremonial life such as scepters, bows and arrows, crowns, ceremonial pipes, ayahuasca vessels, and ceremonial dress.

DISCLAIMER: The following information is intended for general information purposes only. The publisher does not advocate illegal activities but does believe in the right of individuals to have free access to information and ideas. Any application of the material set forth in the following pages is at the reader's discretion and is their sole responsibility.

Rainforest Medicine: Preserving Indigenous Science and Biodiversity in the Upper Amazon is sponsored and published by North Atlantic Books, an educational nonprofit based in Berkeley, California, that collaborates with partners to develop cross-cultural perspectives, nurture holistic views of art, science, the humanities, and healing, and seed personal and global transformation by publishing work on the relationship of body, spirit, and nature.

North Atlantic Books' publications are distributed to the US trade and internationally by Penguin Random House Publishers Services. For further information, visit our website at www.northatlanticbooks.com.

ISBN 978-1-58394-608-4
Library of Congress Catalog Card Number 2013023729

4 5 6 7 8 9 VERSA 25 24 23 22 21

North Atlantic Books is committed to the protection of our environment. We print on recycled paper whenever possible and partner with printers who strive to use environmentally responsible practices.

To those of you who live ardent and committed lives acting out of deep concern for the fate of our Earth and all its species, this book is most dedicated. To the people of the Earth, may it serve to educate and to enrich your lives on every continent. And to the Amazon rainforest, may it assist in your preservation.

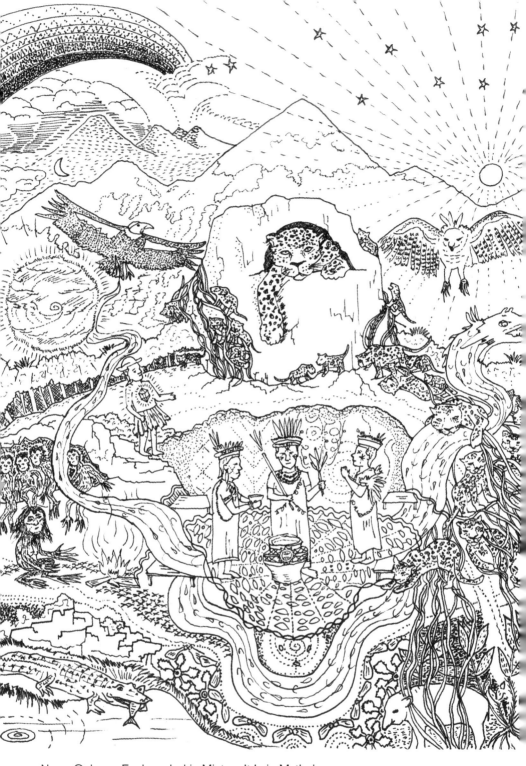

Napo-Galeras, Enshrouded in Mist as It Is in Mythology

CONTENTS

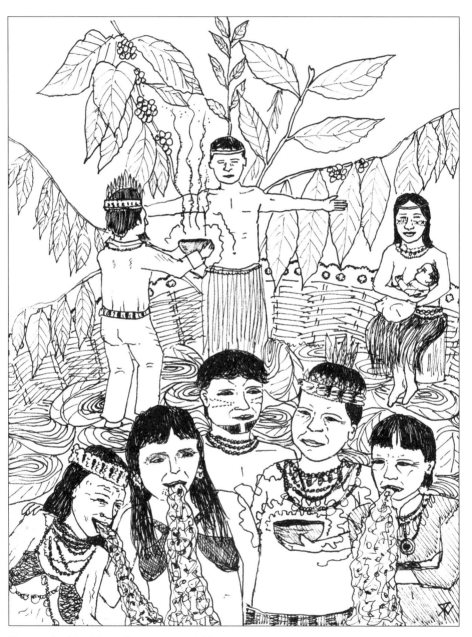

Renewal with *Tzicta*, *Guayusa*, and *Piton*

Foreword by
DANIEL PINCHBECK

I met Jonathon on my first trip to the Amazon in 1999—he was our exuberant, indomitable guide on a visit to the Secoya in their rainforest home. I later wrote about that journey in my first book, *Breaking Open the Head*. I was overwhelmed, deeply moved, by the contrast between the Secoya culture and the visible decimation of the rainforest by the oil companies, who continue to lay waste to our most precious natural resources. Since then, Jonathon and I have deepened our friendship, and, under his auspices, I have had the opportunity to sit in ceremony with the Secoya elders many times. Knowing him as I do, it is delightful for me to encounter this book—full of marvels and legends, jungle rustlings, mystical insights, animated by a gleeful spirit of camaraderie, resurrecting the vanishing knowledge and way of life of a people and a culture from which we still have so much to learn.

Although most people are only dimly aware of it, life is a philosophical expedition into the unknown. If we take our lives as journeys into vast and ever-deepening mysteries, then the true friends and teachers we meet along the way are like diamonds shining in the dark vastness of eternity. Jonathon is one of those jewels for me. We are very lucky to have his extraordinary account of a way of life and a culture so different than anything we in the post-modern hyper-industrial peak-everything West can easily imagine or absorb. We believe we know what is important, yet in our hubris and ignorance we may have forfeited the most crucial, the most meaningful, aspects of being.

Entranced by our technological and virtual spectacles, it is hard for us to realize that we need to stop, arrest our momentum, tiptoe backward to rediscover everything we have lost. Is it too late for us? Are we meant to observe haplessly as the last jungles are absorbed into industrialized wastelands, swallowed by the greedy, insatiable maw of our corporate consumer culture? Let us hope not!

According to the scientific data, within a few decades our unsustainable progress will prove more or less fatal to the planet. We will need a true alchemical miracle to salvage our civilization from the straight road we are building that leads to the abyss. As individuals, we have the opportunity to overcome our cultural conditioning. We can take a new path.

For the Secoya, living their pristine Amazonian dream of plant teachers and celestial confidantes, the miraculous was everyday; the everyday was miraculous. While our culture fixates on transforming the Earth into that short-lived abstract construct we call money, those Secoya still true to the traditional ways explore subtle and esoteric aspects of being.

During a ceremony with Tintin, one of their great wisdom teachers, I saw the irony of the situation. With his culture pushed to the edge of oblivion by the petroleum and palm oil companies, Tintin, like the other Secoya maestros, possesses so little in this world, almost nothing. Yet during the long *yagé* nights, his spirit expands to show itself as incomprehensibly vast, soaring through shimmering astral dimensions with ease and grace. Like the rest of the Secoya elders, Tintin is a king in the other dimensions, yet an orphan in this one. While our political leaders, CEOs, and masters of finance imagine themselves to be the lords of the Earth, ruling the world through their cunning manipulations, they might find themselves to be meaningless specks in the spiritual realms where the Secoya and other indigenous elders are kings and rulers.

It is still conceivable that humanity could awaken to accept our role in the larger community of life. Following the ideas of Buckminster Fuller and other great visionaries, we could use our creative and technical genius to reckon with the damage we have done to our home. If this is going to happen, the sacred medicine of the Amazon will play a crucial role. Over the last decades, when Westerners discover yagé (or ayahuasca), many have personal experiences of illumination, feeling responsibility for the natural world, discovering their solidarity with indigenous people and ancient ways. Often people's lives change radically as a result. They change their career, their friends, their diet, and shift life priorities.

Through my experiences, I accept that most of the miracles and wonders Jonathon describes in this book are true: When we properly align with creator, anything can happen. As dire as our situation now appears, we may be able to transform it, to restore the Earth, once we overcome greed, pride, and ego—once we are ready to learn from the celestial forces who know us so well, who wait for us to contact them.

Rainforest Medicine provides wonderful insights into how we can do this, laying out a path we can follow. As a spiritual primer, it couldn't have arrived at a more perfect moment. I hope you will enjoy it, and take its lessons to heart.

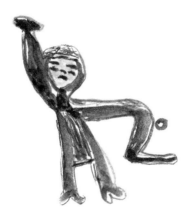

Man Reaching for Knowledge

Daniel Pinchbeck is the author of *Breaking Open the Head: A Psychedelic Journey into the Heart of Contemporary Shamanism* and *2012: The Return of Quetzalcoatl.* He is cofounder of Evolver.net, executive director of the Evolver Network, and executive editor of Evolver Editions, an imprint of North Atlantic Books. He is featured in the documentary *2012: Time for Change.*

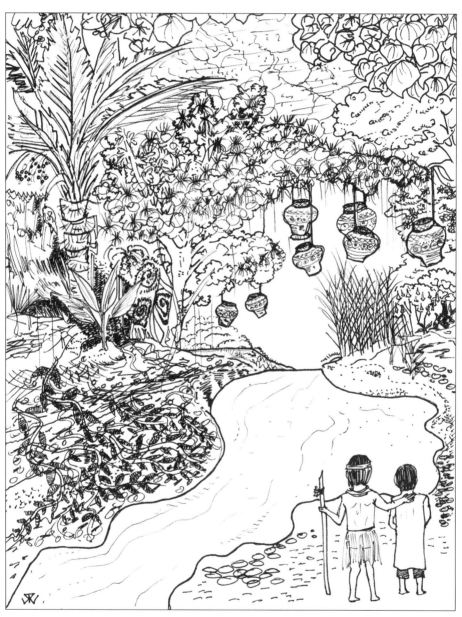

Spirit Vessels Hanging from the Yutzu Trees,[1] from the Kichwa Legend of the Juri-juri

PREFACE

Rainforest Medicine is a synthesis of over twenty years of ground-level experience in ethnobotany, rainforest conservation, and documentation of vanishing traditions in the upper Amazon regions of Ecuador and Peru. The information collected here is intended to impart critical environmental and cultural information, reaching out to enhance our collective knowledge of the essential, vital, and vanishing Amazonian traditions and ecosystems. Through glimpses into the spiritual life and science of the Secoya, Kichwa, and Waorani peoples, their ancient legends and practices surrounding the use of visionary plants, and the rainforest realms in peril, I hope to awaken more interest in this body of knowledge. By shedding light on the diversity and importance of the rainforests and the appropriateness of ancient ways, this book aims to be a meaningful contribution toward safeguarding the forests' perpetual value. I hope it can inspire readers to awaken to a culture of service, an approach to life that benefits the entire web of creation, a humble orientation to others that is capable of shifting the destiny of planetary evolution from the dismal direction of conquest and destruction toward the noble and heartfelt interconnections of sustainability and symbiosis.

All the great time-tested traditions of the Earth urge us to think beyond our own needs. They inspire us to consider the needs of others both human and nonhuman, present and future, as if they were our *very own* needs (which, from a Oneness perspective, they are), and to act upon this. Protecting what's left of Earth's great tropical rainforests and striving to record and understand the collective wisdom of the region's people is among the most valuable legacies we can leave to the future.

Given the transcendent importance of the rainforest for planetary well-being (I refer to oxygen production, carbon sequestration, and the myriad natural processes beyond comprehension that occur there daily), we must view the rainforest as a natural laboratory filled with the fruits of millions of years of evolution. From our human point of view, there are plants that heal certain ailments and others that reveal great secrets; yet above all, the tropical rainforest itself is a great medicine. This ecosystem is a mainstay of the planetary immune system, a perennial stem cell capable of renewal and fertility. It is an ecosystem that all Earth's species need in order to be healthy, to maintain climate stability, and to continue life as we know it.

It can be said that the link between the natural environment and people is the basis of culture. Our cultural heritage unifies people with plants, with our sustenance and medicine, with the elemental powers and the natural cycles. The cultural context is relevant to herbalism, agriculture, and all plant use in all societies, and it is particularly crucial for understanding uses of the so-called "plant teachers." If we are to best comprehend the roles that these sacred plants play in peoples' lives, we must understand the time-tested traditions that have evolved with human use of them. It is precisely these traditional guidelines that have allowed the sacred plants to act as positive agents among people and societies (as opposed to the negative "drug problems" of heedless Westerners).

The indigenous knowledge and fundamental plant-use guidelines that I attempt to convey (though I'm just another outsider) are miniscule fractions of the cultural wisdom accumulated over countless centuries in the equatorial rainforests of the upper Amazon. My idiosyncratic selection of scenes, historical happenings, legends, myths, and stories told to me is intended to illustrate the potent magic and sheer beauty of Amazonia, as well as the importance of protecting these regions of mega-biological and cultural diversity. By depicting imagery and imparting information about plant-medicine traditions and other aspects of indigenous science from several distinct Amazonian societies, I attempt to pass along bits of these societies' wisdom, and to add some critical context and advice for interested novices and contemporary shamanic aspirants.

It is now apparent that a modern style of ayahuasca usage and exploration (a.k.a. "journeying") is being developed among Westerners, and for this process to be authentic, it is crucial to have reference to the principles and core teachings of the ancient ways. Those outsiders who are being drawn to learn more about the plant-medicine science of ayahuasca should take special note of the respected guidelines that have long governed its use. By making the effort to be better informed about all dimensions of plant medicine, including the original beliefs and methods, we can make personal decisions to develop an increasingly respectful, deep, revelatory, and appropriate relationship with these sacred plants and traditions. Only in this way will their secrets unfold to the benefit of humanity and all of nature.

Contained within this ancient mode of science, at its simplest and most practical, are profound methods for contemplating wholeness and reestablishing a personal connection with the whole. These methods rectify critical misperceptions and cleanse the individual of many false assumptions taken today to be truths. When properly prepared and administered, ayahuasca—also known as *yagé,* pronounced ya-HEH, as well as a number of other indigenous names—can realign one's worldview and way of perceiving nature, showing how to find a sense of place within the human community as well as the greater community of all life. In the hands of a master of this plant-medicine tradition, the energies it allows access to can be channeled to help other people regain inner balance, healing, and renewal. The people then may find themselves more aware of their participation in the creative unfolding of the universe, as co-creators expanding the original celestial order.

Some of these indescribably beneficial effects can be obtained even through the truncated and limited experiences of so-called "ayahuasca tourism," as well as more serious experimentation and journeying. Mild doses on a regular basis constitute a church service for some people, a healing purge for others. Such modern uses of this traditional medicine are evolving and spreading across the globe, and may help us find a way out of the ecological and spiritual mess we're in—certainly they're a route worth exploring as we seek to prevent the collapse of Earth's life-support mechanisms. However, in the Western rush for instant gratification, it's vital to try to understand that this science is vast, and its full comprehension requires a dedicated lifetime of study, which few Westerners (and, indeed, few modern Amazon dwellers) are capable of, or have the necessary courage to undertake. Yet it seems that elements of traditional Amazonian medicine can integrate into modern times to help realign people with a more holistic and natural mode of being.

As regards both palliative and preventative care, sacred plant-medicine traditions and the ancestral approach to healing are perfectly tailored to each person's specific needs. Exactly how ayahuasca works to awaken within each person a brand-new opportunity for renewal is a bit beyond rational comprehension. This is why the traditional elders among the Secoya people say, "The yagé knows; we don't know."

Though my intention is not to promote ayahuasca usage, for that is a personal choice (and some say the medicine summons you, not vice versa), it has been my calling to expend great amounts of time and effort to record some of the vanishing traditions of indigenous peoples in their rainforest realms of the upper Amazon, and now to offer this mythographic and ethnobotanical documentation. While it is far from a complete account, readers will obtain a broader and deeper understanding of this part of the world and its rich medicine traditions. The need to understand and respect these traditions is even more relevant now that the "grandmother medicine" is becoming known worldwide.

Furthermore, *Rainforest Medicine* seeks to convey both the profound value and extreme vulnerability of the tropical rainforest, as found in the upper Amazonian and tropical Andean regions of Ecuador, the country I was raised in. I hope readers will sense the urgency of somehow being a part of stopping the blind destruction of native forests and cultures, and looking deeper at the wisdom and healing available from plants, the natural world, and the ancient ways. Herein are offered glimpses, ideas, and visions of how to go about doing this.

I am morally driven to bear witness to the annihilating effects of the expanding colonization frontier and non-sustainable resource extraction occurring in the rainforest, such as oil production, logging, and the expansion of oil-palm plantations on ancestral indigenous lands. The industrial machine is harsh in its erasure of traditional ways of life, and the caustic colonial mentality inhibits the transmission and upholding of ancient or different ways.

I convey a small portion of these rich traditions through my own experiences, stories told to me, and my adventures among the forest people, including remarkable masters of deep knowledge and healing capacity. When I was growing up in Ecuador, I visited the rainforest often. As a young man I became involved in rainforest conservation and cultural revalidation efforts together with indigenous people. Though I now live primarily in Costa Rica, I continue to assist with various environmental and social projects in the Andes and upper Amazon. As a result of working together and becoming close friends with families that adhere to tradition as much as possible in their turbulent new society, I am able to pass on whatever vestiges of the old ways and ancient wisdom I have managed to gather. This knowledge was shared with me from their open hearts, not to create a closed society of eso- teric knowledge, even though in the past this information was for the most part held in secrecy. Today the elders know that we have come to a time where the secrets of nature must be shared in order to facilitate people's awakening.

It's a challenge to find contemporary interpretations and relevant ways to connect these ancient truths to the lives of actual people in the current of modern times, without diluting the meaning or the essence of these truths, especially when they are taken out of their context; this is the challenge I have set for myself in this book.

From 1990 to the present I have been fortunate to participate in various rainforest conservation efforts, some more successful than others. From 1990 to 1994 I worked on the physical demarcation of Waorani territory, during which 130 kilometers of boundary lines were created to delineate their legally granted land title. Our entrance to this territory was the oil boomtown of Coca, from which we traveled long distances to the end of the slippery black oil roads, then walked into the pristine rainforest. Deep in Waorani territory I participated in a process that achieved the indemnification and relocation of thirty colonist settler families, members of the Shuar ethnic group who, following the oil roads, had settled on Waorani legally titled lands. This process of clarifying the boundary lines largely halted a six-year war that had been escalating between these two groups.

Meanwhile I was also working with the Mamallacta family, members of the Kichwa ethnic group, in the outskirts of the town of Archidona, to oversee an initiative to demarcate and protect the Napo-Galeras isolated limestone massif, a project that led to the mountain's inclusion in Sumaco/Napo-Galeras National Park. During these same years I made periodic visits to the Kichwa community of Amazanga outside Puyo, helping channel funds from grade-school "save the rainforest" bake sales and private donations that led to ancestral land reclamation through a process of land acquisition. These efforts helped create the Llushin River biological reserve bordering Sangay National Park, or the *purina tambu,* which means a "place that's walked to," a remote place in the rainforest far from the bustle of village life, where traditional ways and ceremonial life can be upheld.

In 1995 I began working with the Secoya to recoup some of their ancestral homelands at the lagoons of Pëquë'yá (Pëquë: black caiman, *Melanosuchus niger; -ya,* river) on the border with Peru. This effort continued for the next five years and ended in successfully achieving recognition from the Ecuadorian government of the veracity of the Secoya people's ancestral relationship to this place. I had an apartment in the town of Baños, far from the Secoya lands along the Aguarico River, and I traveled back and forth across the colonization frontier. I was fortunate to have the opportunity to befriend many of the elders and the greater community and to work with them on various projects. Another collaborative cultural revalidation initiative led to the publication of several booklets for the local schools on the uses of medicinal plants, both in Spanish and in Paicoca, the Secoya people's language. All the while I collected and documented plant lore and traditions, collaborating at times with some of the best botanists in the field in advancing our understanding of the rainforest.

A more recent initiative is that of Wairachina Sacha, "Rainforest of the Purifying Winds," an attempt to gain maximum protection status for one of the most significant intact stands of Tropical Wet Forest left in Ecuador (and perhaps the world). It is adjacent to the eastern slopes of Napo-Galeras and is at the pinnacle of terrestrial biological diversity. A deeper glance into this magnificent rainforest ecosystem is offered in the chapter called "The Eyebrows of the Andes."

Another long-term project involves collaborating with members of the Costa Rican and Ecuadorian park services to share experiences and enhance the protection of existing national parks and designated wilderness areas. Without appropriate management, these areas remain threatened by colonization and various business interests, despite their protected status.

It is a direct result of these efforts to join in solidarity with the people of the rainforest that I have been able to learn firsthand about many aspects of the indigenous traditions discussed in these pages.

Each chapter of *Rainforest Medicine* explores a different facet of the vast and diverse topic of indigenous plant-medicine traditions. Herein I've attempted to create a composite picture of the rainforest, its diversity, the people, and the sacred plants—one that will stand the test of time as an anthropological account of this place and era. Here are myths and legends and some interpretations, cultural vignettes, accounts of rainforest conservation efforts, plant-medicine lore and practical botanical information, illustrations, photographs, travel stories, personal experiences and those of traditional elders, shamans, and spiritual masters, parallels between ancient spiritual traditions, and much more, boiled down and refined into what I hope is a potent linguistic brew. Readers will deepen their understanding of this unique part of the planet and renew their zest for being part of co-creating a better world.

Chapter 1 is an introduction to ayahuasca, indigenous science, and traditional Amazonian medicine, providing an overview and outlining general concepts that will facilitate readers' comprehension of the chapters to follow. Chapter 2 addresses the shadow side of local medicine practices—the sorcery and superstition that degrade the true spiritual science. Chapter 3, "The Gift of Ayahuasca," is packed with facts about the sacred plant, including sample legends of its mytho-historical origins.

Chapter 4, "Elements of the Ayahuasca Experience," explains some of the key aspects of an ayahuasca healing ceremony, such as the songs that are sung to invite the spirits and relay their energy, and the visual imagery or "designs" brought by the medicine. Chapter 5, "Preparing a Proper Brew," relates the Secoya method of harvesting, handling, and cooking the ayahuasca vine and its varying admixture plants.

The designs turn brightly colored and fragrant in Chapter 6, "The Celestial Summer of the Cicadas," in which I discuss old-school Secoya gatherings where shamanic knowledge was shared and new adepts graduated. Everyone, not just the drinkers of yagé, participated in these annual pilgrimages. Here is revealed the fullness of the ancient shimmering medicine science—the timeless teachings of the *Ñañë Siecopai*, "God's Multicolored People," who gave the Secoya this plant-medicine tradition as a form of intellectual technology to facilitate remaining close to their heavenly origins. The encounter with those celestial beings deeply influenced the traditional ways of the Secoya people. A glimpse into their sacred culture reveals the profundity of traditional yagé usage, particularly during the celestial summer of the cicadas, the season when the heaven people approach the Earth and the drinking of yagé is most auspicious.

Chapter 7 takes us even deeper into the rainforest to visit the utterly unique world of the Waorani, Ecuador's most recently contacted indigenous group, including thoughts on the recent (2013) clashes with the last clans in voluntary isolation. I discuss how I was able to learn about the pulsating heart of their most independent way of life, and their distinct view of *miiyabu* (what they call ayahuasca), which sheds an entirely new light on this topic.

Chapter 8, "The Eyebrows of the Andes," explores the mighty rainforest of the upper Amazon and tropical Andean regions, where we find some of the highest biological diversity per square foot on the planet, particularly in the Tropical Wet Forest life zone found only at the base of the Andes. We learn about geography and rare plants, gaining appreciation of the jungle setting from which this tradition of plant medicine has evolved. While the Waorani, Kichwa, and Secoya communities that I write about have little in common and their languages are vastly different, they all recognize Napo-Galeras as a sacred mountain, here in the heart of this biodiversity stronghold. Enshrouded in mist as it is in myth, Napo-Galeras generates respect. This chapter summarizes some of the efforts and adventures that led to protection of Napo-Galeras as an Ecuadorian national park and discusses current conservation efforts. Halting the blind destruction of this and all precious rainforest bioregions should be among humanity's top goals right now.

Chapter 9, "Lineage Holders of the Ancient Traditions, Deep Forest and Urban," is a compilation of short anecdotes illustrating the life and ways of various traditional elders, yagé drinkers, sages, *medicos,* and *ayahuasqueros.* These lineage holders of the plant-medicine traditions are Kichwa, Waorani, and mestizo (mixed ancestry), and they are my co-workers, friends, and instructors whose wisdom and experience made this book possible. By sharing a little about these remarkable people, I help readers understand their lifelong devotion to knowledge and service.

Despite the tremendous complexity of information and the interwoven tapestry that constitutes the worlds of ancestral indigenous sciences, the tropical rainforest, and the modern relevance of ancient wisdom, I've attempted to at least touch on the different arenas of interest so that this book can appeal to a wide range of experts and laypeople alike.

In reference to my own personal experiences with the medicine, I have been fortunate to participate in ceremonies with traditional elders in many different indigenous settings, through many years of dedication as well as at considerable cost, and I have been able to confirm for myself much of the information in these pages about what the grandmother medicine can potentially teach us. I have had the good fortune of walking the land and living among the people in their rainforest wilderness. My ethnobotanical studies have allowed me to learn about the deep knowledge contained in nature, and my work as a rainforest conservation advocate has allowed me to understand the polemics and complexities behind these issues. Despite having lost my credits at Humboldt State University after the one-year leave of absence I requested turned to ten, I know my time in the field has been well spent. The education I received in the great university of the rainforest has given me a much broader vantage point from which to write about these profound and utterly important topics today.

Although *Rainforest Medicine* is written partly as a personal memoir, I have attempted to not exaggerate the significance of my personal experiences or make it seem that this work is greater than others. Much better writers than I have given us personal accounts of travels and insights from the upper Amazon. And better-funded and more effective conservation groups have tackled greater dilemmas. Still, I feel that my investigations and experiences are worth sharing in the hope of offering yet another perspective, and a further deepening of our understanding of these issues.

I sincerely hope that *Rainforest Medicine* can serve as a valuable tool in the promotion of cultural and environmental education as well as protection and reverence for the mighty rainforest as we struggle toward planetary sustainability. By offering views of the vanishing world of traditional peoples, sacred plants, and the once seemingly limitless rainforest, I hope this text will stand as a record of what was and as an urgent plea to humanity to awaken to what is, as we realize the potential of what can be and thereby ensure that the true treasures of the original Earth shall remain here forever.

Jonathon Miller Weisberger
Osa Peninsula, Costa Rica, 2013

Chapter 1

Introduction to Indigenous Science in the Upper Amazon

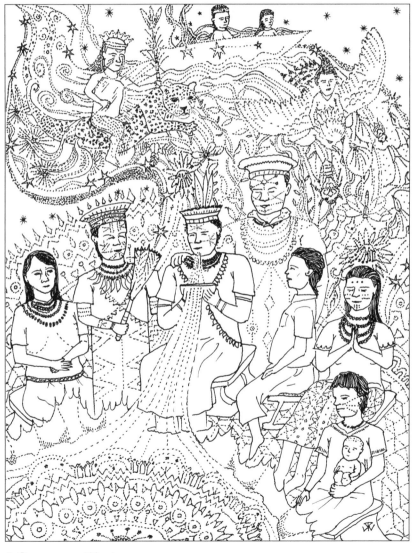

A Ceremony of Yagé

"The principle of the reality of spirits has been tested and supported cross-culturally by shamans for thousands of years. Once
one understands that spirits exist, much that appears impossible
to outsiders is really quite understandable and even may be subject to replication."
    —Michael Harner, *Cave and Cosmos*[1]

If science is defined or understood as a mode of seeking knowledge,
a means of approaching and interpreting nature in a way that can
be demonstrated to others, then the plant-medicine traditions of the
Amazon as they have been practiced constitute an authentic scientific
discipline. Following a systematic methodology, these traditions aim
to build and transmit a common body of useful, reliable knowledge.
It is evident that there is both an "indigenous science of yagé" and an
"indigenous science of ayahuasca," distinct in tradition and lineage;
and for that matter, many more traditional sciences exist that are distinguished by the culture or region, such as the indigenous science
of *miiyabu* (among the Waorani), the indigenous science of *natem*
(as practiced among the Shuar and Achuar), and so forth. Use of this
sacred plant medicine is widespread throughout the Amazon basin
among many indigenous groups, all with their various methods and
names for similar plant-medicine brews. Ayahuasca, the vision vine,
occupies a central position in the distinct branches of the indigenous
traditions that this book explores.[2]

It is important to view the collected knowledge of the indigenous
peoples as a form of science (the modern West's most valued route to
information), and thus to give it the respect it has always deserved. The

practitioners of this science hold it in great respect, and their larger community respects those who pursue this revered body of essential wisdom in the correct manner. In fact, in tribal societies the world over, as anthropologist Michael Harner writes, "The shaman is referred to not only as 'one who sees' but also as 'one who knows' or as a 'person of knowledge.'"[3] Experiential (firsthand) knowledge is clearly the most reliable and concrete in any effort to comprehend both the visible and largely unseen worlds. Shamanism explores an area that contemporary Western science knows little about—the mind. Its archaic techniques are based not on a religious philosophy but on empirically validated methods that produce the experience of ecstasy and educate the student about states of consciousness. In the Western tradition, the term "gnosis" refers to knowledge experienced as self-evidently true.

While most of us will be unable to dedicate this lifetime to learning the deep truths of plant medicine and its advanced methods of steering energy—in other words, full shamanic training—it's still possible to benefit from the accumulated field of knowledge and to have our own experiences of gnosis. This book aims to properly facilitate such learning through insight into the plant-medicine traditions of the upper Amazon. I have attempted to record and preserve a fraction of this fading visionary world and also to intimate what's possible in our collective future if we can expand the myopically material and limited scientific conception of reality that prevails in the West. (I refer to the mindset and actions that are engulfing the planet under the paradigm of scientific materialism and corporate consumer culture, with no acknowledgment of spiritual practices or energetic therapy.) To truly journey with plant medicine, it is necessary to temporarily suspend rational judgment and enter into a non-dualistic, more mythical and thus magical mindset, where supernatural and natural meet as one and the same, in a process of co-creation where there is no separation between viewer and what is being viewed, where thoughts are louder than thunder and adhering to stillness a must—a mindset that the ancestors of the Earth's ancient spiritual traditions knew well but modern philosophy and scientific method deviated from. The latest discoveries in many fields of science are bringing us back full circle, but that's a complex tangent for this limited space.

A non-dualistic paradigm enables complete integration with the veracity of life, leading one toward a balanced and integral conception of self, community, and nature. Having stood the tests of time, the plant-medicine traditions of indigenous peoples must be seen as a true holistic science illuminating a simple and original way of life that helps keep people on track. This spiritual science—yes, the two words go together!—not only addresses healing from mental and physical illness, it enables attainment of complete understanding of the heavenly order; purification and strengthening on multiple levels of one's entire being; and spiritual, physical, and universal integration. The discipline of the science and its spiritual guidance extend to the governing of the self and contributing to the protection of family and community. Through enacting a highly civilized and humane way of life, essentially aligning with and becoming the cosmological order itself, we are able to recognize that we are not separate from it.

A Celestial University

I would venture to call this ancient science the original educational system of the inhabitants of the Amazon region, based on the teachings it imparts and on the fact that it relies on a communion between a master, teacher, or guide and his or her apprentices and students. When adhered to correctly, this system's curriculum provides a complete development of all the aspects of the self—intellectual, physical, and spiritual. Integrating all facets of one's being into one fortified whole is the union of the accumulated knowledge of an adult with the inherent innocence of the child. This new being is a child of heaven and a child of the earth, and few malignant forces can impact it. Of course, nothing is invincible, and the major exception is when this science is misused, as in the workings of sorcery (see the next chapter) or the accidents that can occur when not adhering properly to the guidelines that regulate this plant medicine's use. Nonetheless, many of the noble elders, spiritual masters of this tradition, have lived to great ages, and some have apparently risen from their tombs after death. Others just vanished when their time came.

There are many marvelous stories that illustrate this phenomenon. Here is one about a great master of this tradition, a Secoya by the name of Waosutú. He was an effective healer and well loved by the people, but others were jealous of his abilities and they ganged up to kill him. To their utter amazement he did not resist, simply letting himself get killed. A few days later, no one could believe what they were seeing: there was Waosutú as if nothing had happened to him! They planned another attack and killed him again, and again he let himself get taken, just like that! Some time passed and he appeared again unharmed. This greatly disturbed the crooked and corrupt people who wanted him dead and they planned yet another raid on his home. This time Waosutú maneuvered off to the side, escaping their attack. He dove into the river, and a large anaconda was seen slipping through the water. After this Waosutú was never seen again.

In the indigenous science of yagé as practiced among the Secoya and western Tukanoan speakers of northwestern Amazonia, master and students attempt to reproduce the same phenomena, time and time again, in order to obtain complete understanding (for example, meeting spirits known as Jujupai, "doctor people," also known as Ujá-pai, "immortals who heal," whose energy becomes the healer's resource in bringing about efficacious transformations in well-being). Those who repeatedly delve into this mystery strive to recognize unchanging truths within ever-changing realities, such as the eternal existence of the legions of celestial beings and divine immortals, referred to among the Secoya as Wiñapai (about which more below).

This indigenous scientific method, with its highly sophisticated way of interpreting and relating to the world, enriches life's every moment, especially under difficult circumstances. It enables what can be called miracles. Adepts may receive the ability to heal illnesses, gaining both spirit helpers and a clear understanding of how to offer appropriate guidance in alleviating suffering, achieving balance, and improving quality of life, including complex and apparently incurable cases that involve intertwined physical, emotional, mental, and energetic blockages.

The process begins by training the body to imbibe larger and larger amounts of alkaloid-rich plant medicines, as well as learning the ancient methods of energy circulation. Graduation occurs after one has drunk hundreds of houses of yagé, a "house" being an all-night ceremony where copious amounts of yagé are drunk after being prayed over or "cured" by the *yagé uncucui* (a seasoned drinker of yagé and master of the ceremony). To complete the basic training, students must drink at least five houses of extra-thick *ëo yagé,* also known as *weasiko yagé* (yagé that has been cooked extra thick to a honey-like or corn gruel-like consistency—see the section on preparation); to hone their healing abilities, they must also drink two other sacred plants, *ujájái (Brunfelsia grandiflora)* and at least five houses of *pejí* (an ancestral variety of *Brugmansia suaveolens*). This graduation process can last years or even decades, and merely drinking the plants does not guarantee graduation, because one has to adhere to strict discipline and moral virtue.

There are rare cases where initiates can graduate in less than a year, and if so it is due to their particular energy alignment—in other words, virtues they were born with. The Secoya speak of a Colombian man who came to drink yagé with them in the 1950s. With only a few houses of yagé he graduated as an accomplished master; before he returned home, he healed many people who were ill. But for the most part it is considered dangerous to learn too quickly. In general one must digest the deeper aspects of the teachings little by little. They come through life experiences, or they are passed through the master and the medicine from the spirit realm. To learn yagé's deep truths, one must suffer and undergo personal sacrifice. For in order to achieve celestial visions, one must inevitably undergo many types of anguish and uncomfortable situations, if only from the rigorous *dieta,* which in and of itself is a challenge to uphold.

To follow a dieta, Spanish for "diet," means that one abstains from particular foods and practices temperance, sobriety, and self-restraint. All known traditional cultures that utilize yagé employ some kind of dieta. All dietas include practicing celibacy at the onset, and then, when married, sexual abstinence before and after the ceremonial period. Many also feature exercise routines, breathing practices, invocations, and the learning of sacred incantations and prayers, along with the admonition to adhere to a virtuous life. Considered to purify the body, make it receptive, and capture the attention of the helping spirits, dietas are the internal self-discipline program of the indigenous sciences of the upper Amazon used to acquire spiritual clarity, strength, and power. They are discussed further in Chapter 4.

It is much easier to learn certain peripheral aspects of the tradition, such as the use of medicinal plants to heal, than it is to graduate as a fully-fledged master. Yet there are cures that only the masters can effect. To graduate as a healer in the science of yagé is a life-long devotion of study and experimentation, involving many levels and types of graduation.

According to traditional guidelines from the good Secoya elders, a definitive step-by-step process is required to gain the highest knowledge. First, one must meet the beings of the celestial realms, the Wiñapai (always-new people or beings). This takes time and is accomplished by strengthening and refining every level of one's being, and drinking copious yagé well-cured by the master, all in an effort to see and be accepted by the celestial immortals.

There are legions of these celestial immortals, each with their own provenance, these being the vast and distinct heavenly islands, realms, or celestial abodes—referred to in Paicoca (the Secoya people's language) as *matëmo qiro*. These are energy abodes that transcend time and space, and I like to refer to them as "immortal islands."

Some of these spirits live within the heaven of the water, including the Jujupai (doctor people) and the Ocopai (water people); others reside within the heaven of the air, such as the Sëra Wiñapai (swallow-tailed-kite immortals) and the Wakara Wiñapai (ibis immortals). Some live inside a heaven inside the earth, such as the Jaicuntipai (immortal people of the high hills), who reside inside the sacred mountain of Napo-Galeras. Others are ancient progenitors of life who resided on the Earth eons ago, such as the Ometsiapai (eternally-young people of the summer), the Mañoko Wiñapai (starry always-new people or starry immortals—such as the Usepopai, people from the Pleiades), and the Wiñatsi'bonsë (always-young-and-fresh celestial children).

It is imperative that one meet the celestial spirits first, for if one meets the demons and spirits of the Earth first (the *Watí*), it may be difficult or impossible to see the Wiñapai. After meeting the celestial immortals, then students can meet the earthly spirits, which now will not succeed in tempting them to do harm. After further training, when students enter deeper into the learning, they meet Pai'joyowatí, "People-soul/heart-spirit," the chief of the Earth spirits, the one who ordains all the Watí.[4] Given his status as commander of the Watí, it seems appropriate to refer to this character of the world of yagé as the "Demon King." Despite this name that is my personal tag for Pai'joyowatí, he himself does no harm; he is the ally of the healer.

When the shaman wants to show you this spirit and blows it on your yagé, then you can see it, but otherwise it's close to impossible to find Pai'joyowatí on your own, as a traditional Secoya elder told me. Here is the account he shared: Pai'joyowatí appears and looks at you in the eye, at which moment you need to look right back at it without blinking. Most suddenly it reaches out, grabbing for your heart. In that same moment you need to reach out and grab for its heart, which can be seen hanging in his chest. Both of you are there looking at each other, holding each other's throbbing hearts. You give his heart back and he gives yours back. After this he will never again attempt to harm you and will forevermore help you to heal the people.

From the place of a strong and virtuous physical foundation, the student attempts to embody the celestial knowledge learned through the drinking of yagé. By upholding earnestly the accompanying discipline, he or she makes progress along the path of spiritual self-development. To establish communion with celestial immortal beings and be accepted among them, one must have a master who knows the way, and one must be consistent in strengthening his or her virtue and self-discipline. To accomplish this is far beyond mere intellectual seeking. It is the great school indeed, an authentic university of life. It requires the aid of an experienced guide, someone who has been through the process and knows the path to the "celestial islands"—one who is wise and has slipped past the multiple traps. Having embodied these "designs" (visual messages and pathways), the master can make them known to the student. The master can introduce and even "marry" the students to the beautiful heavenly beings. Of course the master can only go so far, he can only show the way. The students must have the highest respect for the tradition and adhere firm in their discipline; they must strictly follow the dieta outlined by the master, a self-challenge program that is intended to help one accomplish the refinement and concentration of energy until it becomes piercing and pure, enabling the students to see the truth of the nature of life. Only thus can the student receive the energy designs of heaven, brought forth by the celestial beings that are revealed to the student by the master. Once the student is initiated, he or she can learn directly from the heavenly spirits.

It's possible to meet the heavenly spirits on one's own, but it is much more difficult. To succeed at this one must be generous and diligently uphold selfless service to others. One must maintain a predominantly calm disposition, while holding no discriminations, being supportive and non-judgmental, and keeping to this as one's sole purpose, ready to serve at all hours of the day, even in the middle of the night if called upon, or need be!

Above all, from the most traditional perspective, to be accepted among the celestial immortals was to prove to oneself the unity of all existence, visible and unseen. By obtaining a calm and poised disposition and a generous and round character, one secured and served— embodied and lived—this unity. This approach to every moment was seen as the most transcendental of life motives—it was life's meaning and truest purpose! To sway from this was to court disaster and bring about destruction not only of oneself but also the world one is part of.

It is evident that this process reinforces the vital importance of adhering to a celestial moral order, to universal principles and universal law.[5] When one is in alignment with this cosmological order, then one can tamper in the destiny of things and know that one's actions are appropriate. One builds a spiritual foundation with the accumulation of many virtuous acts as well as a precisely accurate body of knowledge and experience. The practices are then transmitted intact to the next generation, thereby ensuring continuity.

In contrast to Western scientific protocol where the quest for knowledge is primarily intellectual, relying on sophisticated devices, the indigenous scientific method has never drifted from the fact that it must be a complete and integral self-delivery—that is, a full integration of intellect, body, and spirit. Practitioners understand that to know the material sphere completely one must first strive to know the hidden, more esoteric spheres of life, considered to be much larger, several hundred trillions of times larger, which is just another way of saying that it cannot even be measured. Spirit is larger than the human mind can comprehend, and too vast for it to invent. We must make ourselves sensitive enough to discover it.

When properly approached, the indigenous science and the sacred way of life revealed through the teaching of the plant-medicine traditions allow for an authentic communion with the entirety of the spiritual realms. One does not need to go anywhere to discover this truth. It can be found in the here and now of one's very own body, and this then sets the tone for life in the human world. Maybe this is what Secoya grandmother and traditional elder Matilde Payaguaje meant when she said, "There is no need to look elsewhere. This is the people of wisdom's most ancient tradition. Here all knowledge culminates. There is no other greater wisdom. This one covers all humanity and encompasses the entirety of the universe."[6]

Despite the chaos of social structures in collapse and the devastating daily encroachment of the "modern-day machine" into the primal rainforest, the students must stay steadfast in their discipline all the way to the very end, and then discover that there is no end, and no beginning either, only the moment, the exact felt presence of the immediate now and the need to be awake to this, as a caring person in every moment of this existence. . . .

It's beyond ironic and bordering on tragic—almost as if the cosmic serpent has actually eaten its own tail—that the part of human culture rejecting symbolic modes of knowledge for pure rationality (i.e., Western civilization) must rediscover DNA and other confirmations of ancient knowledge thousands of years later. At long last and in multiple disciplines, indigenous knowledge and modern science are meeting face to face, yet it is precisely now that this ancient knowledge is disappearing almost faster than the rainforest itself.[7]

A Unified Worldview and Way of Being

Visionary plant medicine in its ceremonial context is a portal to unseen realms, one that was made known in order to help the temporal maintain its connection to the eternal. Countless generations of people worldwide used this portal before it opened in our modern societies. Ayahuasca was given to humanity in the mists of prehistory in order to maintain or, when necessary, regain an essential balance, back when the people lived in total intimacy with nature, when the human spirit was still pure enough to commune with the spirits.

In cases of the original peoples of the Earth it meant alignment within the celestial energy ray of their stellar origin.[8] To understand indigenous science we have to try to understand their unified non-dualistic perspective. The closest I have come to observing it embodied in living humans is when I spent time among the Waorani people, deep-forest dwellers. I was able to befriend many of the old Waorani when I collaborated on a four-year initiative from 1990 to 1994 that accomplished the physical demarcation of 130 kilometers of boundary lines indicating portions of their government-acknowledged ancestral lands. (I write more about this project and the Waorani in Chapter 7.) The Waorani people's outlook has evolved as a singularity, with no outside human interference, only the unhindered workings of great nature. Their language has no known linguistic affiliation to any other. They developed and survived within and alongside the evolution of the rainforest and its thousands upon thousands of species, which the Waorani say they themselves helped sing into existence.[9] In a traditional context up to about the 1960s, the average Waorani would know no more than seventy or so people in their entire life. Members of this ethnic group have their own unique approach to indigenous science. The Waorani do not pursue the famous DMT-related visions and purging of the yagé brew. Yet they nonetheless have a deep association with both nature and spirit and live a life in which spirit upholds matter, where spirit guides and matter follows. Among the Waorani, and still to this day, the actual use and knowledge of miiyabu (their word for ayahuasca, the *Banisteriopsis* vine) is restricted primarily to the families of *iroinga*, the spiritual masters—the ones who embody, as the Waorani say, *"Duuuuube Waorani bai,"* the "good way of the ancestors," the most ancient ways of the people.

One of the memorable Waorani elders was an old warrior named Mengatue, who became my mentor. Given Mengatue's reputation for shamanic knowledge, when I first went to his house I asked about miiyabu. He reached up into the thatch above his fire pit area—many Amazon residents keep their medicinal herbs above the fire to stay dry in the humidity—and pulled out a dried-out, rolled-up little leaf. He said, "With this, I can see my enemy's image in the smoke of the fire. When I blow, that person is dead." He then told me that the Waorani don't use sorcery and are adamantly opposed to it. "When you touch this plant," Mengatue clearly stated, "spirits come to your side as if they were your children. If you get angry at someone, they can go and kill that person. This is why it is very dangerous to touch this plant. If you are touching this plant you must not get angry. This way no one will be harmed and your life will not be ruined."

Mengatue also said that a lost Waorani can find his way back home if he or she rasps with a sharp knife some powder off one of their own teeth and mixes it with one leaf of ayahuasca. The mix is consumed and the Waorani will remember how to get home. You might see this as a metaphor for us modern people, where "home" can be defined as an original state of pure consciousness that allows for living an undivided life with the whole.

In this light one can understand the Waorani use of miiyabu as a type of homeopathic association. In this approach, less is more and more is less. But few can be as sensitive as the ol' Waorani who have spent their entire lives in the deepest and most remote rainforest regions.

The Waorani knowledge of miiyabu goes far back in their oral history. Mengatue said that in ancient times the ancestors of the Waorani came to Earth from a constellation called Namocapoweiri. The Earth's first people, who were called the Monakageiri, lived on the leaves of the miiyabu mashed with the fruits of the *petohue* palm *(Jessenia bataua)*.[10] This oily, highly nutritious drink rich in alkaloids was their only food source, their very staff of life. It is likely that human beings and the sacred plant-medicine vine of ayahuasca have been in intimate association for a very long time. Knowledge of the Waorani people's rarified approach to miiyabu broadens our own understanding and gives a different perspective on the distinct avenues of indigenous science and ancestral plant-medicine traditions.

In modern times, it is perhaps the Secoya who have taken the drinking of yagé to the furthest possible limits. From their spiritual science we learn of an approach to this plant that is different from that of the Waorani yet equally deep. The Secoya people's rich ceremonial curriculum was woven into the traditional way of life wherein each individual strove to prove and embody the truth and the cosmology of the ancient spiritual science, with their entire lifestyle revolving around this. People once aimed to become the living cosmology itself and to "wear it on their bodies," as Secoya traditional elder don Cesareo Piaguaje says.[11] This is symbolized by the *sehué* necklace, a traditional adornment of the Secoya people and of the yagé drinking tradition. It corresponds to a constellation called Sehue'wë, and by wearing the necklace one is symbolically placing a part of the sky upon one's body. To me, in my way of interpreting the ancient traditions, this can mean nothing less than yet another heartfelt way of aligning oneself with universal law: by "wearing the cosmology on one's body," one becomes the cosmology. It is yet another beautiful way of confirming that we are not separate, that we are one, unified and indivisible, with the living, breathing universe.

Many people I have met from traditional indigenous villages in the upper Amazon were raised in the presence of regular yagé ceremonies. They heard the elders singing at night and sharing their wisdom early in the morning, day after day. They understand the significance of the tradition—its grounding in spiritual truths—though some of them may never have drunk yagé.

There are always some families that hold true to tradition despite all the changes and difficulties they are obliged to undergo. The indigenous people who follow the traditional ways, whether they drink the medicine or not, are for the most part quiet in their demeanor, steadfast, and generous—early to rise, free with their smiles, community-oriented, and always ready to help. In fact, the oldest and most joyous people as well as the most realistic and grounded community members in all the traditional villages I have lived in and visited are the drinkers of yagé and their descendants, and it is thanks to these spiritual guides and their families that many aspects of traditional Amazonian medicine have survived into the present.

Despite the traditional use of ayahuasca presently vanishing, certain peripheral aspects of the cultural heritage and the healing arts can still be seen among Amazonian peoples.[12] This includes an intimate knowledge of nature, natural cycles, biodiversity, local medicinal plants, dietary traditions, and work and exercise ethics; methods of fasting for gaining spiritual strength and accomplishing purification; creative endeavors such as traditional music, art, community sports and games, string games, and riddle solving; mythology, cosmology, storytelling, face painting, and ceremonial life; and a contemplative mode of practical work such as agriculture, house and canoe building, and the making of utensils for everyday need, such as hammocks, nets, sifters, and baskets. Another noteworthy aspect of traditional life is the symbolic mode of viewing existence through legends, dreams, metaphor, and mythology, as will be detailed in the coming pages. Underscoring all, the indigenous wisdom continues to uphold the culture of service and to promote morality and integrity as requirements for a happy life.

Though traditional ways can still be seen in practice today, many of the deeper aspects are vanishing among the Amazonian people as they are subjected to exploitation and Western-style poverty. Can the ancient ways coexist with modernity? Can they adapt, can they triumph? Can we rescue these practices and somehow remake them anew in a new age?

Good Masters Are Hard to Find

In the collision between the remoteness and purity of the rainforest realms and the crassness of consumer culture, the difference is so extreme that for the most part there has been no authentic or practical method for this medicine system as traditionally practiced to integrate and adapt to the changing times. Consequently its normal transmission has been interrupted or completely severed. The youth are drawn to the jobs and debauchery of the colonizers, and the discipline to maintain a strict diet and other forms of abstention is largely lacking.

And, sadly, many of the good elders' time has come and they have left this plane of existence. Worse, many have been prosecuted for their practices and some outright murdered, even by their own people. This has occurred on many occasions since the advancement of colonization, and one can only conclude that such acts result from fear and ignorance. One of my esteemed friends, don Esteban Lucitante of the Secoya community, was brutally clubbed to death in 2005 with his own oar by drunken youth from a neighboring Siona village on the Rio Aguarico. They lured him with a false story about a child in need of healing. He went alone in his canoe, in full ceremonial regalia and with yagé, to help. Then, as he was tying up his canoe, they attacked him. He was a selfless healer loved by many.[13]

I shared many laughs with Esteban, nicknamed "El Mágico." Yagé drinkers tend to be dynamic characters who love to laugh! I was able to participate in ceremonies with him between 1995 and 2004. This was during a period when he started drinking yagé again after many years practicing Evangelical Christianity. He realized that as an evangelical he could not heal; after his nephew died and he hadn't been able to help, Esteban felt frustrated and sad, and chose to reawaken his earlier practice of drinking yagé. He returned to Colombia for a while, where he studied again with his older brother, a Cofán master living in the mountains. (Esteban was a half-Siona, half-Cofán married to a Secoya.)

In 1997 Genaro Yiyocuro, the last graduated Siona yagé drinker along the Rio Aguarico, was shot in the head early in the morning while resting in his hammock after a ceremony. He was killed by another community member whose aged mother died in their canoe, possibly from heat stroke. The son blamed it on the yagé drinker and without question or pity walked up to his house and shot him. Similar incidents have happened to other traditional masters and their disciples. Cecilio Piaguaje was a great drinker of yagé who is said to have walked over the surface of a lake one early morning after a ceremony; he was poisoned by colonists in the 1970s. A similar fate has befallen several of the traditional masters and their students of the Siona, Secoya, and Cofán peoples just in the last fifty years.

Maybe the path these masters follow is so pure that it highlights the darkness that is purged in the course of the medicine's constant work. The corrupted people who commit these crimes have taken it upon themselves to see that this light no longer shines, affirming the dismal notion that there is no room in this now-corrupted world for this type of purity. Of course there is also a (displaced and mainly superstitious) fear of *brujos* or sorcerers, people who acquire spiritual power and pervert it for evil ends.

Ultimately the practitioner of this science has little to talk about and for the most part will not be understood by the majority of people today. It is difficult to even begin teaching if a student doesn't have time and patience. Whether one is a local youth or an eager foreigner, there are few opportunities to enter and sustain this learning process, one that is loaded with obstacles and can last for decades. In order to fully understand and embody the ancient science at a level that would allow one to teach its continuation, there needs to be the opportunity for transmission.

Like the burning of the ancient library at Alexandria or the supremely ignorant incineration of stacks of invaluable Mayan codices, the loss of knowledge we are experiencing as the last of the traditional elders pass from this physical plane of existence without heirs to their knowledge—as well as the very environment in which sacred plants grow—is a tragedy occurring right now as you read these lines, one that could well be beyond redemption.

Many of the last living traditional elders and spiritual masters are getting too old to drink yagé, and their time to teach has passed. For all these reasons, good masters are hard to find today. If you have the great fortune of finding one with whom you wish to study, please respect the following advice. Never be a burden on the master; rather, find ways to lighten his or her workload so that you can be supportive of this person's ability to be an anchor for heavenly energy on the Earth.

Despite the difficulties of getting on a spiritual path and staying there, the sincere seeker should not be dissuaded. Many spiritual traditions remind one to follow nature not man, and the universal subtle law is present everywhere, as are spiritual resources for those who seek them. The truth can be found and cultivated—one needs nothing more than a sincere heart, a willing hand, and an appropriate level of self-determination, time, and patience!

Humans must follow nature, since nature follows the true way of heaven. Nature follows the way of the celestial immortals, the never-failing source of inspiration, the eternal masters of this and all sacred medicine traditions. From the Taoist teachings comes ancient confirmation of this:

> "My divine nature is as pure as the nature of Heaven.
> The constancy of my strength is like the Sun
> The lucidity of my mind is as bright as the Moon
> My tolerance is like that of the good Earth
> My forwardness is effortless, like flowing water
> My calmness is like the mountains."[14]

A Show of Power

Several elders I have met attest that the following account is true. The story was initially told to me by Fernando Payaguaje's son-in-law, who was also his assistant and yagé cook, my good friend Reinaldo Lucitante, a witness to the event.

Among the Secoya, at the time of graduation, the newly coronated master will demonstrate his powers for the sole purpose of making it known that "I'm ready to serve." Don Fernando Payaguaje, a graduated drinker of yagé whose words are preserved in the book *The Yage Drinker*,[15] is said to have gathered the people at the lagoons of Cuyabeno the morning after a ceremony of yagé. He was ready to reveal his powers so the people could see that he could be trusted as a guide. At 9 AM he held his hands up and said, "There is a mirror that holds all in place as we know it. I am going to turn this mirror around just for a moment." Shortly afterward the sky went dark, as if nightfall had come prematurely; a few minutes later the sun again shone in the sky. Did don Fernando have exact astronomical knowledge that enabled him to calculate the moment of a solar eclipse? Is there a mirror that holds all in place, as he said, which can be tampered with by the hands of a person of advanced spiritual development? Either way, one thing is for sure, Fernando had deep knowledge of nature—in all regards he was a highly advanced practitioner of indigenous science. When this great master died in the village of San Pablo de Cantesiaya in 1994, there was an earthquake and several people saw two large jaguars loping off into the forest; their tracks were seen by everyone, right there in the village center.

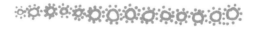

Hakë ("father" in Paicoca) Cesareo Piaguaje, my great friend whom I love like a father, is among my best informants and teachers of the traditions of yagé. He is an elder of the Secoya people, a healer and guide, and a friend to all who come with a good heart and clear intentions. Thanks to his generosity and patience, I was able to gather a large amount of the information I convey regarding the traditions of yagé among the Secoya people. He often talked about his grandfather, *Yai* (Jaguar) José. "When Yai José graduated," Cesareo enthusiastically told us, "he tied a sewing thread between two balsa trees and stepped up onto it. His body was light and he started dancing and singing, back and forth along the thread, which didn't sag even once! In one hand he was holding a gourd of yagé, in the other the *matipë* [ceremonial scepter]."[16]

Did Yai José achieve union with universal forces to such extent that he could pretty much levitate, defying gravity? It seems as though he did. Is this not an advanced form of science? Cesareo himself never failed to be impressed by this event and would relate the story with pride that he was the grandson of this great man.[17]

The masters demonstrated fantastic realities such as these on very rare occasions, as they believed that if they did so too many times the drinkers could become sorcerers. Perhaps such a show of power would only occur twice—once when the healer was ready to show the people that he or she was ready to selflessly serve the community, and once at his death.

Obtaining Healing Plants from the Celestial Realm

One could make a case that the indigenous scientific method does a few things that modern-day science can't, such as bring back objects from other dimensions. Consider, for example, the yagé drinkers' accounts of retrieving healing plants from their visits to the celestial realms, the matëmo qiro or "immortal islands," abodes of the Matëmopai and Wiñapai. (These terms refer to the heavenly people and always-new divine immortals, respectively. As on Earth, there are multitudes of beings in other realms, each group with its own name.) Certain of these plants, kept and cherished by the elders and their descendants as botanical treasures, seem not to be found anywhere in the wild, despite the presence of thousands of plant species growing in the surrounding rainforest.[18]

For example, the Cyperaceous sedge (genus Cyperus) called *watí nuní* in Paicoca is cultivated by the elders and said to be the gift of an ancient yagé drinker. It is known to ward off negative spirits. Another example is the *ñumí*, in the genus Piper, whose leaves are used to alleviate babies' growing pains. The fragrant tubers of the watí nuní or the aromatic green leaves of the ñumí are used to make *ocoraca*, sacred water cures. They are slightly mashed into some water contained in a small gourd and infused with a specific energy pattern through singing and blowing. These remedies are effective for rebalancing a wide array of disorders related to the central nervous system, in addition to the specific uses just mentioned. The songs employed for making cured water are called *ocoraca jujuyë*, and this constitutes a sacred art practiced only by the yagé drinkers, who have the energy to properly cure the water and make it effective for healing. These songs are the ageless melodies of divine immortals, stretching from the dawn of creation, from the place where the primordial energies conceal within themselves their shimmering wisdom.

Some of these sacred plants are family treasures. One such plant is named *pai saye nuní* (people-departure nuní, *Cyperus* sp.) from the custom of mixing it with *bonsa* (*Bixa orellana*, known in the West as annatto) to make a paint to use on the body of a deceased person so that the spirit is seen by the celestial immortals and guided to the eternal heavenly abode. In the words of Celestino Piaguaje, nephew of the accomplished drinker Fernando Payaguaje,

> Nuni is an herb that is born from a tuber, which is what a healer received, in one of his visions, from the hands of the angels. My uncle Fernando takes care of that plant and no one has it but him. He doesn't give it away. And if anyone stole it from him, it would have no effect, because it only acquires its power at the will of the healer. When I was a child, he gave some of those roots to my mother, but when she later became an Evangelical, she let them die off. Nuni is employed in the following way: you dig up the roots, wash them and grind them into powder, and then mix them with a little achiote and paint the body

of someone who has just died. The healer paints only his deceased relatives in this way. I saw Fernando do that in Cuyabeno with my two grandmothers. He painted two lines on their faces, on their nose, also on their arms and feet. Sometimes people who are not relatives can be painted, if they have requested it. On other occasions, nuni is employed as a curative. Then, you split the roots and let them drip their juice into water, which is then drunk.[19]

Celestino's aunt, Joaquina Piaguaje, Fernando's younger sister, has said about nuní:

My father acquired that plant, which came from a family of Canteya [River of Wild Cane, or Putumayo] people who had reached the sky and lived along the banks of the river of eternity. That's why my brother Fernando knows about it now. If you put it on someone who is dying in their hammock, the nuni will bring him back to life; you'll put him in his grave but he'll go out from it to the great river. When the sky people see him coming, they'll go down to the healer and ask, "Where did this man come from, who has come to us?" "I sent him to you, because he's a relative of mine." "Well, if that's so, he can stay."[20]

Master yagé drinkers have received sacred plants in visions so that they may confirm their communion with the celestial immortals and refresh their varieties. They then plant them near their homes. Other species obtained from the realms of divine spirits include yagé *(Banisteriopsis caapi)* and yagé ocó *(Diplopterys cabrerana)* as well as sugar cane *(Saccharum* spp.), chili peppers *(Capsicum* spp.), and other medicinal and fragrant herbs. The latter include such species as *uncuisí,* meaning "to drink" or "to make soup from"—it is *Renealmia alpinia,* a cultivated and cherished ancestral heirloom of the Secoya people. There is an intriguing story of its domestication, and here I offer only a portion. The account reveals the depth of indigenous symbolic imagery.

After a long saga of a battle between human and supernatural forces, the head of Wanteanco, the Jaguar Mother, is carried to the high branch of a towering *imigëi* tree *(Ceiba pentandra)* by a large white-headed laughing falcon called the *macawá*. The skull, dried to a bleached white from the hot sun, remained there, rolling back and forth along the branch, singing. One day a wind blew the skull from the branch. Upon hitting the ground it shattered, splattering the small seeds inside. These seeds grew to be the first uncuisí plants, but because the plants were surrounded by snakes from their earliest appearance, they could not be approached. Some people with a long pole got hold of some fruits and planted the seeds elsewhere. Again snakes were ever-present around the plants, but this time there were fewer of them. Again the fruit was taken with a long pole and the seeds planted in yet another location. This time the plant grew without the snakes and the people were able to continue to cultivate it, and some Secoya people grow it until this day.

There are many more plants that the elders attest were brought back from the celestial realms, as well as a great collection of ancestral cultigens obtained through mythic encounters. I have documented more than 120 varieties of ancestral cultigens, plants found nowhere in the wild, and many accounts of their supernatural origins.[21]

More Mysterious Affirmations from the Yagé

Other affirmations of the existence of the celestial realms include what can be called miracles that occur during the inebriation of yagé. In the Secoya village of San Pablo de Cantesiayá, my friend Maruja Payaguaje, the daughter of the late Fernando Payaguaje (the great yagé drinker mentioned above), displayed to me a necklace with celestial charms tied to it that was given to her by her father. I have also been shown celestial palm nuts brought back from the world of yagé by the late Esteban Lucitante. They are in all regards similar to those of the *sidá (Astrocaryum murumuru)*, yet in different shapes, like little trumpets or small circular bells, shapes not found on the wild sidá palms that grow in the forest. Don Esteban said, "Whenever I use my yagé necklace and meet new Amazonian ethnic communities or even modernized native communities, the natives, particularly the elders, always look especially attentively at the yagé trumpet-seed around my neck. After a few moments of looking at it carefully they are always astonished by it, because they know it does not come from the material world; it comes from one of the spiritual worlds of the people of yagé."[22]

The elders shared stories with me about other phenomena brought about by the "people of yagé" such as profusely aromatic smells that fill the ceremonial lodge as a sign of the arrival of the Wiñapai, or when objects sought in visions appear in 3D reality. For example, one tale involved a ceremony in which all participants were in a deep meditative trance at dawn after having drunk thick ëo yagé that night. A disciple's spirit reached the celestial realms. Then at the conclusion of the ceremony when the man woke up and raised his head, at that moment a sound was heard like cloth ripping, and bunches of celestial palm nuts began falling onto the ground. In anticipation that this would happen, since they had planned to attempt it, the ceremony leader had woven a new basket in order to gather the nuts. This he did—most of the others still being held in trance and deep in their visions. He gathered several handfuls to fill the small basket, then blew on them to cure them, and covered the basket. Shortly afterward, the nuts that had bounced and rolled across the floor vanished as suddenly as they had arrived, but the nuts blown on by the elder drinker were still in the basket. Each of the drinkers was able to take a few to craft their necklaces with.

On another occasion, the ceremonial lodge was filled with flying swallow-tailed kite hawks called *sera wiwé* in Paicoca, the Secoya language. The master reached out and grasped one of the birds. Then he most unexpectedly broke open one of its wings. He raised it to his lips and through the hole in the bone he blew a marvelous song that echoed in piercing reverberations. Then he threw the bird in the air and it flew away unharmed! The same thing could also been done with a fish: The morning after a ceremony, abundant fish would be swimming upriver. The master who had summoned them would go to the river's edge and take one in his hands. He would break it open like the bird's wing and blow a marvelous song through a vertebra, then throw the fish back in the river and it would swim away unharmed.

Such phenomena both confirm the integrity of an eternal celestial order and serve as a response to humanity's deepest desires for proof of the existence of the immortal abodes. The notion of a celestial realm, of a spiritual land with no sin or suffering, has always been at the heart of all people, together with a desire to simply live in peace and dignity. In countries where social and government structures are failing and ecosystems are being strained to their breaking point, the knowledge of these realms offers hope in deeply troubled times and, as in the past, provides impetus to adhere to a virtuous way of life including non-impulsiveness, generosity, patience, genuine happiness with life's every blessing (even the smallest ones), and a high level of tolerance to the hypocrisy that fills this modern world.

Meeting the Chiefs of the Animals

"The Indians communicate, individually or through their shamans, with animals and plants; this communication is not meant to be with the zoological or botanical species, but with energies the Indians believe to be inherent in wildlife. Daily shamanistic and personal practices and understandings link people's health, food, sex, social interaction and metaphysical experiences into a coherent belief system in which man is inseparably joined to nature."

—Gerardo Reichel-Dolmatoff, *The Forest Within: The World View of the Tukano Amazonian Indians*[23]

The role of yagé as a trans-dimensional energy portal is illustrated by a plethora of accounts from the elders of today and yesterday—and who are we as Western skeptics to say they are not factual? The Austrian anthropologist Gerardo Reichel-Dolmatoff was told many anecdotes that relate to our topic, such as the following passages from his book *The Forest Within:* "Shamans claim that they visit the masters' abodes, and penetrate into their interior during their narcotic trances. This they have to do in order to talk to the Master of Game, and convince him to release some of his charges for the hunters and fishermen, so the people may eat." He expands on this theme a few pages later:

> Two energy circuits are involved here: One is the cosmic circuit of cosmic *bogá*. (In Tukanoan understanding, the organizing principle of the universe is the life force called *bogá* which produces semen/pollen leading to insemination, growth, and maturity, followed by death and the regeneration of semen/pollen, in which all living beings participate.) The other is the local circuit, which links the hunter to his prey, the fishermen to his catch. *Vaí mashë's* (the master of the animals) houses, be they hills, pools, or whatever, are imagined as repositories of energies represented by game, fish, and fruits, womb-like storehouses and breeding grounds from which the surrounding environment has to be constantly replenished. In order to achieve this, new energies have to enter *Vaí mashë's* domains, and these consist of human life forces.

Later he writes, "In speaking of this topic [the Tukano Indians] always emphasize that '. . . when drinking yagé we see our *maloca* [house], our gardens; we see our forests and we see the fish and we see the game animals.' Another shaman said: 'with yagé we see the abodes of the game animals, of peccary, deer, curassow, we see them all.'"[24]

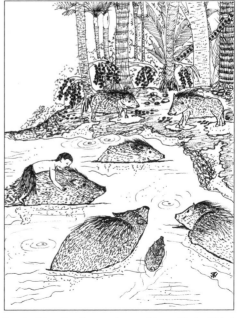

Here is an example from the Secoya people that is both entertaining on its surface and mind-blowing in its depth (if you are open to yagé's reality). For starters, we'll accept the word of those who assert that each animal species has a spiritual leader. One of these leaders is the Sensetañe, a

Carried by the Peccaries to Meet Their Chief

Wiñapai who is chief of the peccaries (wild boars) that live in a spe-cific region inside the earth. The Sensetañe is known to have his own yagé, used among the peccaries to bring animals from under the earth onto the surface, and then to bring them back inside where they are protected. This enables them to enjoy their paradise even more after having refreshed themselves with a change of food and environment. The paradise of the peccaries is a place where their favorite palms hang thick in fruits, always ripe and low to the ground. In joyful ease they eat and lounge in the mud pits.

After one has passed the temptations of sorcery and learned to heal, the next step in traditional Secoya yagé drinking is to achieve the ability to summon animals, and first among these are the wild boars and the fish. Through the inebriation of the yagé, the graduating disciples and master drinkers enter into the realm of the peccaries and request per-mission from the chief. Then the Sensetañe may temporarily open and close the portal between the peccaries' realm and the humans'. The pec-caries come running out onto the earth, stumbling close to the village, at times even walking right up to the home sites, giving of themselves so that the people may live. Often, though, when the peccaries come near the lodge, the people in the yagé ceremony may be immobilized in their hammocks, so drunk that they are not able to hunt or kill them. Other villagers, recognizing why these boars are so close to the village, take the animals and later give meat to the yagé drinkers, knowing that they were too drunk at the time to acquire any for themselves.

I once actually saw this occur, at a ceremony with several traditional elders who agreed they would call the peccaries because they needed the food. Sure enough, the following morning just behind the yagé lodge were the peccaries! Soon several had been killed and gutted by the Secoya elders and were being smoked on our little fire.

When summoning animals is being practiced for the first time, dur-ing the inebriation of yagé the body of the student whose spirit went so far as to enter this realm thrashes on the ground; maybe he is even screaming. He might have fallen from his hammock and possibly been placed back and tied in by family members or helpers concerned for his safety. The elder master, singing until dawn, maintains the sacred space. I have been told by the last elders who know this art that they now, for the most part, refrain from this practice. Today, with so many colonists nearby, and with the youth having converted to Christianity and often now working with the logging and oil companies, the disadvantages of revealing these skills are too great in the face of new lifestyles not sensitive to the ways of spirit. The practices are ridiculed, feared, or not respected. Or perhaps if the Earth's true abundance were recognized by the wrong people, such as the colonists, they will kill too many boars and sell the meat, or maybe some Secoya are no longer as generous as in the past and will hoard the meat—all of which can bring on negative retributions from the spiritual chief of the wild boar who delivered them, possibly bringing harm to the shaman. This is but one small example of how the rapid, often overwhelming changes of modernity have smothered the ability to uphold this spiritual art and science.

The following narrative was imparted to me by Cesareo Piaguaje. A Secoya village was moving locations. A very sensitive young boy felt shamed by an incident with some other youth, and when the village left, he vanished into the wilderness and lived alone. He began to follow the wild boars. At first they were scared of him, but then they got used to him, eventually accepting him as a friend. They crossed a large river and encouraged him to hold onto their backs while they swam him across (see illustration on page 25). On the opposite bank were abundant palms with fruit bundles hanging low to the ground—they had reached the paradise of the peccaries. Suddenly their chief appeared, the Sensetañe, who held the boy in his arms and transformed him into a celestial being.

Yagé drinkers in the village saw in their visions that the missing boy was still alive and performed a ceremony to call him back home. Many people held hands in order to form a net, and he came running through and they caught him. The yagé drinkers healed him by singing magical incantations on him and shaking the leaves called *mamecocó* (made from the broad-leafed grass *Pariana radiciflora*), and it was not long before he adapted to village life. He became a skilled drinker of yagé, proficient at summoning peccaries. He was able to call the red peccaries, which have an especially thick layer of fat (a prized characteristic), right up to the peoples' houses. Sadly, though, he was killed by jealous sorcerers.

With these types of reports in mind we can begin to see how truly profound is the world of yagé to its original inhabitants.

Raising and Lowering the Mythic Underworld Nets

Don Cesareo shared with me the following. In order to protect their territories from others and to make the land rich for themselves, drinkers would hold yagé ceremonies to raise and lower the underworld nets. The people called the fish and wildlife out from inside and simultaneously hid large jaguars, snakes, and dangerous caimans underwater and within the underworld. They would then fish and hunt and live well. When they were ready to leave, in order to deter other settlers from their rainforest paradise, the masters and students would again drink yagé ceremonially to raise and lower these nets—this time hiding the fish and wildlife back under the world and taking out the jaguars, poisonous snakes, and large black caimans to protect the cherished land. In such ways relatively few people maintained large rainforest territories. This sounds like nonsense, but it is the truth of these people, and something that still occurs to this day. (See illustration on page 33, "Raising and Lowering the Mythic Underworld Nets.")

Cloth, Thread, and Needles from the Crab Jaguar's Store

Another intriguing entity from the world of yagé is the Camiyai, the Crab Jaguar (see illustration on page 29). This entity lives inside the dimension of the water, where his house has a room with variously colored cloth, twine, and sewing needles, all neatly stacked up like goods for sale. This deity of the earth does not actually sell these goods but rather gives them as gifts to the yagé drinkers who with their wisdom and dedicated service make our world a better place. If a person can concentrate his or her spiritual energies enough to even arrive there and enter the Crab Jaguar's store, he or she will receive these gifts. In his house the Camiyai is like a person, and if you visit he is generous, benevolent, and kind. There, under the water, one can breathe as if in the air.

Cesareo told me that when he was a child he wore a white cotton tunic that his grandfather Yai José had brought back for him from the store of the Crab Jaguar.

Crab Jaguar also has a fierce side. He sometimes puts on a particular magic tunic that transforms his human form into a big jaguar with crab claws. In this state, he is capable of sinking canoes and even snapping them in half. In the past he would do harm, because he is an ardent defender of the wilderness and doesn't like it when a lot of boats go over his abode. Eventually it gets intolerable for him to live where there is too much human activity, and he departs for more remote wilderness regions, his existence known by few.

Spiritual masters of old were able to obtain these valuable items from the Camiyai, once again proving the existence of this reality by bringing back completely dry cotton cloth, twine, and sewing needles from inside the realms of the water. The Secoya tell of a true occurrence, not a legend, of a Spaniard named Ligerio who proved the truth of the Camiyai and retrieved a ball of dry cotton from inside the realms of the water.[25]

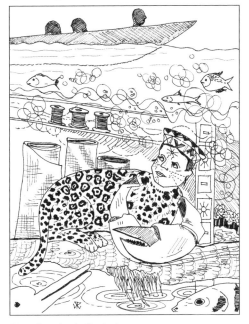

The Camiyai, Crab Jaguar

It's not possible to list all the phenomena spoken about by the drinkers of yagé—for instance, the Menkoyiyi, like a giant anaconda with splotched patterns decorating its ears, and long fangs like a jaguar and long whiskers, who embodies control of the weather through the power of electricity (lightning), protects wilderness regions, and expedites universal response and retribution; its name can be translated as "electric-eel water-dragon." Then there is the Añapëquë, whose name means "boa caiman." Cesareo calls it the "freshwater whale," also relating to it as a giant catfish with an extra-large mouth. This creature with its magical powers has been known to suck down boats passing over its underwater abode, usually at the locations of giant whirlpools and remote lagoons. It is believed among the Secoya that this mythic beast swallowed up the Spanish conquistador Francisco de Orellana, whom they attest disappeared at the mouth of the Amazon.[26] Also in the realms of the water are the Tsiayapai, the "River People," and Ocome, who is a divinity of the water—he is the husband of Waitsantsame Nomio, "Half-fish Half-woman," who is a mermaid. On land there is Wanteanco, also known as Yai Hakó (Jaguar Mother) or Yaipai Hakó (Jaguar People Mother). She is beautiful and kind during the months of the celestial summer and appears as a wretched old hag during the rainy season. Today she is a deity or immortal elemental power of the Earth, but long ago she had a body, until she was killed by a shaman. Her brain transformed into the seeds of the uncuisí, an important Secoya food used to add flavor and nutrients to soup. The Ocoyai, the Water Jaguar (who is the Jaguar Mother's sister), has a short neck and a flat tail, and it travels through underground passageways that allow it to move effortlessly from one river system to the next. All these mythic creatures and more the yagé drinker must learn about and see, and in some cases pacify, for they are intimately associated with obtaining complete knowledge of their realms.

The Future of Ayahuasca

It is a sad truth that despite ayahuasca's great potential to steer humanity and the benefits it has granted many people in the past (not to mention its straight-up and barely-believable magic), this art and science is fading fast in its traditional context. Simultaneously we see that it is passing to the West, in a new form of syncretic ayahuasca use that is developing among interested people the world over. It seems as though as one door starts to close, another opens, and one could reckon that the medicine is moving to where it needs to go, striving to offer people the ultimately satisfying challenge of awakening and becoming a conscious human being. Although this may be the case, any conscious human being cannot help but be saddened by the tremendous loss of biological and cultural diversity taking place today.

Despite all this, while the traditional modes of transmission crumble, hope for the future of the yagé tradition comes, ironically, from outside the rainforest—from elements within the very cultures that seem bent on destroying it all. Globally, as more and more people seek reconnection with original nature and their true identity, they are participating in ayahuasca healing ceremonies and/or seeking health through the use of various botanicals from the Amazon rainforest. The ability of indigenous science, traditional Amazonian medicine, and ayahuasca to assist people in attaining insight, balance, and wellness has been proven on countless occasions. Due to the effectiveness of this medicine, it is inevitable that we will see it gain in popularity, and this will—in ways beyond imagining, as ayahuasca assists people in their personal journeys—help salvage both the medicine traditions and the rainforest environment itself.

In a world governed by corporations and driven by profit margins, even the knowledge of top scientists is not respected, let alone that of feathered masters. Nevertheless there will come a time when indigenous science and modern scientific methods will merge their strengths to help steer humanity back on course. The spirits, deities, and immortals revealed through the drinking of yagé want this more than anything else. This includes enacting sustainable alternative economies and appropriate progress on local levels (as opposed to massive development), opportune education and loving upbringing of children, protecting the sources of pure water and air, caring about the methods used to raise our food, and immediately protecting Earth's mighty rainforest and wilderness areas, home of these great traditions and most diverse terrestrial ecosystems.

Meanwhile this knowledge will continue to help people and communities as it expands beyond the jungle, and I want to believe that nothing can stop it. It is evolution at work, the constructive cycle of the universal energetic flow manifesting itself, gaining momentum and daily getting stronger. More and more sincere Westerners are studying with *maestros* or joining a type of church that honors this medicine, and more and more books are being written on it. I sincerely hope that the information and anecdotes in *Rainforest Medicine* will promote this beneficial phenomenon. The ripples reach far beyond the plant-medicine traditions, which ultimately are simply tools for our awakening.

So despite the loss of much of the original body of knowledge, peripheral forms are being passed along. From these seeds, there can exist a future when the vines again flower, and these arts and ways are respected and able to flourish anew in the rainforest and the world over.

Chapter 2

Degradation of the Spiritual Science:
Sorcery and Superstition

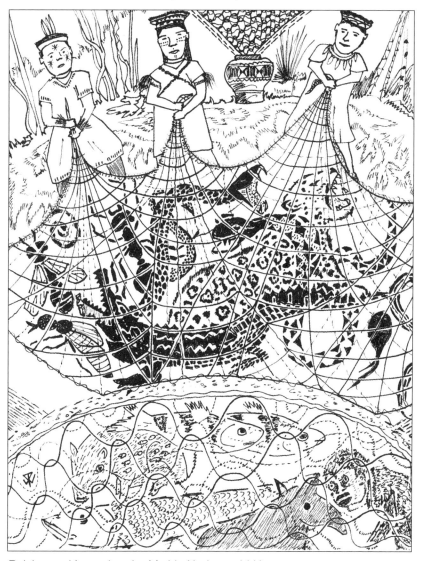

Raising and Lowering the Mythic Underworld Nets

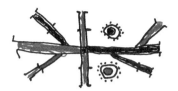

"We don't realize the point at which we become evil."
—Bessie Head, *A Question of Power*[1]

As one learns to transcend the relative dualistic realms, the master drinkers of yagé and their students clearly distinguish between good and evil, a necessary prerequisite for opening the way to any form of effective communion with divine immortal spirits. Thus, choosing to always follow the path of goodness, selfless service, and virtue is at the root of the authentic and original form of this spiritual science. However, some practitioners of these arts and sciences—often lacking appropriate training and a good ceremonial guide, and possibly having experienced many negative incidents in their lives due to hardship and despair—have deviated from the spiritual path and operate with a nebulous distinction between good and bad. They will do both, or essentially whatever circumstances and people request of them.

This tendency can be aided and abetted by earthly spirits, because they are much easier to see and interact with than heavenly spirits. Thus witchcraft requires less skill and personal discipline than healing. Furthermore, earthly spirits need humans in order to enact both their negative and positive traits. These spirits bring out the best when working with advanced healers firm in their convictions and virtue who use them to heal, and they bring out the worst in weak people, manipulating their lower impulses and leading them to act out convoluted fantasies of jealousy or vengeance. This is how ayahuasca becomes associated with sorcery and malice, a tendency the good elders strongly advise students to completely avoid.

The potential to use plant medicine to manipulate and do harm is one of the initial traps presented to novice drinkers of ayahuasca. Of course anything potent is like a double-edged sword, and the effects often depend upon the hand that wields it. The present book tries to share fundamental guidelines not only to caution readers who are experimenting with ayahuasca, but also to illustrate how sorcery and superstition have contributed to the decline of the true indigenous spiritual science.

Sadly, sorcery and witchcraft are and always have been prevalent. When we consider the sometimes-predatory or simply unhelpful nature of many of the earthly spirits and the ignorant weaknesses of humanity, we can see how the dark side arises and degrades the spiritual science that gave birth to it. The deeds of sorcery offer short-term gratification, including gifts or money from ill-willed people who request favors or other shortcuts and benefits. These earthly rewards make shouldering the burdens of a shaman much more attractive, but as the Peruvian ayahuasquero don Solon Tello once said, "The most attractive things are also the most dangerous things."[2] And so it is that wayward shamans eventually suffer retribution for their actions.

As discussed in the previous chapter, investigating this spiritual science is an arduous lifestyle that requires great virtue, effort, and discipline. It feels like one is always a little hungry, or as if one is barely holding on. For this reason the great Amazonian sage Pablo Amaringo spoke of the "trail of heaven" as being a narrow and winding path, elusive and harder to follow than other paths.[3] Yet it is undeniably the correct way, even though it is not recognized by most people in the world—it is the Taoist Way of Heaven; the Secoya *Wiñapai ma'a*, Path of the Ever-New Ones; and the Waorani *Waaponi durani bai*, the Good Way of the Ancients.

Cesareo once told me, "The deep satisfaction that one can feel when in the presence of the Matëmopai [sky people] is unlike any other."[4] With this type of experience, one's commitment becomes more firm, and what once seemed a narrow and winding path becomes the only way one knows or wants to follow. Such conviction alone gives great joy. Even just the notion—and much more the experience—of the existence of the legions of heavenly immortals is enough to keep practitioners on the right path, in hopes of basking in their presence. And once the acceptance and support of immortal spirits are achieved, one finds it easier not to sway into the temptations of greed and selfishness. Then the winding narrow path no longer seems thin or precarious; it reveals itself right here and now as the only path, and it is as wide as the universe and as glorious as the celestial realms.

It is for this reason that all the authentic drinkers of yagé in the Amazon that I have met share a great love for nature and all humanity, and they are outspoken protectors of the rainforest and the good way of all that is right. In *The Yage Drinker* Fernando Payaguaje differentiates between good and bad practitioners of yagé:

> The sorcerers only know the lower levels of the cosmos. . . . They know the sky only up to the house of the sun. They have never seen the celestial people, the ones who live well, the loving people. Instead they make contact with inferior beings, including the spirits of sorcery. For their part, the healers don't linger at low levels of knowledge, but drink more and more yage. Not for the pleasure of doing it, because it's a great sacrifice, but because they desire greater knowledge. They try all the varieties of yage, boiled down thick and strong, until they're able to meet the healing spirits, the celestial people, contact with whom makes them reject all sorcery and stay forever in their friendship. Thus they acquire the power to heal.[5]

To give the benefit of a doubt to some of those wayward practitioners, perhaps they consider helping someone to be an act of goodness even though what they are colluding with may be evil. (Remember that some medicine men and women are simply trying to make a living, not see God. . . .) Many ayahuasqueros in the Amazon have fallen into the trap of colluding with impure motives: They do good at times by helping some people get well, and they do bad at times by fulfilling inappropriate requests, such as casting spells and setting traps on innocent people. Thus they tend to attract many kinds of demented and obscene clients and help them achieve their desires regardless of the object. These sorcerers or *brujos* curse people with illness, death, and misfortune, interfere in marital relationships, manipulate people financially and psychologically, help lonesome individuals fulfill their lust with minors, knock sincere individuals off track and interfere with their studies, et cetera. Such low-level spiritists cause all kinds of confusion and sorry consequences, especially on the spiritual level. When shamanism strays from its original path, it brings nothing but sad results.

Fernando again: "The sorcerers unite themselves with those demons [*mawahopai*, morpho butterfly people] and then they fly. The demons whistle to trick and lure the chosen victim. When that person appears, the sorcerer fires off his magical darts. If the person is a healer he can tell that it's demons that are whistling in the air, and he'll be able to defend himself. In any case, the flight takes place in an instant. The sorcerer can be in his home, reclining in his hammock, smoking a hand-rolled cigar. The tobacco burns while he flies with the demons, and he returns without anyone noticing."[6]

When Fernando says, "In any case, the flight takes place in an instant," he reveals how delicate is the path and how critical it is to be clear in one's intentions and firmly dedicated to the highest values. The Secoya attest that it is at the beginning of setting out upon a spiritual path that one is most vulnerable to getting manipulated into associating with these potentially malignant spirits. This is why Cesareo often says, "When you hear the Watí [spirits of the earthly plane] calling your name, do not go. In the visions of yagé or in your dreams when the Watí want to hand you something, do not accept, for they get you to entangle with them by offering you wonderful-looking things that attract your attention, and if you show interest, they have succeeded. In their presence, stay still and quiet as if you were dead. Ignore them totally. Then they will leave you alone."[7]

Spirituality vs. Spiritism

These are words of counsel from don Pablo Amaringo, the great Peruvian healer and artist:

> We must understand the difference between spirituality and spiritism.
>
> Spiritism leads to damaging and malicious things—
> to panic, terror, and madness.
>
> Reject low-level spiritism that attracts negativity and sorrow.
>
> Spirits often try to offer you things—do not accept.
>
> Celestial beings bless with their calm presence.
>
> Merge with only the highest universal spirits—the celestial beings.
>
> Spirituality leads us to just, saintly, and pure things.
>
> It unites us with the highest spiritual origin, with justice, rectitude, and service.
>
> Justice, rectitude, and service bring peace, and peace allows for all highest things to manifest.

The elders assert that in the past there unfortunately were lineages of sorcerers in the Amazon who never had good intent and did not simply stray into nebulous territory. The elders recall stories of sorcery by corrupted power-hungry people who used plant medicine to ruthlessly kill without fear, shame, or pity. Such people have for the most part finished themselves off, but their brutal tactics are remembered.

In order to avoid the shadowy pitfalls of sorcery, true students on a path that supports life strive to reach for and embody the ultimate designs, the most profound knowledge and beautiful representations and manifestations of that understanding. In the broader conceptualization of the science, good and evil can be easily understood. It is in the gray areas where the novice is vulnerable to falling. One needs to develop common sense and intuition, along with piercing and unfailing discrimination between good and evil, knowing how to respond to each. The moral order of things and the most ethical approach become topics of intense searching and discussion. Successful students eventually gain a deep universal understanding that seals them from ever going down the path of doing harm. They graduate as healers, and they are rooted in a unified perspective.

No Tolerance for Sorcery

The Secoya delineate four basic levels of spiritual achievement as a result of drinking yagé. The first and simplest is being able to do harm and falling into the temptations of sorcery. The second level, with one's knowledge and awareness, entails learning how to heal; the third, calling the animals; and the fourth, direct communion with the creator.[8]

The Secoya reveal their varying degrees of tolerance for evil-doers in the following saying: "If someone is stealing from your home, invite him to a meal. If someone is killing through sorcery, the person's own father is obliged to kill his son in order to put an end to the harm-doer who has passed the final limits of tolerance."[9] In essence this means that low-level petty crimes are handled by showing a higher, more generous way of being in the hope that the morally questionable person will carry out some self-reflection and will change, bringing back the natural order of things. On the other hand, if the transgression has gone beyond repair, such as in the case of taking a human life, the evil-doer's own father is obliged to find him and kill him. Whether this has actually ever happened I have no documented anecdote, but the saying puts a pretty heavy responsibility on appropriate parenting!

It's much easier to pass spiritual tests and avoid falling into the traps of sorcery when drinking under the guidance of a proper master. Cesareo spoke of his time as an apprentice with different elders and masters. After sufficient training and cleansing through a combination of drinking yagé, sustaining a specific diet, and upholding *ñuñerepá paiye,* the Secoya code of upright living, there would come a point when the youth were put through a spiritual test in order to cleanse themselves of all temptations to carry out sorcery. These temptations can be attributed to two different factors: one is lack of understanding and the other is bodily contamination or ill health. "Contamination" refers to unclear motives and unresolved personal matters that sway the novice from giving undivided attention to the cause of seeing and being accepted among celestial immortals. The novice might fall into self-aggrandizement, while possibly leading to thoughts that one is seeing the ultimate truth—a dangerous combination.

During the months of the celestial summer, the sap of the *wansoka* tree *(Couma macrocarpa)* would be gathered. Just before drinking a ceremony of yagé, and when the master deemed it to be the right moment, he would splash this sap over the youth, who would be delicately dressed in new tunics and freshly made ceremonial ornaments and abundant aromatic *maña,* the fragrant leaves and tree barks used to adorn oneself in the ceremonies. At dawn, the sticky sap that under normal conditions takes several days to get off one's skin and is very difficult if not impossible to remove from clothes would be completely gone, as if none had ever been there. This was a sure sign that the Jujupai, the doctor people, had responded to the ceremony. When the spirits take away the sap, they are also removing any final contaminations within the bodies of the students that could potentially block their clarity and lead them to cause harm or even become sorcerers.

On one occasion during his training, don Cesareo was shown how easy it is to do harm. (I will mention here that Cesareo has a ceremonial name, Camporazá, which he said is the name of a fragrant medicinal bark. I will sometimes use this name or Fragrant Medicine Bark when discussing Cesareo in a ceremonial context.) He was already firmly committed to the higher path and had seen many celestial visions, but his teacher wanted to give him a powerful incentive to never cause harm, never, not even once. His master rubbed Camporazá's hands to pull out from within him any potential to do harm that still lingered. Then the master said, "Now you rub your hands some more." When Camporazá looked at his hands after doing this, there on his palm before his eyes was the *virote,* the harmful spiritual projectile or dart that becomes physical. He had heard about it but never actually seen it before.

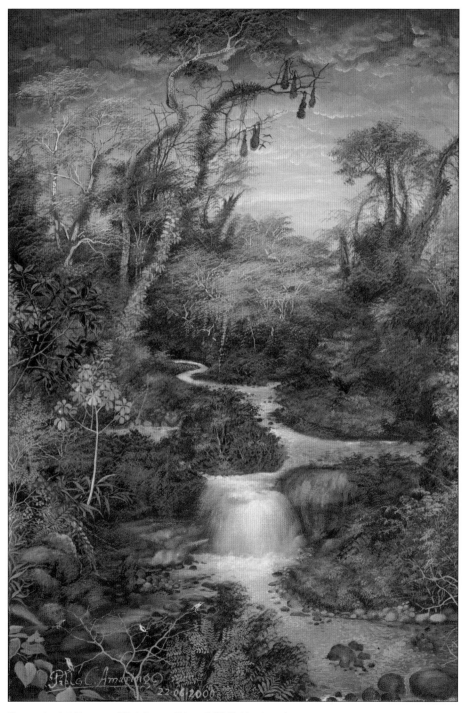

Cascada del Bosque, "Rainforest Waterfall," Pablo Amaringo

Note: All photos unless otherwise specified are from the Ecuadorian Amazon and have been taken by the author, JMW. Dates represent year taken.

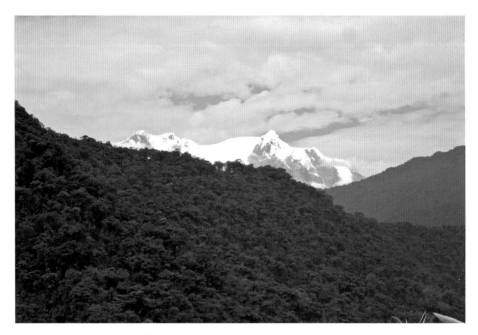

Antisana, clothed nearly to its snow line with vegetation

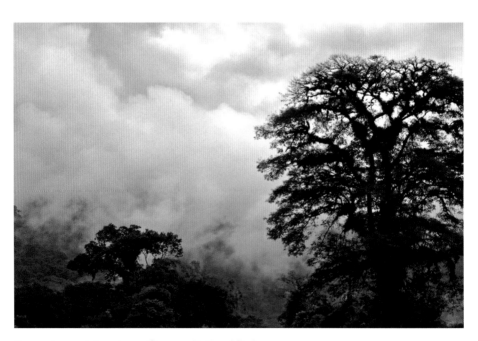

Premontane rainforest near Sumaco National Park

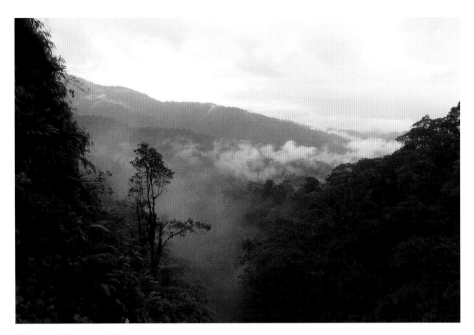

Slopes of Sumaco Volcano

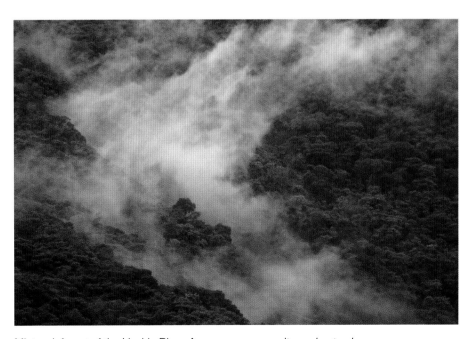

Misty rainforest of the Llushin River, Amazanga community *purina tambu*

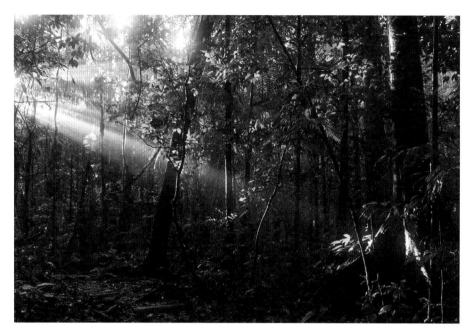

A shaft of morning light in the Tropical Wet Forest (by Murray Cooper)

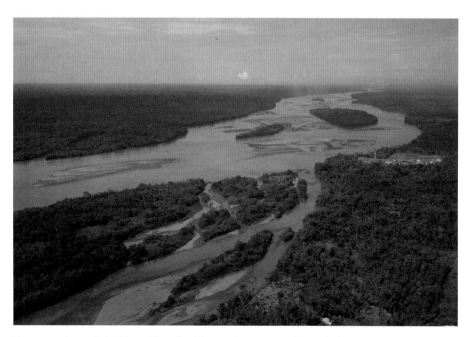

Upper portions of the Napo River (by Murray Cooper; see his website at
www.murraycooperphoto.com)

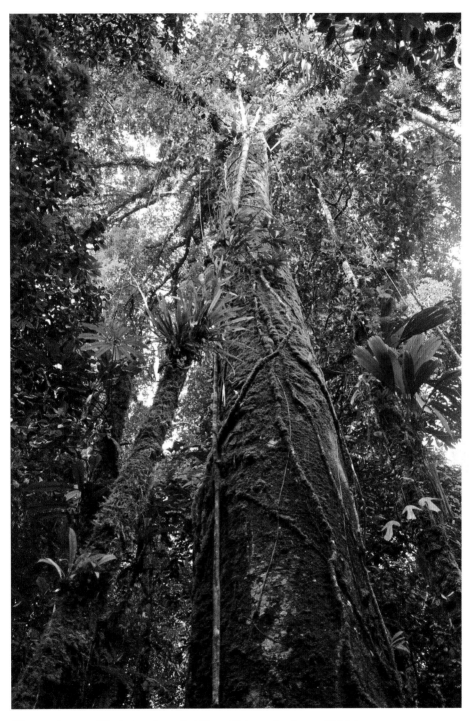

Giant cedar tree *(Cedrela odorata)* at Napo-Galeras (by James Ficklin)

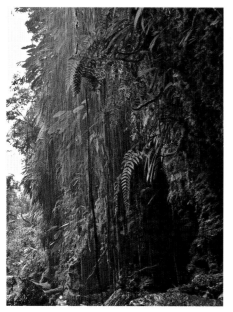

Limestone cliffs, western slopes of
Napo-Galeras

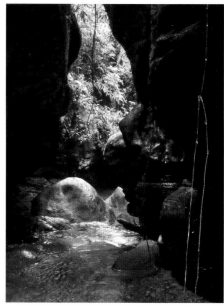

Faces of ancient masters?

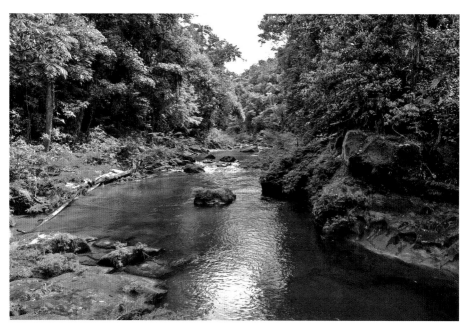

Pusuno River, Napo-Galeras, at the Mamallacta family *purina tambu*

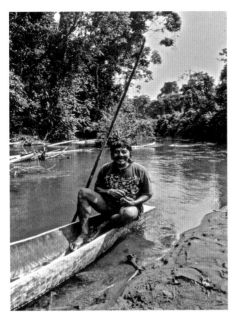

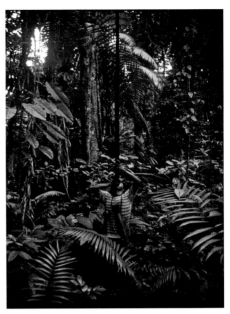

Mengatue on the Shiripuno River,
Waorani territory, 1992

Moi Enomenga near Queweiriono, 1992

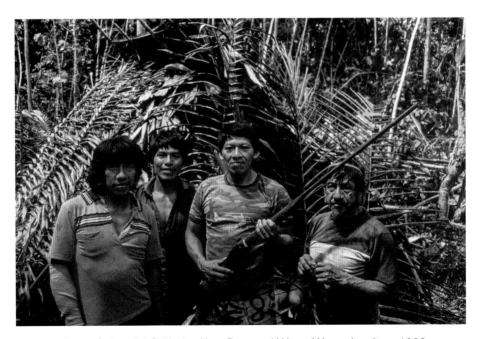

Wepe and sons (left to right): Nanka, Kue, Owe, and Wepe, Waorani territory, 1992

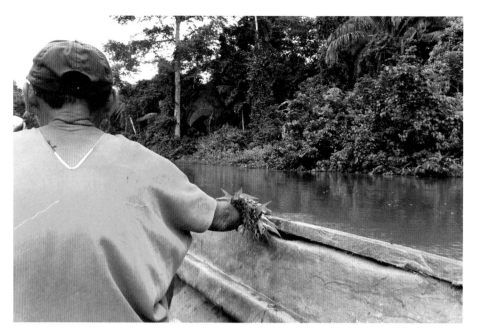

Among the Secoya, Aguarico River, Sucumbios Province, 2009 (by James Ficklin)

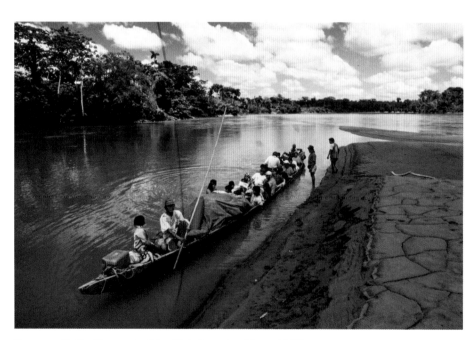

Voyage with the Secoya to Pëquë'yá, Aguarico River, 1996

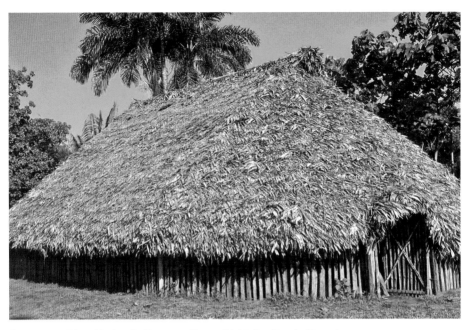

Secoya traditional lodge in Sewaya village, 2011 (by Sarah Chase)

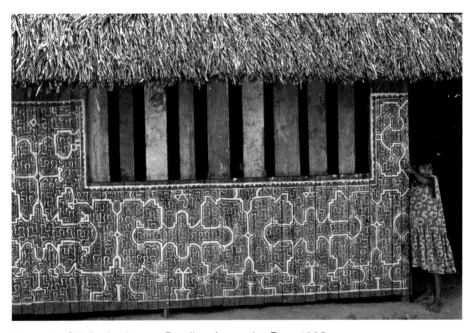

Home of a Shipibo healer near Pucallpa, Amazonian Peru, 1998

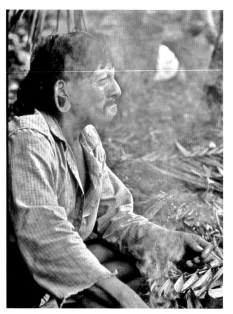

Mengatue, Waorani, 1993

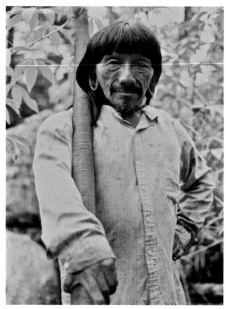

Koba, Waorani, 1993

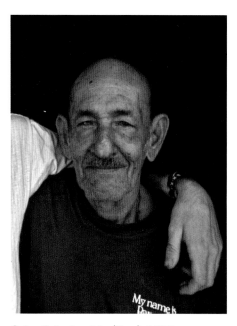

Solon Tello, Lamista (Peru), 1998

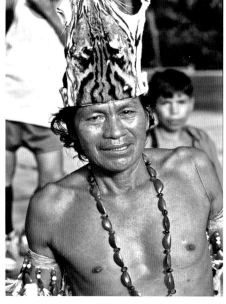

Casimiro Mamallacta, Kichwa, 1994

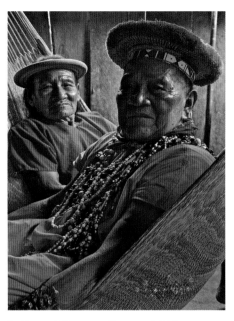

Delfin and Cesareo, Secoya, 2011
(by James Ficklin)

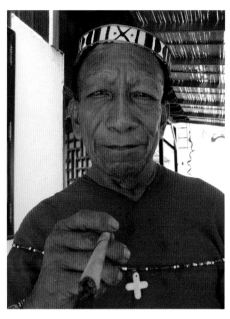

Agustin ("Tintin"), Secoya, 2011

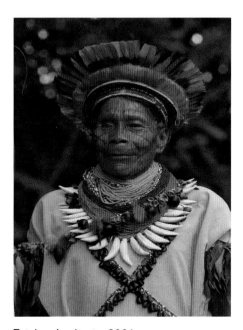

Esteban Lucitante, 2001
(by Murray Cooper)

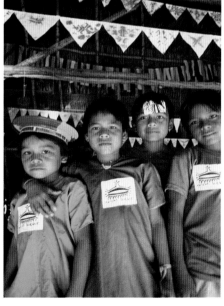

Secoya youth, 1997

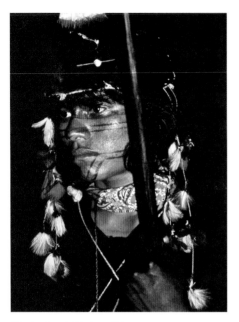
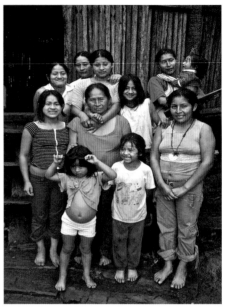

Flavio Santi, Kichwa/Shiwiar, 1994

Mama Lucila and family,
Amazanga community, 2006

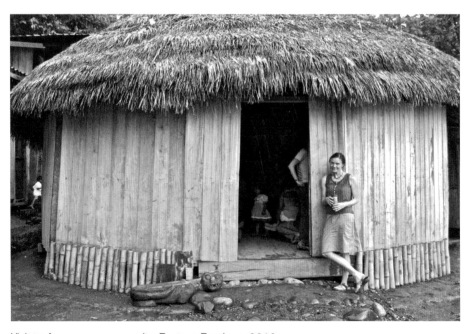

Visit to Amazanga community, Pastaza Province, 2010

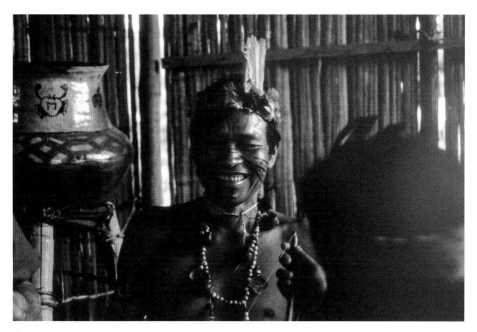

Casimiro Mamallacta at his home in Archidona, 1994

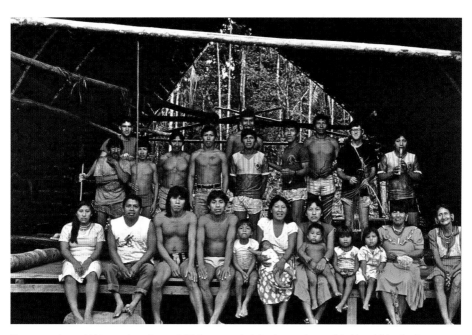

Demarcation of Waorani territory, 1992; at top left is the author, with friend Mashuri Waite to the right, in a black t-shirt

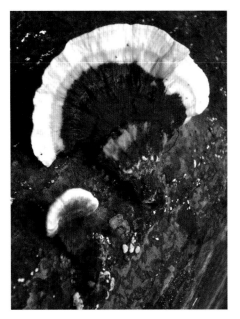

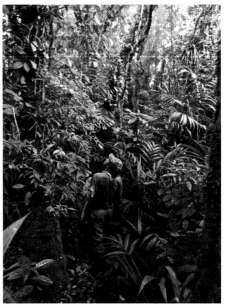

Fungal splendor: wati su'u, "spirit axe," a medicinal mushroom

Eastern slopes of Napo-Galeras, 2010 (by James Ficklin)

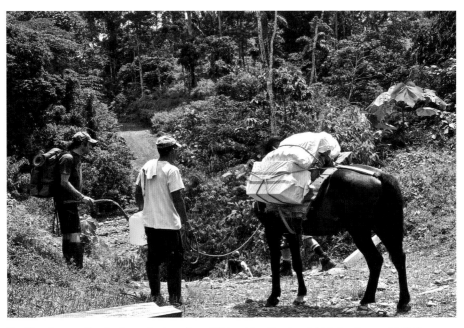

Packing in supplies for botanical study at Wairachina Sacha, 2010 (by James Ficklin)

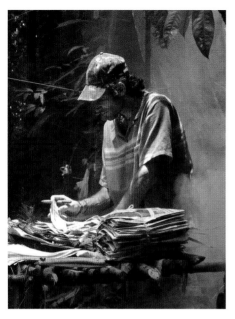

The author collecting plants
(by Bruce Harlow)

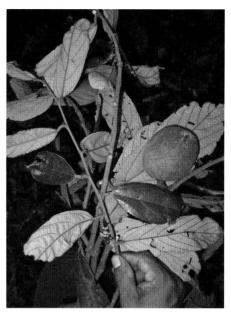

Wild cacao relative,
Theobroma subincanum

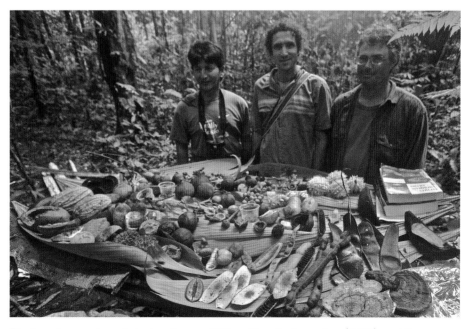

Biodiversity sample and plant gatherers: William Poveda, the author (JMW), and Bruce Harlow, Tropical Wet Forest, eastern slopes of Napo-Galeras, 2010 (by James Ficklin)

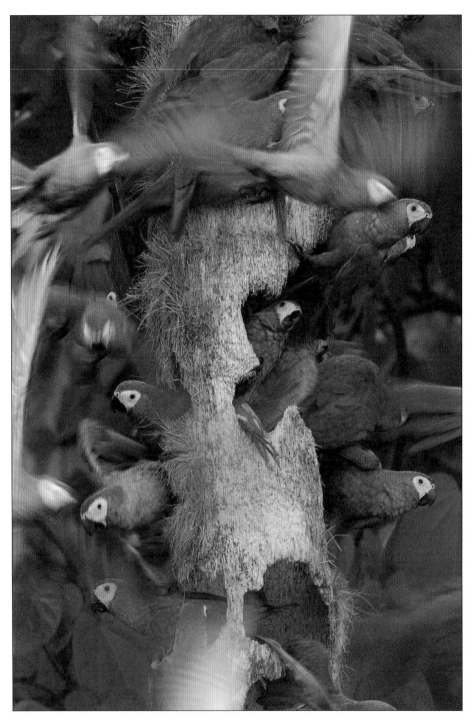

Guacamaya manilata / Red-bellied macaws *(Orthopsittaca manilata)* (by Murray Cooper)

"Now blow it into that wansoka tree," his teacher said. Young Camporazá aimed his hand at the tree in front of their camp and blew on the back end of the dart, as instructed, which went flying off at high speed then lodged deeply into the tree trunk. He was startled to see this and was even more shocked when within a few days this tree began to die. By week's end the leaves had turned yellow and fallen off. Within a month the tree was rotting and then got toppled in a windstorm. Camporazá's master said to him, "You see now that sorcery is real and the perils are grave." Young Camporazá reflected deeply on this and saw how the wansoka tree sacrificed itself for him so that he could see and learn and commit to never letting the ways of sorcery tempt him. Again he pledged to stay on the highest path, firmly rooted in the way of heaven.

Cleansing Temptations of Sorcery on the Sun Canoe, a Secoya Practice

The Sun Canoe, Ënsë Yowë, cruises far from the planet Earth; on its deck ride celestial immortals of a peculiar and unique nature. This cosmic boat is said never to come between the Earth and the sun; it always stays far from the Earth on the opposite side of the sun. In the old days this boat could be seen in visions when the people underwent deep-level ceremonies, after months of dieta in the wilderness.

Don Cesareo related the following account of the Sun Canoe. I was able to record this at his home in August 2006 and translate the material from Paicoca to Spanish with the help of Alfredo Payaguaje, the elder's nephew.

> In my youth, my grandfather brought me to the Sun Canoe in order to be cleansed thoroughly of all traces of contamination that could potentially lead to my becoming a sorcerer and to the inevitable abuse of power. All this occurred deep in the trance of yagé, with a pure setting and the precise following of ancestral ways, which enabled us to see these wonders as clear as day.

Upon arriving, we stood on board. The men of this boat ride at the front and the women at the back, and they all inspected me. My *wiñapai maro* [heaven-people crown] was taken off and handed around to be looked at, and my beaded sehué necklaces as well. Then the commander of this tremendous boat placed heavy necklaces on me that were loaded with artillery of many kinds. He placed on my head a heavy crown of sorcery, then he loaded onto my body a multitude of highly sophisticated weapons and warfare devices, all in dark and heavy tones. All the while my master was nearby, standing among them in his ceremonial regalia with his azure blue, red, and yellow heaven-crown, and his beaded sehué necklaces, and I could see that my master had not been touched.

Then I was sent over to the side where the women were. I was handed over to them by the commander of the boat, to the queen goddess among the women. There the women, instructed by their queen, proceeded to take off one by one all the weapons and items of sorcery that the men had loaded on me. Other women were holding my wiñapai maro and my heavenly sehué necklaces.

After it was all removed, I was standing there before the divinity, who said to me, "We can see that your discipline has been courageous, and you have contained yourself well." Then, instructed by their queen, the women adorned me with my beaded necklaces and then my crown, which shimmered even more than before. Their colors were brighter and now took on a light of their own.

After that his grandfather brought him back to the ceremony where they had been sitting in concentration. From then on Camporazá's authority as a healer and his ability to tap into heavenly energies for this purpose were confirmed. For this to happen one must have no traces of negative energy whatsoever. The Sun Canoe is an advanced vision, one that few aspirants have been able to witness, let alone board.

Perils and Pitfalls on the Path of Shamanism

According to the Amazonian beliefs, another peril of shamanism is that the sorcerers oftentimes attempt to kill the healer. They do this because they see the healer as an interference. The magic used by the sorcerer can be removed and released, and it then flies back to its owner, hitting him or her most unexpectedly in the back. The sorcerer gets ill and takes revenge, dedicating his ceremonies to "seeing" who is the healer that is interfering in his doings, and then trying to topple that healer. The healer must proceed with care, as noted by Fernando Payaguaje in *The Yage Drinker:* "To heal the victims of an attack like this, [the master] calls certain spirits, combining himself with them so as to locate the darts which are causing the illness. Once the darts have been taken out, he hands them over to his guardian spirit, who will keep them from returning to the sorcerer."[10] Wise healers know how to dispose of the sorcery in appropriate ways that disintegrate the malice and help avoid awakening the revenge of the sorcerer.

Sometimes several sorcerers gang up on a good healer to test his strength. This is among the perils and pitfalls of the path of shamanism, and such incidents still occur in the Amazon. This type of evil retribution is the main reason my good friend Pablo Amaringo was forced to abandon his ayahuasca healing practice. Despite witchcraft attacks on him, he never swayed from the path of service and dedicated his remaining years to teaching art and giving free spiritual tutelage to many local youth of the impoverished neighborhoods and riversides of his native Pucallpa region (Peru). He accomplished this through his Usko Ayar School of Amazonian Painting, and his consistent devotion to education and teaching.

Secoya elder Basilio Piaguaje explained to me the following in relation to shamanism and sorcery. He said that there are spiritual traps called *pitayari* in which the entire body of the brujo dies and his heart gets taken. These are traps the yagé drinkers have learned from the celestial people to spring on sorcerers in order to put an end to the sorcery. If a healer places this trap on a brujo, the brujo will look everywhere for a place to hide in order to avoid his destiny. His spirit tries to hide inside roots, under the earth, and in crevices, but he knows that there his evil intentions will be discovered, so he doesn't stay long and goes from place to place hiding. Eventually he tries to hide in heaven, but before entering he comes to a bridge. When he crosses it, the bridge falls out from underneath him. He falls and loses his heart. Within three months he gets weaker and weaker. No one can heal him and he dies.

There are four traps of this sort that have been employed in order to put an end to sorcery. That one is *pai pitayari,* described as "the checkpoint on the spiritual bridge to heaven" or "the time of midnight." There is also *campo yariwá,* meaning "where the sun is at 9 AM," and *weku yariwá,* "where the sun is at midday," and *wigonza yariwá,* "where the sun is at 3 PM." Only people who have not caused spiritual harm can pass over these bridges; a brujo who has killed people and then tries to hide in heaven falls to his demise. The Secoya always warn against entering into sorcery because they have seen that when people follow this tragic path it brings only misery, first to others and then inevitably to the perpetrators.

Don't assume that tourists and dabblers in ayahuasca from other cultures are exempt from the potential influence of sorcery, either. Sorcerers often come off as virtuous and friendly individuals, yet they secretly abuse innocent foreigners during ayahuasca ceremonies, going into their souls without consent to see what their home cities look like, satisfying their desperate personal needs to see and know more at any cost, as a vice and for mere superficial satisfaction.

Some brujos are said to be able to see inside the bodies of their victims, where they can confiscate spiritual possessions and sever relationships with helping spirits that this person may have acquired or been born with—helpers and other internal qualities that are still young, tender, and weakly rooted from lack of spiritual training. These sorcerers can see virtues in human beings as if they were strands of yarn linking them to their heavenly origin, and when they sever these threads it leaves the people orphaned from this source, sending them into depression without ever knowing the root cause. Things a person may have never felt, like jealousy and greed, begin to creep into his inner feelings, which confuses him even more.

There are accounts of jealous yagé drinkers who have stolen the *pinta* that crowns a young disciple, this being the heavenly "designs" or virtuous energy that facilitates fluent communion with the celestial immortals. The young student no longer sees visions and can be driven into an amnesiac depression. This type of spiritual damage can only be cured by an advanced drinker of yagé, someone who is a true doctor of the original medicine school and embodies its tradition and spiritual development. Such a healer is someone who truly knows how to heal and to fix major imbalances—someone who associates with immortal spiritual medicine doctors, as well as with the Demon King[11]—and sadly, few of these skilled healers remain in the world today.

Another harsh phenomenon occurs when the teacher turns against the student. Many times the student surpasses the teacher, and the teacher can become jealous and attempt to kill the student. Once in Secoya territory I met a Colombian by the name of Jaro Muñoz who had spent thirty years of his life wandering the Amazon, moving from tribe to tribe, living among many deep-forest peoples. He had just come upriver from Peru where he had been living for a while in a remote Secoya village. They recommended that he visit don Cesareo in Ecuador, so to his house Jaro arrived. Not long after, Jaro began to share his stories. I was there at the time, and his powerful and heart-wrenching experiences would be shared with me after the day's work helping the old man in his garden. Jaro told us how his entire family had been killed by guerrilla drug lords in his home valley and how this had instigated his wanderings in the hopes of healing his broken heart.

At one time he lived among the blacks panning gold. While he was there, a black he-woman (someone who is biologically a woman but acts like a man) put a spell on Jaro and made him into his wife. Jaro would cook and clean the house and wash the clothes, all the while under a terrible spell, an episode that lasted well over a year. His friends informed his father of this, who, with the help of a shaman, came to rescue Jaro. They grabbed him and ran, one on each arm, holding him tight. After they left the place of his imprisonment his body started twitching in agony—there was something holding him back. But they kept running as Jaro screamed. The whole while the shaman was invoking helping spirits, and blowing on Jaro as they dragged him against his will farther and farther down the path, until finally the sorcery "popped out of him," as Jaro put it. The spell or the bad spirit that had him like that popped off and he recovered his senses. He ran with his father and the shaman. Later they camped and the shaman cured water for him to drink, and blew on him and healed him with plants. This was how Jaro escaped. This occurred in a remote rainforest area of Colombia's Chocó region on the Pacific coastal slopes of the Andes.

Jaro studied with a shaman master in a remote region of the Colombian Amazon who tried to kill him when he saw that Jaro began surpassing him in his spiritual authority. He wanted to cut him short in the process. Jaro barely escaped with his life. Here is his account. He had been going to great lengths to help the family of the shaman he was studying with. He even brought the shaman's wife to the hospital and got her healed, paying for it himself by making beaded necklaces and bringing them to sell at a tourist shop. He also worked hard through agriculture and some selective logging of fine woods that had been blown over in a windstorm to acquire the money to buy the master an outboard motor.

The shaman master agreed to coronate Jaro with his shimmering wisdom designs, passing their energy to him so he could truly see after nearly two years of providing support. They had already drunk some yagé but the master had not passed on his power yet. They cooked the yagé and the shaman master blew over the cup and blew on Jaro too, and Jaro drank. He saw immediately that he was being enrolled in a large university. He received an identification card and went off to his first class, but stopped to buy some grapes from a sidewalk vendor lady. When he opened the door to his class he noticed that everyone was already seated. He looked at his watch, and he was exactly thirty seconds late on account of the grapes. Before the auditorium of hundreds of students, the elder teacher, whose beard reached nearly to the ground, spoke to him by name and said, "Jaro, you will not be allowed to attend class next time you are late."

He went on to tell me that every night afterwards, he visited this university in his dreams. Every night he entered the classes and participated in many sessions on topics that ranged from distinct types of healing to advanced esoteric studies of nature, electromagnetism, and many other quantum realities. He and his teacher drank several more ceremonies, and each time he was allowed to explore deeper and more mysterious teachings, when the teacher realized what was occurring—Jaro was progressing further than he. Not even the teacher had been able to see such tremendous visions. Losing sight of all the help Jaro had given him, the teacher turned on his student and planned to put a spiritual trick on him, so that Jaro would get killed and never know where it came from. Jaro was informed of this by his new helping spirits, which is what allowed him to escape in the nick of time. The shaman master sent out giant peccaries from under the earth that aimed to stop Jaro and pound him into the ground, but he had escaped moments earlier and was able to pass from the area just before this occurred. He left, never to return.

Reining in Sorcery

Many transgressions have occurred and continue to occur from the abuse of ayahuasca. The indigenous societies themselves wrestle with this dichotomy of good and evil, but not until the Christian evangelical missionaries began preaching generalized negativities about all shamanic activities did the entire practice of shamanism and the drinking of yagé in particular come under attack from the outside. With their narrow Western religious mindset, many missionaries past and present have undermined true shamanic pursuits and cast all practitioners into disfavor, influencing young people to choose a different course of spiritual endeavor and all people to view illness and misfortune in an entirely different, more "rational" way. Granted, the historical facts of colonization and penetration of the rainforest for industrial purposes exacerbated native superstition and intertribal warfare, and the missionaries' work did contribute to alleviating much of the endless retaliation for deaths believed to be caused by witchcraft from neighboring sorcerers when they actually were a result of previously-unknown foreign diseases to which the natives had no immunity.

So while the evangelical missionaries helped halt intertribal warfare in some areas (such as the Waorani territory), they simultaneously worked diligently to put an end to what they considered sorcery, demonizing the traditional life of the people and of course the drinking of yagé, as it was practiced among the Siona and Secoya, for example. The missionaries witnessed the deep trances of the drinkers and the often bizarre scenarios that occur under these conditions, and evidently the amount of energy released by ceremonies and the degree of chanting was astonishing and crazy to them. Even if they did not outright chastise the ceremonies of yagé, they were successful in turning many of the people against the ceremonies, especially the women, who were the first to follow the evangelists in the hope that this would bring peace. While others were sleeping, the yagé drinkers would be up all night, maybe even several nights in a row (as during the months of the celestial summer). But the missionaries noted that the yagé drinkers were kind and genuine people, and when questioned about where or how they acquired these customs, their response was "From God, the one and only God, the same God that you adore."[12]

What the missionaries didn't know was that the good-hearted traditionalists of the people were diligently upholding the ancient ways through their customary yagé ceremonies, and they were not the ones causing the sorcery. Nonetheless, the intruders severely curtailed the authentic spiritual life of the people by marginalizing their ceremonial practices. This naïve and judgmental approach fails to understand or respect any of the traditional indigenous wisdom and contributes to the loss of an immense body of human experience and knowledge.

Because the Christian teaching carries a strong sense of judgment based on good and evil, traditional life became associated with evil. The holistic, non-dualistic nature of the indigenous approach to life was not grasped by outsiders, and they yanked the people's roots. Evangelical work is in many ways the tip of the spear for the penetration of oil companies and other exploiters, and in some cases they work side by side, the smiling face of the ruthless beast that is consumer culture.[13] However, it should be noted that some missionaries such as those from the Capuchin order (which stems from Catholicism) have a very different and much more sensible approach. They have encouraged indigenous people to uphold their traditional ways and values and have been true friends and guides to the people during challenging times of transition.[14]

Ultimately it was not the evangelical missionaries who reined in sorcery. They may have put a stake in its soul body, but it was not the end, as they might like to claim. The native people themselves had techniques for grappling with out-of-hand sorcery, and one particularly effective technique eventually became sufficiently widespread to counteract the damage. To understand how this knowledge came to the people, it is important to note that in the past, before the arrival of the rubber barons (the first resource extractors to turn the rainforest of paradise into an unendurable hell for its residents[15]), the Amazonian people enjoyed great intercultural reunions and festive gatherings, when many tribes came together to share in peace and enjoy one another's company. One popular site was the wilderness lagoons of Pëquë'yá (Black-caiman Lagoons), along today's eastern boundary between Ecuador and Peru, where tribes from distant regions, particularly of the Tukanoan language group, would gather during the summer to drink yagé for approximately three months when the weather was fine and the cicadas singing. This phenomenon occurred there since ancient times, and a great deal of knowledge was shared during these encounters. From different places people would come and set up camp to learn and to enjoy each other's high-spirited company. Deep, lasting friendships and new family ties arose because sometimes marriages would occur. Such great intercultural reunions/exchanges were dedicated to the arts, to the good and pure life on the land, and were a part of most Amazonian societies. They came to an end with the disruption of traditional and ceremonial life, though the yagé drinkers continued to frequently depart for adventures to far-off lands to enhance their body of experience and knowledge, to make friends and allies, and to trade plant lore and ancient ways—a conference of sorts but no longer a full-on tribal happening. The following is a powerful account that is but a small piece of this shared knowledge, and it relates how one yagé drinker's voyage and sharing was the silver bullet that eliminated sorcery from many regions.

At some time roughly around the 1930s a yagé drinker of the Koreguaje people from Colombia came to a gathering. He imparted a secret related to the elimination of sorcery learned by another Koreguaje yagé drinker from the celestial spirits. The secret is effective beyond compare. If the death of a person was truly caused by sorcery, then the sorcerer will die within several days of others carrying out this tactic.

Should a family member die suddenly and unexpectedly, no one in the family was to cry, and everyone was to act as if the person had died a natural death, only mourning the loss *after* the secret tactic has been carried out. Without touching the dead body, one cuts a small amount of skin from the palms of the hands and soles of the feet, as well as some hair. Four clay pots are acquired for this process, two small and two large. Inside the small clay pot the victim's skin and hair are placed, with strong tobacco juice. It is covered with the second small pot. This in turn is placed inside a larger pot that is then filled with some water as well as gasoline or diesel, and all kinds of toxic and poisonous plants—for example, long black palm spines and irritating plants such as the caustic seeds of a certain palm and the caustic sap of certain aroids. Then the last pot is placed on top as a cover. Under this a fire is made and the entire container brought to a boil. The elders say that in some instances the container was known to actually mention the name of the person responsible for the death: The culprit's name would be pronounced through the frothing gurgling boil, bubbling up out of the pot. As soon as the pot starts to furiously boil, it is smashed onto the fire with a long pole. Diesel and more dry firewood and palm leaves are thrown on to create huge flames, emitting a deathly black smoke.

This smoke, containing the witchcraft that caused the death, must now find its owner. The witchcraft that caused the malice is "orphaned," and with nowhere to go it goes looking for its "owner," the sorcerer, the brujo who sent the magic venom. The smoke circles around for a while over the trees and eventually drifts off in a certain direction. The sorcery goes looking for its source. It finds the witch and quickly and unexpectedly strikes him (or her). He will start coughing blood or fall over in agony as his stomach swells until it bursts. He will be found by many witnesses, lying there dead the following morning, with a long hairy tongue hanging out of his mouth.

One such account dates from as recently as 1995, and it was perhaps one of the last times this tactic was carried out, though the elders tell of having used this on many occasions. In this particular episode a young girl died suddenly, so the secret practice was performed and smoke rose up into the treetops and drifted downriver. A few days later word came that a notorious brujo living among one of the colonist Shuar communities had died.[16] This brujo was feared among them and was believed to have caused a lot of harm and sorrow among his own people as well. The Shuar that brought the news were relieved that finally he had died.

If the cause of death is not sorcery, then no one will die from this tactic. Sorcery is viewed as a thing—though it is invisible, it is a substance, a projectile that causes harm, and this malice when released in this way returns only to where it came from, taking the life of the sorcerer who caused the harm as a precise retribution.

Cesareo would say about sorcery and the need to dodge the endless retaliation, "What for? It's too much work, hauling water from way down in the creek, hauling firewood all day, cutting yagé and pounding it for hours and hours, while withstanding thirst and hunger from fasting all day—just to do harm! I don't think so!"

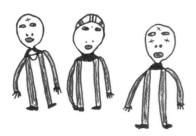

Chapter 3

The Gift of Ayahuasca

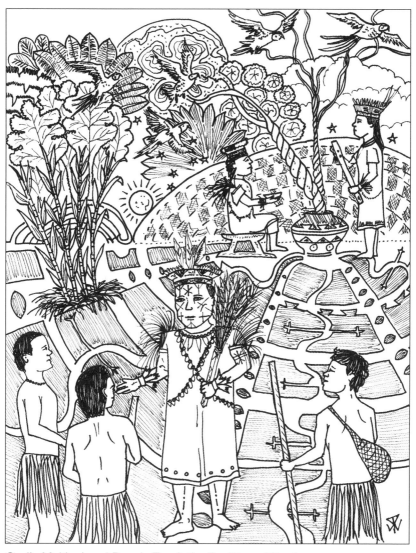

God's Multicolored People Teach the Tradition of Yagé

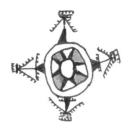

"The plants involved are truly plants of the gods, for their power is laid to supernatural forces residing in their tissues, and they were divine gifts to the earliest Indians on Earth."
— **Richard Evans Schultes, Albert Hofmann, and Christian Rätsch,** *Plants of the Gods* [1]

Properly understood, traditional Amazonian medicine and the vast body of knowledge it encompasses constitute one of Earth's great holistic systems of natural healing. Contained within this collected ancestral wisdom are methods for curing most if not all physical ailments, allaying disturbances of the mind and soul, attaining energy, visiting unseen realms, corroborating the veracity of divine beings, and achieving balance with the environment and one's community. Essentially, the practices aim to ameliorate and elevate the challenging experience that is life on planet Earth.

In the Amazon, a bioregion where cultural diversity is as rich as biological diversity, a broad array of methods contribute to this system of achieving knowledge and spiritual development. In some cases they have been practiced for millennia.[2] Among the oldest and most traditional approaches is the consumption of alkaloid-rich, sacred plant medicines and adherence to a dieta prescribed by one's master or (when a practitioner is more advanced) suggested by a plant spirit itself. The most prominent plant medicine in the upper Amazon and currently most intriguing to Westerners is ayahuasca (yagé). So far-reaching is the scope of this sacred medicine vine—a fundamental pillar of the South American plant-medicine tradition—that it has touched or shaped almost every part of the life of the indigenous societies that use it.

The botanists quoted above in *Plants of the Gods* concur: "The drug may be the shaman's tool to diagnose illness or to ward off impending disaster, to guess the wiles of an enemy, to prophesy the future. But it is more than the shaman's tool. It enters into almost all aspects of the life of the people who use it, to an extent equaled by hardly any other hallucinogen. Partakers, shamans or not, see all the gods, the first human beings, and animals, and come to understand the establishment of their social order."[3]

Though there is little archeological evidence, practical applications for this sacred jungle vine likely have been known by native peoples since antiquity. In 1851 when *Banisteriopsis caapi* was formally brought to the attention of the West by English botanist Richard Spruce, its use was already widespread throughout the Amazon basin and western slopes of the Andes. Use of ayahuasca has been documented among seventy indigenous societies and more than forty language groups.[4] In all cases, oral tradition (the only deep history we have of rainforest peoples) holds that its use was taught to the inhabitants' ancestors through direct encounters with divine spiritual beings, supernatural entities, and mythic ancestors, and this fact or belief—call it what you will—is not to be underestimated. It is important to note that it is the yagé drinker's personal relationship with divine beings, powerful spirits, trans-dimensional ancestors and/or plant spirits and other spiritual entities that enables him or her to work effectively in this human realm—in sum, to work what others might call miracles.

Ayahuasca is most popularly consumed as a mixture of two principal plants, one being *Banisteriopsis caapi* (ayahuasca itself) and the other a variable admixture plant, depending on the region and cultural background of its brewing, often either *Diplopterys cabrerana* (known in indigenous languages as *yagé ocó* by the Secoya, *chagropanga* in urban Peru, *yají* among the Achuar and the Shiwiar of Pastaza Province in Ecuador, and *chali panga* among Kichwa speakers) or *Psychotria viridis* (*chacruna*[5] in the Iquitos area of Peru and *amiruka panga* among the Napo Runa Kichwa in Ecuador—two of the many names for the same plant).

The woody portions of the ayahuasca vine represent the energies of the earth, the bringer of harmony and strength. Admixture plants represent heaven, the bringer of light, clarity, and wisdom. While there may be variations among plant species and sub-species, the alkaloids are generally consistent. Yet a proper brew is much more than alkaloid soup. A true batch of ayahuasca or yagé—one considered drinkable by the traditional elders—must unite the heavenly and earthly energies, spirit and matter, light and strength. A beautiful hymn from the União Vegetal, an ayahuasca church of Brazil, eloquently portrays the combination of these two plants as the "Divine Union." When this brew is imbibed, one experiences many kinds of bodily and psychological sensations.

The particularly interesting aspect (especially to scientific-minded Westerners) of combining ayahuasca with the leaves of either the *Psychotria viridis* bush or the *Diplopterys cabrerana* vine is that a vital chemical synthesis takes place that results in the striking or even astonishing effects that can ensue—said and known to be among the most profound of entheogenic experiences (a term referring to an enabler of divine visions). These plants do not have remotely the same result when ingested separately.

To break it down chemically: a proper ayahuasca brew contains both beta-carboline and tryptamine alkaloids—the former (harmine and harmaline) obtained from the ayahuasca vine *(Banisteriopsis caapi),* and the latter (N,N- or 5-MeO-dimethyltryptamine, a.k.a. DMT) from the admixture plants chacruna *(Psychotria viridis)* or yagé ocó *(Diplopterys cabrerana)*. DMT is not orally active unless combined with a monoamine oxidase (MAO) inhibitor; and the harmala alkaloids in ayahuasca are potent short-term MAO inhibitors that synergize with the DMT contained in the admixture plants, allowing the DMT to reach the brain and not be inactivated in the stomach.[6]

The active ayahuasca alkaloids can be felt on a bodily level as they temporarily inhibit the function of the acids in the stomach, acting on the place of the root source of the body's strength, the area allied with earth energy. Meanwhile, the admixture plant(s), containing DMT—a molecule that acts temporarily in the brain—represents heaven in that it affects the head and sensory perception. The head is considered in many traditional worldviews to be the body part symbolizing heaven. Here we encounter the first of many incredible facts about this medicine tradition: This synergistic combination was "discovered" independently by numerous tribal groups throughout the upper Amazon and Orinoco basins, societies that live in a rainforest wilderness comprised of a hundred thousand different plant species. The odds of this being a coincidental trial-and-error process are impossibly high, and knowledge of the molecular properties of plants and the art of combining them chemically is a recent scientific discovery in the West. The alternative explanation, and the one given by all native people, is that the knowledge was imparted to them through direct encounters with celestial immortals, such as the Secoya encounter with God's Multicolored People, who delivered the first yagé vines and taught this plant-medicine tradition. Among the Shiri and Inca, their forefathers underwent transubstantiation after dying, their wisdom preserved within the very tissues of these plants, so that their people could achieve and understand their wisdom upon imbibing them. Other ethnic groups then learned about this lineage and the knowledge was passed on. (These legends appear later in this chapter.)

Simply to accept that supernatural spirits really exist and/or that a plant can have intelligence is to make a huge break with rational scientific method as practiced in the West. This is precisely what ayahuasca demands of us. This can be understood when, in order to embody, understand, and be the truth, one integrates all the elements of one's being in the quest for knowledge as opposed to a merely intellectual pursuit of certain concepts and topics.

As one writer and seasoned psychonaut put it: "There is far more to this business than left-brain logic would suggest—as 'sophisticated' Westerners we dismiss the entities of the imaginal realm and are, to our extreme disadvantage, dismissed by them in return."[7]

The imbibing of these medicines and related activities such as gathering and preparation of plants and specifics of the dieta are accomplished under the tutelage of an experienced guide or mae-stro who has already undergone the process and "knows the path"—someone who has safely reached the other side, so to say, and has returned and can now show others the way.

The level of advancement that the maestro or maestra has made, revealed through the kind of spirits he or she associates with, will largely determine the level that the student achieves. If students are very good and self-determined, they will take it further, surpassing their maestro and forging new spiritual frontiers in the seemingly unlimited realms of discovery and study. As Secoya traditional elder don Cesareo Piaguaje said, "Once the student is initiated, the designs continue to open and expand and you can learn directly from the heavenly people." These "teachers" are the progenitors and protectors of all life.

While there are cases of students learning on their own, for the most part it is capricious and fraught with peril, especially at the outset, when aspirants can be presented with spiritual tests that they may not yet have sufficient wisdom to pass. Another pitfall is the existence of trick-ster spirits (that are in most cases within oneself) who attempt to block students from achieving their highest goals. Without proper training or the firmest convictions, neophytes can be tricked into becoming a sorcerer and doing harm. Then one runs the risk of incurring adversar-ies and being forced into conflict, and for this reason the medicine is a complex and arduous path, with few contemporary takers.

Various Approaches to Ayahuasca and Yagé

Ayahuasca is known by many names, including the widely used term *yagé* (pronounced ya-HEH), originating among Tukanoan peoples of present-day northwestern Amazonia. "Tukanoan" refers to a language group named after one of its representatives, the Tucano tribe of Brazil and Colombia. The Secoya people are classified as members of the west-ern Tukanoan language group. As touched on in Chapter 1, the yagé tradition of the forest can be distinguished from an ayahuasca tradition and science that was handed down originally from the Incan forefathers of the Andes highlands; this esoteric knowledge made its way to other tribes in the Peruvian Amazon. Within the rapidly growing mestizo (mixed indigenous and European and/or African ancestry) religious groups in Brazil centered on the plant as a sacrament, it is called *daime,* and the Church of Santo Daime has gained a legal foothold in the U.S. as well. And these are only three main branches of this plant-medicine tradition; there are many. This book uses *yagé* and *ayahuasca* somewhat interchangeably, the main two monikers that have passed into English usage. I must explicitly state, however, that each word relates to a quite different tradition and background that govern the medicine's use and administration, so I tend to use the name of the plant specific to the tradition I am writing about at the time.

The name *ayahuasca* can be traced to the Inca, and several Ecuadorian and Peruvian tribes. In Ecuador and Peru this word and tradition were passed from the Incan patriarchs to the Kichwa people.[8] In Peru the Incan heritage passed to tribes such as the Amahuaca (who among themselves are called the Huni Kui), who taught the Shipibo, who then taught the mestizos, who then taught the later waves of foreigners.[9] The traditions of ayahuasca (today spelled among the Kichwa-speaking people *jayawáska*) thus stem from many lineages and indigenous groups, which could be one reason that the vine today accommodates new circumstances in a syncretic mix of traditions and cultural practices.

One of the more visible differences in the relatively recent development of the traditions is that ayahuasca and daime tend to be used among urban or town people more frequently and in lesser dosages for regular sessions of health maintenance and spiritual renewal (like an enema or possibly for others a church service). Ayahuasqueros, also called *medicos* or *vegetalistas* in Peru and *yachac* in Ecuador (those who are proficient with using this medicine) frequently incorporate multiple admixture plants and specialize in journeying with those plants or treating particular conditions with them, usually serving as broad-spectrum medicine men and women for their neighborhood and beyond. Ceremonies conducted by the Santo Daime, União do Vegetal, and similar Brazil-based ayahuasca churches conduct the drinking in a congregational setting devoted to Christ, where they wear uniforms and sing hymns and songs of religious piety.

Yagé, on the other hand, is at the center of a forest-based tradition and incorporates more intense training and higher-dosage extended ceremonies than what takes place in an average União Vegetal or Santo Daime church ceremony. A typical ayahuasca ceremony in an urban setting (such as is common in Iquitos, Peru) could be said to fall somewhere in between full-blown yagé jungle journeying and the Brazilian-style church experience. It's often easier for a curious foreigner to find an ayahuasquero in a town or city in Ecuador or Peru than to encounter a properly trained shaman among the forest and river dwellers in the Amazon headwaters. And few modern ayahuasqueros have attained the spiritual skills of an old-school *yagé uncucui*. This is the term the Secoya use to refer to what we would call a shaman. It is translated into Spanish as *bebedor de yagé* (drinker of yagé). Such a person is devoted to a truthful path of service and spiritual development. Note that in any culture or language, "shaman" is generally a term earned by acts of actual healing; it is not self-claimed but rather bestowed by others on a person with spiritual knowledge and proven healing abilities.

As might be expected, shamans in the yagé tradition undertake healing a range of human conditions when requested (which remains the primary focus of an urban ayahuasquero). In addition, the yagé drinkers are known for their scientific investigations of how far the medicine can take a human being into other realms. The Secoya and other western Tukanoan speakers have taken the drinking of yagé to the furthest extents possible, drinking more and stronger yagé than most probably any of the Amazonian peoples. Following the ancient celestial transmission, the sacred plant touches every part of their living and breathing culture, traditions, and spiritual science.

Important Differences in the Traditional Consumption of Ayahuasca and Yagé

Although the names *ayahuasca* and *yagé* both refer to essentially the same potion made from similar plants, the approach varies greatly between ayahuasca of Kichwa and Incan origin, and yagé of lowland Amazonia and western Tukanoan origin. Ayahuasca (Kichwa and Incan style) is usually prepared leaving the bark on the vine and is only slightly rasped and pounded. Like this the vine will be boiled, thereby leaving more tannins in the brew and gaining a more powerful purgative effect (i.e., it makes one vomit). Yagé (Secoya and Tukanoan style) is prepared by pounding off all the bark and leaving only the woody bone of the vine to be boiled. Consequently these brews have far less tannins and cause less vomiting. I have met Kichwa ayahuasqueros who admit to having learned from deep-forest shamans the technique of pounding off the bark and using *Diplopterys cabrerana* as the admixture plant instead of *Psychotria viridis,* and they attest that the brew is much better.

Ayahuasca is prepared with the chacruna or amiruka panga— the admixture plant *Psychotria viridis* that contains N,N-DMT. Yagé is prepared with yagé ocó, or *Diplopterys cabrerana,* which contains 5-MeO-DMT and is believed to offer a more primal experience and be more effective in revealing the inner dimensions.

Among the Secoya, before drinking yagé the participants consume the yagé leaf emetic. Then, some days later, when they are ready to drink proper yagé, the body is prepared for the ceremonies to come. Participants will be able to absorb without vomiting the strong yagé medicine that has been sung to and prayed over by the master, who infuses into it the sacred designs, ranging from the plants' supernatural origin to any of the vast themes to be explored as part of the great learning process that drinking yagé is.

Ayahuasca prepared with the bark makes one vomit more during a ceremony, and thus it is difficult to hold in enough of the brew to gain its full effects and see the celestial visions. Perhaps this difference in preparation can be attributed to a process of cultural erosion. In the past the Kichwa prepared their ayahuasca similar to the way the Secoya do now, always far from the house, while fasting and never allowing menstruating or pregnant women to come near. But the old-school guidelines for handling these sacred plants have been forgotten or ignored for several generations, and bark removal could be one of customs that fell away as the tradition was taken up by the average urban ayahuasquero. So while new demands for providing the experience as a result of increased ayahuasca tourism have revived this tradition, important aspects of the ancient approach are often neglected.

Other notable differences in these two traditions include the fact that a typical ayahuasca ceremony begins at sunset and ends after midnight, with the healing work occurring from 10 PM to midnight, whereas in a ceremony of yagé the drinking begins just after sunset, but the fullness of the ceremony really takes place after midnight and closer to three in the morning. From 3 AM to sunrise is when the healing occurs. Based on personal observation and conversations with the elders, between 10 PM and midnight is when the primal energies of the Earth and the earth spirits are present; from 3 AM to sunrise is when the celestial spirits descend. Therefore one could generalize that for the most part ayahuasqueros work mainly with earthly spirits, while yagé drinkers call the Yagémopai (the people of yagé), which are celestial immortals, also known as Wiñapai (always-new people) and Matëmopai (heaven people).

There are some differences in the songs as well. The songs of yagé are for the most part higher-pitched and sung at a higher frequency and faster tempo—sometimes merging into an oooing, an elongated high-pitched oo-oo-ooing—while those of the ayahuasca tend to be slower, melodic, and more melancholy. This is because the songs of yagé invoke the celestial immortals, whose energy emanations are highly refined, whereas the songs of the ayahuasca invoke the spirits and deities of the Earth, which are more familiar and tangible. This is a simplified generalization, and the songs of both traditions are deeply moving, as they both evoke profound spiritual realities. They share an emotional quivering-jaw singing style whereby the singer transmits the precise energetic reality taking place at that moment. Through song it is brought forth, presented and made known, a skill honed by the shamans.

This difference of working with celestial spirits more than earthly ones is also revealed in the origin myths of the two traditions. The first ayahuasca vine and chacruna bush grew from the grave of Manko Cápac, an ancient master and founding father of the Inca people. We can surmise that it is an earthly tradition because it grew from a tomb; on Earth death is an inevitable part of this physical realm. Yagé, on the other hand, was a gift from the Ñañë Siecopai, God's Multicolored People, a tribe of celestial immortals.

Both traditions have profound cultural significance and value. It is important to recognize that the earthly spirits dominant in the tradition of ayahuasca can be associated with both good and bad, as that is the nature and propensity of the terrestrial spirits (generally referred to as *Supai* by the Kichwa or *Wati* by the Secoya). In my experience the Secoya are much more versed in the different kinds of spirits and their qualities and virtues. The drinkers of yagé are well aware of the potential perils of association with the earth spirits, and it is done only after firmly establishing a relationship among the celestial immortals, as previously discussed. One type of earth spirits is the Mawahopai (morpho butterfly people), which the elders say can help the advanced healer accomplish difficult cures. Yet these same spirits can confuse inexperienced drinkers, making them cause damage to other people. Another terrestrial spirit is the Jurí (a wind spirit), a group of which taught the Secoya all their weaving skills, but also sucked out the eyes of some people who fished in their lake without their permission. Yet another is the Wí'watí (growth spirit, known as a hairy spirit with two faces), who regrew the Amazon jungle after the great flood simply by speaking his name. . . . The list is long of the spirits you never want to meet, unless you have confirmed your relationship with the heaven people and are ready to take the next step and advance as a healer.

The tradition of yagé encompasses all the spirits, but it is governed by the celestial spirits, who are much harder to see because they require enhanced discipline. These celestial entities cause no harm, they are pure medicine through and through, they are concerned about the fate of the Earth and humanity, and it is within their ability to bring all humanity and all of nature toward an integral salvation, toward healing and unity.

The Meaning of the Names Ayahuasca and Yagé

The names of these plants alone are rich in meaning that reveals their unique place in society. The most appropriate English translation of the Kichwa term *ayahuasca* is "vine of the soul," since *aya* means "spirit" or "soul," and *huasca* is "vine." Calling it *huasca* is descriptive since the plant is a vine, and it is symbolic because a vine is something used to tie things together, to yoke or unite two distinct parts. As we shall see, indigenous languages are deeply symbolic in the Amazon. And in this light the plant can be seen as a bridge for crossing from one side to the other, or one reality to another, in order to gain an obstacle-free approach to the voyage that is life—the voyage we all inevitably must embark on, for the mere fact that we are alive means we must die. Therefore by calling this plant *ayahuasca,* it is understood that it joins one to one's own soul, allowing one to cross the bridge over from ignorance to clarity, from unconsciousness to knowing oneself—and like this the turbulent waters of life become manageable. You might say it helps each individual to find god, spirit, or the divine, whatever the name. In this light the term "entheogen" that is used to refer to these plants could not be more appropriate. It means a substance that can allow one to see God, not merely imaginary visions. Ayahuasca is an agent that reveals one's inner divinity, and one can understand the name as meaning just that from the indigenous perspective.

Jáya(c), a different pronunciation of the same basic word, translates as "bitter." Among the Kichwa-speaking people in Ecuador, the plant's name is pronounced *jáya(c)'wásca,* "bitter vine." In the Kichwa way of perceiving and naming things symbolically, the bitter flavor is associated with the liver (bile is bitter). It is believed that drinking bitter herbs helps maintain health; and that the bitter taste enhances life—a tenet of traditional Chinese medicine as well. Therefore I think the most accurate literal interpretation of the word *ayahuasca* is "bitter vine," though "vine of the soul" is more eloquent. "Health-enhancing vine" and "spirit-catalyst" are also indicative of its multiple meanings. Due to the plant's salubrious effects and the respect it generates, it is often referred to as *abuelita,* grandmother, a term that symbolizes connection to the nurturing spirit of the Earth. Love flows when there is authentic communion—something all human beings need to live a life of health and well-being. All of this is contained within the word *ayahuasca.*

The vine itself is more than just a vine—spiraling like the twin helices of DNA, it is a repository of all information, wisdom, and realities. Elder Secoya yagé drinkers relate that upon accomplishing long periods of training, they see the vine "open"—what seems like a thin twining vine "peels apart" to reveal the magnificent limitlessness of the universe. Engulfed in energetic flames and emerging from the canopy of the flowering vine comes the *Toyá Uncucui,* the boa of designs, which allows one to see the entirety of the celestial realms and the multitude of divine immortals, who descend down along the designs path it lays out. Known by the people as a doorway, yagé gives passage to the greatest of mysteries, allowing one to see that they are not impenetrable mysteries, just secrets of nature revealed to those who have not drifted away from her.

In order to accomplish a justifiable English interpretation of the word *yagé,* I will need to bunch some words together in order to ensure that I do not contribute to the dilution of its true meaning. With this in mind, *yagé* can be translated as "a universal revealer of the inner dimensions" or "doorway to the supernatural realms." *Yagé* also refers to "a mystical passageway between realms."

Among the forest peoples, the symbolism of the word *yagé* (regardless of the language) applies to every part of the plant and its life cycle, as well as its people and their relationship to their ancestral territories, to the extent that the vine is seen as a person who extends through the land like the river, its head the source, the body the main trunk of the river, and the arms and legs the tributaries. This symbolic imagery clearly indicates the use of yagé in helping the people maintain a knowledge of and union with their rainforest homelands (see illustration on page 137). The plant's flowers are the "trail of the heaven people," facilitating descent from their celestial abodes to the Earth, in order to teach and fill the yagé drinkers with their supreme immortal energy.

The word *yagé* also refers to a kind of trans-dimensional energy vortex or transmitter that allows humans to communicate with high celestial beings and thereby receive spiritual energy and nourishment.

As you can see, the word *yagé* means a lot, and it still means a whole lot more. It is certainly much more than a drug or hallucinogen, and to refer to it as such is vastly undermining.

The term *yagé* was passed down from the Secoya people and other Tukanoan tribes such as (to name only a few) the Coreguaje, Tama (from the Caqueta; strange types of sorcery there), Payaguaje (greasy-face clan, from the Napo River, known as Jaiyá in Paicoca), Piaguaje (bird clan from the headwaters of the Siecoya River), Macaguaje (they were from the Putumayo River; famous for the advanced knowledge of animals and management of animals, and they had abundant game in their forest due to this reason), Yaiguaje (jaguar clan; they were from the Putumayo and are Cantëyapai—in Paicoca the river Putumayo is called Cantëyá, meaning "river of cane"; these people were close relatives of the Siona), Emubain (howler monkey clan), Angutero (Secoya relatives who live in Peru along the Yubineto River), Queyëbain (a deep-forest tribe from the headwaters of the Angusilla River),[10] Oyoguaje (bat clan), Senseguaje (peccary clan), Oyobai (bat people), Siona (who today live upriver from the Secoya and also at the Cuyabeno lakes), Ocoguaje (water clan), and the Yiyoguajë (glass-bead clan). Other clans whose names I have not been able to acquire an interpretation for are Zeoqueya, Icaguate, and Sayë clans.[11] All these peoples were drinkers of yagé, and of course last but not least, the Secoya who are composed today primarily of two family groups, the Piaguaje and the Payaguaje. The western Tukanoan clans, possibly the Secoya themselves, several generations in the past taught their sacred science to the Cofán and the Kamsa, who in turn taught the mestizos in Colombia.

There is no literal translation for *yagé*. When asked about its origin and meaning, traditional elder don Delfin Payaguaje of the Secoya community responded, "The name was given by Ñañë, the creator, in times of antiquity. Ñañë gave the yagé to the Ñañë Siecopai so they could renew themselves and be close to him."[12]

A Medicine Capable of Inspecting the Innermost Vibrations of Mind

"One wonders how people in primitive societies, with no knowledge of chemistry or physiology, ever hit upon a solution to the activation of an alkaloid by a monoamine oxidase inhibitor. Pure experimentation? Perhaps not."

—Richard Evans Schultes, "An Overview of Hallucinogens in the Western Hemisphere"[13]

"In the Amazon and other places where plants hallucinogens are understood and used, you are conveyed into worlds that are appallingly different from ordinary reality. Their vividness cannot be stressed enough. They are more real than real. And that's something that you sense intuitively. They establish an ontological priority. They are more real than real, and once you get that under your belt and let it rattle around in your mind then the compass of your life begins to spin and you realize that you are not looking in on the Other; the Other is looking in on you."

—Terence McKenna, *The Archaic Revival*[14]

We are beginning to understand why ayahuasca—yagé or "Grandmother Medicine" (a modern name that indicates respect)—is considered to be an entheogen, a substance that "reveals inner divinity." This differs greatly from a hallucinogen or a psychedelic, in that visions and experiences under the influence of ayahuasca (as well as other known entheogens used in ceremonial context) can provide deep and meaningful—oftentimes uninhibited—insights into the nature of life, illness, and well-being, including revelations about the very fabric of existence itself. Experiences are seen and felt as "real," as opposed to flat-out hallucinations, which ultimately are of little or no consequence, as they are mere mental stimulation, no matter how amusing. It is as if upon drinking the medicine a window to other worlds is opened to realities that exist right here and now, closely alongside our own. Boundaries and egos crumble. It is without doubt a shift of viewpoint, an extension of experience beyond ordinary consciousness. Nonetheless, regardless of how "real" the experience may be, or how accurate a reflection it allows of both outer and inner "reality," there still exists the great risk of misinterpreting these "otherworldly" experiences and how they might relate to one's life in the everyday world.

To journey with ayahuasca is to literally inspect the deepest levels of mind, though not every drink will produce an intense vision or lasting effect, as there are many variables. For example, the results are proportional to the discipline demonstrated by the student, especially when one continues drinking. Also, the variation in experience among people consuming the same brew gives credence to the notion of "plant intelligence"—it works on each of us differently and demonstrates a limitless range of action (as compared to pharmaceutical drugs, which have a somewhat predictable and standard effect on most people).

It's said that the medicine gives you what you need, not what you want. Sometimes it's all about purging: vomit, shit, old stuck energy, negative thought-forms. . . . All of it must be purged. This is why aya-huasca is called *la purga* by the mestizo ayahuasqueros of Peru. Deep purging or, stated otherwise, purification of toxins on multiple levels and the opening of energetic blockages, is the front line of any effective and long-lasting healing. At the peak of the experience, one may feel constricted and awkward; it is in these precise moments that the alkaloid-rich ayahuasca is squeezing out, on an emotional level, all kinds of impurities and toxins. When this occurs the traditional guidelines are to stay still and quiet and let Grandmother Medicine do her work. This is when people of weak disposition or with little experience in the ways of the sacred culture can literally flip, run off screaming, or start thrashing on the floor. This is not (as it may seem) "spirit possession"—this is simply the powerful medicine of the yagé awakening one's latent energies. Blockages have been overcome and what was once constricted is now flowing freely.

As for its ability to heal specific ailments, ayahuasca is most effective for the following conditions, among others: psychosomatic illness, depression, childhood traumas, abuse recovery; imbalances of the central nervous system; weakened function of the heart, pericardium, and the body's thermo-kinetic system; as well as intestinal disorders and colonic illness. I would not venture so far as to say it is a panacea for all of humanity's woes. It does, however, put people on the path to wellness, leaving the patient with a significant assignment of personal inner homework, so to say, in order to attain health and clear understanding. Not to be underestimated is the ability of this sacred plant medicine to assist in the rediscovery of one's unadorned and true self. Today many people have let themselves become indoctrinated into a conditioned mode of existence that does not encourage optimal health or enjoyment of life's greatest simple pleasures. A good strong dose of this medicine can help a person get back on track.

In the hands of an experienced guide, when well prepared and adequately administered, ayahuasca enters one's heart and mind to remove all that is in between one's true being and the celestial immortals, integrating all the scattered aspects into one new and whole being that is like a reborn child of heaven. Due to this spiritual and physical health regime, many drinkers of yagé have lived long and productive lives despite the challenging conditions of being completely self-sufficient in the remote rainforest. A shining example for me was the woman I knew as Ñeñco ("Grandmother" in Paicoca) Luisa Payaguaje of the Secoya community of San Pablo de Cantesiayá. She was the last elder woman yagé drinker. She left this physical plane of existence in 2008. I was fortunate to meet her, and even more fortunate to have participated in a ceremony with her, where she drank the medicine with us. She painted our faces before the ceremony, drank several stiff doses, and stayed still as a rock all night. At dawn she was clearing the patio with her machete and smiling.

Origins of Ayahuasca

It can be argued that many if not all so-called myths are actually real on different levels of reality, just as dreams, visions, and other experiences of consciousness have their discrete realms of actualization. This may be why they are such rich mines of symbolic wisdom and insight. Themes and archetypes that crop up repeatedly in the oral histories of widely dispersed peoples can make us sit up and notice that something more is going on than make-believe.

The legends relating the origin of ayahuasca and other sacred plants vary greatly among the distinct indigenous communities that populate the upper Amazon, yet there is a common thread of belief that these medicines were gifted to humanity by supernatural divine beings to assist us in recuperating our original nature and reconnecting with the entirety. Many of the myths document a change in the people's relationship to nature—if not exactly a fall from grace as in the Judeo-Christian mythos, this shift put the Earth's people a bit further away from the spirit world or led to the spirits pulling away and being more difficult to perceive. Thus we must work to refine our essence and ways of approaching life in order to attain something akin to the state of unity we had before, and the communion we enjoyed with the non-human world. The ayahuasca medicine helps us see and remember and return. The transcendental message of the plants and the myths is an essential truth for humanity.

A Kichwa Legend of the Creation of the First Ingandu (Ayahuasca Vine)

Casimiro Mamallacta Mamallacta, a Kichwa traditional elder, shared the following origin legend with me. He attests that *ingandu* is an old, possibly pre-Kichwa name for the sacred vine. Among the elders of the Napo Runa, the Kichwa-speaking people of the upper Napo River, this legend can be heard about the ayahuasca vine as well as a few other medicinal plants and foods. I present it as related to me by *Taita*

("Father") Casimiro. Remember that this account comes from a people who live in a tropical rainforest at the eastern base of the Andes that is particularly rich in biodiversity—likely the richest on Earth (see Chapter 8). It is where Atacapie, the seven-headed boa, slayed Shiu-amarun, the glistening silver-scaled fertility boa. According to traditional elders, the events described in this story actually occurred.

A big storm raged for over a week. The rivers rose to a dangerous level and carried away entire farms and homes. In their meditations, some *yachackuna* (sages) saw that a battle was taking place between Atacapie and Shiu-amarun. After the weather changed and the rains ceased, they went to see. They walked for several days to the location of their vision and, sure enough, there was Shiu-amarun, its body slain on the bank of a lake. Growing in its decomposing heart were seven plants. There was ingandu (ayahuasca, *Banisteriopsis caapi*), amiruka (*Psychotria viridis,* also known as chacruna, a DMT-containing ayahuasca admixture plant), *iru* (a sugar cane variety), *palanda* (a banana variety that doesn't perish in abandoned overgrown garden sites), *dunduma* (a medicinal cyperaceous sedge), *pajujinjibri* (a potent variety of ginger), and *uchu* (a kind of chili pepper). According to these accounts, Atacapie still lives. (See illustration on page 239.)

Interpretation

Whether or not the beings in this account are mythic creatures or "real" creatures in a neighboring reality, their status as magical explains why they are monsters and epic beings not actually found in consensus reality on the Earth. The seven-headed boa, the shimmering fertility boa, the fire boa, the rainbow boa all symbolize phenomena that can be observed to occur on both the microcosmic and macrocosmic levels, the personal and social levels, the earthly and cosmic levels of existence.

Let's look at Atacapie, the destructive boa with seven heads. To me it seems evident from the material of the story that this creature represents many things, including the unfavorable disintegration of the energy centers of the body, understood in yogic philosophy as the chakras, with each one acting on its own terms, not in cooperation with the others. This assumption is not difficult to come to, given the violent and destructive tendencies of Atacapie. Even though they share the same body, the multiple heads reveal the loss of nature's unifying and constructive force. My interpretation of this legend is that essentially Atacapie represents chaos, creating mayhem in the land and among the people, who become impulsive and cannot discern wisdom and right action (for example, what we see happening today in the Earth's big picture).

Ecuador's modern governance is like the seven-headed boa in that its many agencies and institutions act with little or no coordination, yet they are part of the same body that is supposedly one unified government, one that shows little or no continuity with leadership changes, an essential trait for a prosperous nation. The result has been havoc and poverty for the people, and great destruction and contamination of the environment. I believe that the dominance of Atacapie symbolically represents a time of disintegration, where the unified and righteous governing force has been weakened. According to the Five Elements theory of traditional Chinese medicine, this can be seen as the constructive universal cycle being overpowered by the destructive universal cycle of energy flow, and thus the colonization and corporate invasion of the upper Amazon. For without the central unifying force and adherence to the constructive cycle of life, no type of truly beneficial local sustainable development can easily occur. How is the unifying force and the constructive cycle of universal energy re-established? By each person integrating their bodily energy centers, seeing their unity with the integral whole, and acting upon this.

While Atacapie symbolizes destruction, Shiu-amarun symbolizes creation. Its glistening silver scales tinkle and jingle like harmonious chimes or the tintinnabulation of coins cascading down a metal sheet. Along each scale is a razor-sharp ridgeline. Shiu-amarun is said to have lived under the ground, yet not as we think of it, because for Shiu-amarun the earth was not dense but as insubstantial as air!

Elders relate accounts from their elders, who could hear Shiu-amarun jangling like chimes under the earth when the yachac called it to their gardens. It traveled underground to make the earth fertile; where it passed, crops would grow with incomparable abundance.

My personal interpretation is that Shiu-amarun represents the shimmering wisdom that comes from within and allows one to tap into a life of abundance and serenity. The sharp ridges along its scales reveal that no lower energies can attach to this glistening energy vibration. The fact that it is metallic indicates Shiu-amarun's dominance over the effects of climate. Because its metallic scales emit beautiful sounds when brushed together, Shiu-amarun represents harmonious integration of the Earth's most pure and high-energy vibrations. We could say it represents the great realms of purity of the Earth—it represents the heaven that is Earth. Its slaying by Atacapie foretold that a time of disintegration was to come upon the region, where the governing powers would be a tangle of uncoordinated forces, represented by seven separate heads. With this event the people lost their integral relationship with nature that enabled limitless abundance.

The legend also represents the end of unlimited life, which is the beginning of life as survival and the oral history that delineates the present era. This is a time when intermediaries are needed to maintain balance and reconnect with the cosmic forces that can make the Earth a heaven, and this is why powerful magical plants grew from the heart of Shiu-amarun. To ameliorate this loss of connection to the unified whole, and to demonstrate the infinite compassion of the Earth and the celestial beings for humanity and their desire for us to rise above the lowly condition we have proven capable of falling into, we were given the collection of useful and sacred plants that is a memory of Shiu-amarun—a gift of its heart: entheogenic ayahuasca and the admixture plant amiruka, sweet cane, a hardy banana variety, a spicy chili pepper, an anti-parasitic medicinal sedge, and a powerful small ginger bush used to ward off negative energies, ease the stomach, and balance the personality. That these plants originate from this mythic creature shows the need to follow nature, not humanity, as the Shiu-amarun is representative of the purest non-corruptible elements in nature.

Another legend relates the battle of Atacapie and Nina-amarun, Fire

Boa, representing the energy of the Andes mountains. Fire Boa lost an eye in the battle but successfully dislodged Atacapie from Papallacta Lake, where it had been residing, allowing those in the village of Papallacta to live peacefully. Atacapie slithered off to Sumaco Volcano, where it is believed to remain today in a lake near the summit. It's possible that these mythological events represent real empirical changes in the Earth's evolution such as the receding of intense volcanic activity in the Andes, millions of years back, during the main era of the Andean orogeny.

A Secoya Legend: Meeting God's Multicolored People and Receiving the First Variety of Yagé

In the wilderness of the Amazon's headwaters country, near the border between Ecuador and Peru, there is a river known among the Secoya people as the Siecoyá. In its upper tributaries lived Ñañë (also known as Paina), the creator of the human race and many animal races as well. His home, when he lived on the Earth, is considered a sacred region by the Secoya, who call it Ñañë Jupo, "Creator's Paradise," or Mai Hakë Jupo, "Our Father's Garden."

In times not long past, there was not such a wide separation between the realms of the Earth and those of the supernatural celestial heavens. It was easier for mortals to know or visit these places, and the celestial beings would sometimes live on the Earth itself, or descend in their cosmic canoes to bathe in the wilderness lagoons. Don Cesareo, with whom I lived during my five years among the Secoya, visited the paradise of Jupo as a child with his grandfather, and these are perhaps his fondest memories, shared only on days when he awoke in the best of moods. "To arrive there one had to go praying," he would say, "and with sincere and earnest intentions." Like this he was brought as a child. It seemed to have taken them much longer to get there than it did to return. Elders say that people who are impure or who go there with corrupted intentions will never find the location. They will walk for days and get lost in the wilderness, and few people to this day know of its existence.

Just as in the stories of old, when Cesareo's party arrived, large green parrots, the *Ñañëpai hueko* ("God's people's parrots"), appeared to greet them. They screeched in delight, "Eat the apples from that side, but not from this side!" The family was followed by a middle-aged Secoya man who was a little mischievous. They had arrived to where the pillars of the house of Ñañë still stood; two waterfalls cascaded nearby in the river. The man lifted his machete and slapped it against one of the pillars. They are made of *këhna,* a type of celestial metal not found on the Earth, and the machete broke in half. Before they could tell him not to behave in this fashion he had lifted the machete, holding both pieces together. Suddenly, before their very eyes, as if it had never broken, the two parts fused together. He also threw a stick at the guardian parrot and broke its wing. The parrot fell to the ground screeching, then it ruffled its feathers, shook its wing, and flew away unharmed.

Many things they saw there. A *kënjé* tree (copal) was loaded with fragrant sap for making torches. Custom holds that at Jupo, as an offering, one must first bathe these copal trees with *chucula,* sweet banana gruel, then the sticky sap will flow effortlessly off. This they did, and the sap dropped down into their baskets. Legend has it that if the sap is harvested without first splashing chucula on the trees, then blood flows from the tree. Everything must be done with reciprocity and respect in this sacred area.

The legends of Jupo and the miraculous energy of this sacred land are held closely in the hearts of the Secoya people, rightful ancestral stewards of this place—an actual place on Earth. The fundamental teaching is to live always in reciprocity and respect as if the celestial immortals were watching each move, thought, and spoken word.

According to Secoya tradition, the ancestors of modern humans had tails and lived underground. One day at Jupo, Ñañë met a Secoya man who had come to the surface to gather vines. He asked the man, "For what purpose are you pulling those vines into the underworld?"

The man replied, "To make a rack to smoke palm fruits for our daily drink."

Ñañë responded, "What are these palm fruits?"

The man said he didn't have any with him. They agreed to meet again the following day. Ñañë would show the man his palm fruits, and the man would show Ñañë his.

The palm fruits Ñañë was talking about were growing in the garden of Repao, his wife. She was not in agreement with his plan and did not want him to take the fruits. Ñañë was so determined that he transformed into a *toama,* a scarlet macaw, and like this was able to enter her garden unperceived. When he and the man met again, they showed each other the palm fruits they had brought. The man's were just lumps of clay, but the ones Ñañë had brought were delicious. He gave some to the man and said, "When you return back under the earth, many other tribes will smell the palm fruit and eat from this bundle I am giving now, but try to see that some remains for your own people." This is because Ñañë knew that they lived deepest down in the center of the Earth.

After sampling the fruits, the tribes began drifting up, looking for better food on the surface. As the people emerged, one after another, from the Earth, Ñañë cut off their tails and flung them away. The bodies transformed into members of the human race, and the tails became monkeys. Each human tribe produced a different species of monkey, and it is believed that all the human tribes were created here in this fashion, and simultaneously all the monkey species too. The Secoya were the last of the tribes that emerged from under the ground, and they were left in this beautiful region to care for it.

A young Secoya woman who was menstruating came out as well. Ñañë turned her into a deer and she ran off. Then the door closed (possibly so others would not tread on her trail), leaving many tribes of underworld people inside, unable to emerge to the surface. This is one reason why the Secoya traditionally did not eat the deer. Another reason is because it is the food of the jaguar. In the days of old the jaguars were much larger and more ferocious than today, so it was a wise decision and form of self-protection to leave the jaguars' food source alone.

Some generations passed, and it was time for Ñañë to leave the Earth. He pleaded with the people to leave him a disciple, someone he could take with him to celestial realms and teach his knowledge to, someone who would then return to help humanity. Legend has it that none would give up a child. He then said, "If you can listen to me speak until the dawn of day, you will be allowed to renew yourselves." People were falling asleep during his ceremony so he relented somewhat and said, "Those who can hear me until midnight will be allowed to renew themselves," and still by midnight almost all the people had fallen asleep. Only an elderly woman, the *socó* or *capirona* trees *(Calycophyllum spruceanum),* the *siripë* (iguana), *aña* (snakes), and spiders stayed awake to hear the final words of Ñañë before he departed the Earth, followed by multitudes of Wiñapai, Matëmopai, and Mañoko Wiñapai.

Just before departing, Ñañë sent Cunti Cou (the land tortoise) upward toward heaven; it climbed into the sky to achieve salvation along a vine called *cou pinzi* (turtle vine) that grows in an undulating wave-like, stair-like pattern—this is *Bauhinia guianensis,* a medicinal plant useful for ailments of the kidneys. The vine's shape commemorates this mytho-historic event, and whenever seen in the forest reminds the Secoya of this legend, one that confirms an important part of their cultural history. This common vine, seen almost daily in the forest, serves as a continual reminder of their rich oral heritage.

Because of the elderly woman, animals, and trees that remained attentive to Ñañë's last words on Earth, older women who have had many menstrual periods—as well as the socó trees that shed their bark, and the iguanas, snakes, and spiders that can shed their skin—can more easily obtain renewal on the Earth than other mortals. The Secoya believe that they are able to live a fresh life, more similar to that of the immortals where each moment is like a new life. They are not hung up on the many tribulations that people let themselves get caught up with, thus compromising their immortality.

Once Ñañë left the Earth, humans and animals became mortal. Only nature in its holistic perpetuation maintains the ability to self-renew. That's why, as the Taoists say, we must follow nature, not man, in working to attain an integrated original essence.

After Ñañë's departure, the grandmother went to bathe in the river.

She shed her skin and transformed into a young woman. Her old skin, removed like dirty clothes, lay limp in a pile on the riverbank. A child came to look for her but upon encountering the pile of old skin he scurried home and died of fright in his father's arms. His father, outraged, ran to avenge the death and encountered the young woman bathing in the river. He saw the pile of old skin and, frightened by this mystery, he killed her.

A different version of the myth related by other elders tells that the newly-young woman returned to her village. Her grandson did not recognize her and fell in love with her at first sight. He pursued and pursued her until succeeding. She bore him a child. Then one day when she was blowing on the fire, her grandson/husband saw her blow like she used to blow when she was an old lady and he her little grandson. He realized in that moment what had transpired. She said to him, "Yes, I'm your grandmother." After that the youth left her and moved to another village.

Generations after Ñañë departed from the Earth, in the same region of Jupo, hunters of an ancestral Secoya clan, the Piaguaje, encountered a group of people living there. They dressed in multicolored tunics and crossed necklaces made of sehué seeds; their crowns sported an iridescent blue band topped with a ring of red in front and yellow on the sides. They wore fragrant bundles of leaves on their wrists. Decorative lines on their arms and legs were made with a sticky paint that held a white fluff, and intricate designs on their faces were painted with an aromatic substance. Their energy was contained and supreme. They called themselves Ñañë Siecopai—"God's Multicolored People."

The Secoya began periodically visiting the Ñañë Siecopai, who showed them some of their sacred culture and traditions. Here is where the Secoya learned to drink yagé (including the cleansing process of vomiting with the leaves and the methods of preparing extra-strong ëosiko yagé—see Chapter 5). Secoya elders attest to this day that in their visions they see the Ñañë Siecopai drinking copious yagé. They can be seen vomiting regularly as well, which they do in order to maintain their energy level as shining and active.

The Ñañë Siecopai taught the Secoya to drink yagé to recuperate their original nature, so that they could bring heaven to earth, and so that when their earthly time was over they could easily find the path to their original immortal abode where their good ancestors live, along the banks of the Matëmo tsiaya, the "River in Heaven." The Secoya as we know them today still sustain many of the traditions and manners learned during this period.

It was after this encounter that the river where these mythic-historic events occurred came to be called Siecoyá (Multicolored River). During this same period the various clans began calling themselves the Siecopai (Multicolored People), celebrating the profound significance and cultural magnitude of the new way of life and teachings adopted from the Ñañë Siecopai and continually confirmed through the drinking of yagé. They were a semi-nomadic tribe of swidden (slash and burn) agriculturalists before this encounter, and afterwards came a period of cultural renaissance among the people. Many clans, each with its own family name, joined in celebrating the sacred culture and upholding this celestial transmission as their way of life. When the Western missionaries and first settlers moved into the area, they began calling all these people the Secoya, a simpler way to pronounce Siecoyá, the name of the river. Later this river came to be called Wajoyá, "River of War," as here the cultural hero Wajo Sará valiantly fought off the first Portuguese settlers. Today many Secoya still live on this river, known on most maps by its Spanish name, Rio Santamaria.

Among the Ñañë Siecopai were advanced ceremonial leaders who were the holders of the matipë, the ceremonial scepters. One Secoya got too self-righteous and began touching these ceremonial objects. He was politely notified that not even among the Ñañë Siecopai does everyone touch the ceremonial items. The Secoya man thought that he had become immortal like them and that he was sufficiently privileged to touch these items, but by doing so he stepped out of bounds and into his own self-aggrandizement and self-importance. It had become more important to him to touch the ceremonial items, to break the guidelines they had laid down and the naturally respected hierarchy, than to humbly learn from them through participating in their way of life and volunteering.

Secoya elders relate that too many people started coming too close to this area where the Ñañë Siecopai were living, and while they were happy to teach and generously shared the tradition of yagé with the Secoya, they politely requested that when the women were menstruating, they not come near. Among the celestial immortals, the women do not menstruate, and none of them can be anywhere near the smell of this earthly phenomenon. However, some women did come too close, and one day, most unexpectedly, the celestial people were gone. Only the cane bushes were left, but no longer did iridescent blue birds fly from their tops as they had when their masters were present. Some Secoya people took the cane to recall the profound events, and still to this day some grow this striped cane. It is used to treat earache and can also be used to pole canoes. At one time the Secoya had the special variety of yagé called *Ñañë Siecopai yagé*—"God's Multicolored People yagé"—but that has been lost over the passage of time and migrations.

I heard a different yagé origin story from don Delfin Payaguaje. He told me that in ancient times there was a spiritual master with a special affinity for honeybees, which he kept with great joy. One day he ate too much honey and entered a trance. He met a celestial being from the heavenly realms who gifted him a variety of yagé.

According to the elders, yagé has come into human use in many different ways, because there are various types of yagé that over the ages have squeezed through, or somehow passed through, from the unchanging immortal realms to the physical realms bound by constant changes. Often these are varieties that have been gifted from the realms of spirit to the human realms. Many of the ancestral varieties have been left behind in migrations or lost in the overgrown gardens of deceased shamans, such as the Ñañë Siecopai yagé as well as another variety called *nuitu yagé*, which grew thick but not too high, only up to the first branches of a small tree.

Today the most common variety is the *sëño yagé* or *tara yagé*, a yellow variety. It is from a wild vine that was domesticated. There is also the *wai yagé,* a small vine that grows more like a bush than a vine; some strains have leaves with mottled yellow spots. These varieties were obtained by an ancient yagé drinker in his visions, as a gift from the heaven people in response to the earnestness and sincerity evident in his self-discipline. There is also the *tzinca yagé,* a variety with swollen nodes that is said to be governed by the wind, such that those who drink of this vine attest to experiencing visions related to the wind; this variety is used for healing and learning to heal. Other varieties known and cultivated among the Secoya are *tutu yagé* (the "strong" variety), *nea yagé* (the "black" variety with undulations on the edge of its leaves, a variety governed by the power of the water), *jëesaipë yagé* (the "iridescent azure blue" variety), *Usepopai yagé* (the "people from Pleiades" variety), *sense yagé* (the variety of the peccaries), and *yai yagé* (the jaguar variety), among so many more.

Interpretation

The Secoya legend of their encounter with God's Multicolored People deeply affected Secoya customs such that one could probably say that Secoya culture was formed by this event. Other tribes such as the Cofán adopted yagé traditions from the Secoya. This all occurred in the sacred region of Jupo, many generations after the creator accomplished his deeds and departed from the Earth. The Ñañë Siecopai offer a celestial example of refinement and perfection. They dress elegantly, representing a life of discipline, poise, and grace, a life in total integration. The fact that they appeared in the wilderness to hunters pursuing game indicates the need to protect the wilderness and to ensure that great nature, including sacred places like this, survives into the future. That they wear tunics of different colors and lived near the region of Jupo, the location where many of the human tribes originated, indicates that their guidelines transcend racial and cultural divisions. They are immortals, and they came to the Earth to teach the tradition of yagé as a means to align oneself with universal subtle realities. They taught the safe uses of yagé as a vehicle for transformation and protection of self and community, and for obtaining spiritual enlightenment—not through merely understanding a concept but rather by merging completely with the true origin energies of life.

In my attempt to best understand these mythologies, it seems evident that the iridescent blue birds that flew from the tops of the striped cane bushes represent the glistening heavenly energy of these celestial beings, since azure blue is the color that symbolizes heaven in the Secoya cosmology. Stripes on the cane reveal that their energy was uninhibited and freely flowing, like that of the energy of the celestial realms, because one way of attempting to describe these energies is "rising," and the vertical stripe represents energy rising, like a person who is standing.

It is also interesting to note that the Ñañë Siecopai reportedly drank copious amounts of strong, well-refined yagé. It would be difficult to match them in their drinking standards. This indicates a continual devotion to universal alignment, self-refinement, and purification.

The yagé origin myth of the Secoya resonates with human nature as we know it today when we learn of the disapproval of the heaven people when a human became arrogant and self-important. This indicates that the universal hierarchy of subtle laws must be understood and respected. We can see the prophetic nature of this incident playing out today as people learn from other cultures without showing appropriate respect for this knowledge or experience or gift. An obvious example of this is treating ayahuasca as a recreational trip or an experience to simply be ticked off one's bucket list—an ignorant approach that can actually be hazardous. In addition to the danger and insult of disrespect, we have the result that only a portion of the potentially available instruction can be passed, so the tradition gets diluted, often distorted or transmuted. And of course people with partial information hungry for power will corrupt it even more. That's one way sorcerers emerge in the world and evil spirits manipulate humanity for the sole purpose of destroying all that is beautiful.

How then can universal will be respected by modern people and societies at large? By each individual striving to abide by the guidelines imparted by the celestial beings. By attempting be a part of the forces of good that enhance all that is beautiful on our precious home, planet Earth.

Summary of Interpretations

These legends come from distinct indigenous communities, living in relatively close proximity within the Napo River watershed. Despite this proximity, their languages, traditions, and worldviews are completely distinct. The Secoya, who only migrated upriver from Peru into Ecuador in early 1940s, had little contact with the Kichwa, whose language is of highland origin. Yet both mytho-historical accounts can be interpreted to reveal universal truths. We can see that each eloquently portrays a distinct worldview while relating the common theme of this sacred plant-teacher coming forth to counter an imbalance and to give humanity another chance to maintain its relationship with the supernatural energies of Creation, through granting each individual the opportunity to be reborn as a divine child of heaven.

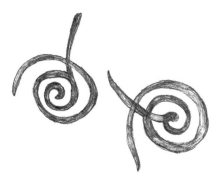

Petroglyph, sacred valley of Cotundo, Napo Province

Chapter 4

Elements of the Experience

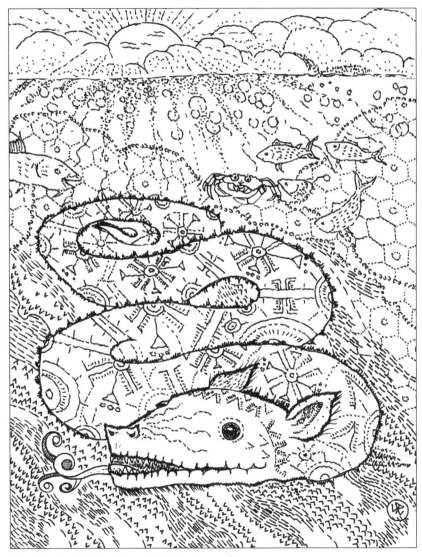

The Menkoyiyi (Electric-eel Water-dragon)

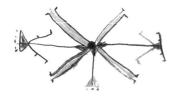

This chapter is an introduction to a few of the fundamental and more unfamiliar (to Western readers) concepts associated with this rainforest medicine. It is not a complete account of the "elements" of an ayahuasca experience, which is a complex, very personal, and largely indescribable event that cannot be broken into analyzable pieces. Many things combine to create a successful ceremony or "experience," including a lifetime of self-development and study of basic principles and universal law, as well as meditation, selfless service, and other consciousness-expanding practices that are known worldwide. In this sense the indigenous science of the Amazon is similar to many of Earth's great wisdom traditions.

Sacred Songs of the Medicine

"Through ayahuasca music—songs, chants, and whistled tunes—a subtle form of control develops; important elements of the vision progress and establish their own key melodies. Each natural object, be it animal, plant, stream or even rock, has its own melodic progression. By means of these sequences, one can examine or enmesh himself within that object for a detailed examination of its nature and its properties."
—Manuel Córdova-Ríos, *Rio Tigre and Beyond*[1]

"Many cultures talk about the songs that come through the plants. If you listen well to a plant that you have solicited medicinal aid from, they say you can learn its song, and its song will be as effective a medicine as the plant material itself. That's when you've

taken that plant in as your deep ally: when you can invoke its medicine without even necessarily touching or finding the plant. At that point you have access to the spirit of the medicine."
—Kathleen Harrison in *Visionary Plant Consciousness*[2]

The normally unseen world is made visible through song, and it is through song that the medicine work of yagé is carried out. These ceremonial songs have come to be known today generally by their Peruvian name, *icaros*.

A wide array of icaros serve as intermediaries between the world of spirits and the common everyday material reality of human life. The songs allow one to enter deeply into a state of concentration in order to gain knowledge and understanding. They are used to accomplish healing work, to invoke the aid of spirits, and to communicate and interact with the spirits who respond to the song. This allows the singer to bring forth the energies necessary to accomplish complex cures or to travel in the spirit realms, and even to take others there. An icaro that comes from a plant transmits power for healing activities directly from the plant, which is like a house for the particular teacher/healer—the spirit of the plant. Other icaros may provide connections with other spirits. With these songs, the healers tame and harness the energies of the natural and supernatural realms.

The Secoya distinguish several types of songs for different purposes. The ceremonial songs are called *yagé hë'hë'ñé* or *wiña caye*. Interestingly, the word "to heal," *juju* (pronounced hoo-hoo in Paicoca), sounds similar to *hëhë*. These words are onomatopoeic, representing vocalization patterns, energetic emanations that produce healing magic and ceremonial atmosphere. *Ujáye* is the term for another type of song, a canticle of glossolalia that spontaneously bursts through when the yagé uncucui—the drinker of yagé—meets any of the legions of celestial immortals. Some contain rhythms that have been channeled by ancient shamans and mythic melodies that invoke the divine beings that govern the tradition. They are also used for healing. The root *ujá* means "to heal": the Ujápai are supreme healer immortals invoked during the ceremonies of yagé. Another plant in the Secoya psychopharmacopeia is *Brunfelsia grandiflora,* ujájái, meaning "great healer." The ceremonial songs called wiña caye are employed when the ceremony leader and the students or participants sing in a call-and-response fashion. Other types of songs used by the Secoya if needed during a yagé ceremony include the *watí ujá,* invocations to ward off negative spirits in order to accomplish healings and protection (these correspond to *arkanas* in the Peruvian shamanic tradition). To culminate the ceremony near the dawn of a new day, the *ocoraca jujuyë* ("preparing healing water") is sung over a gourd of aromatic water containing the leaves of the fragrant cultivated ñumi bush (*Piper* sp.) and/or the tubers of one of the numerous varieties of nuní (ancestrally cultivated *Cyperaceous* sedges).

The words of all these songs may be in the singer's language or in a celestial language that is entirely unintelligible to the singer under normal circumstances. It is believed that spirits communicate through song, as humans communicate through speech. Among societies that allow spirit to guide matter, song is an essential part of ceremonial life. All things have a song; indeed, in the realm of spirit, everything is pure song. Song is the eternal continuum, it is what holds together the creation. Although the world is ever-changing, evolving, passing through its great cycles, it is unified through song—from the most remote past, to the felt presence of the immediate now, to the infinity of the future. Our human ears are not designed to easily hear these songs, and if we heard them all the time we would go mad. To open one's celestial ears and hear some of the songs of heaven and earth one must practice spiritual concentration.[3]

The World Was Created through Song

According to the Waorani, the world was created through song, in their language called *amotamini.* In the Waorani worldview, song is synonymous with creation and is the essence of creation. It animates and gives vitality to the world that itself is song. Song is all and all is song. In the beginning there was song, and song is all that there will be in the end. All that exists is held in place by song. The subtle energy transmitted through song makes known the non-dual reality of no beginning or end.

Softly chanting to the flickering light of a waning fire, some Waorani elders are singing:

> *Uhn kayahue, uhn kayahue*
> *Abukitawenano, kayahue kayahue*
> *Oboyomo, kayahue kayahue*
> *Uhn kayahue, uhn kayahue*

I ask my informant and friend Niwa Enomenga what they are singing. He replies with an interpretation:

> *This is a timeless song, this is an ageless song*
> *The parakeets are circling around the tree-top singing*
> *The children are jumping and sucking the red oboye*
>   *fruits, singing*
> *This is a time-honored song, this is an ancient song.*

The song ends with an enigmatic *Monomemeiri amotamini tíííiiiiiiiií*, "The way our ancestors sang, we sing."[4] From talking to various elders about the meaning of the word *kayahue*, I have concluded that *kayahue* is a gigantic word encapsulating a vast amount of wisdom and phenomena. In a nutshell, it means the most ancient, time-honored, ageless, timeless. The concept includes the notion of what was here in the beginning, what is here now, what will be here in the future, and what will be here in the end. *Kayahue* means song, that which permeates all existence and all ages and, as such, unifies all in the present moment.

A traditional Waorani village never stops singing. I witnessed this when I visited the Waorani village on the Yasuni River[5] in 1992 and many times in Quehueiriono village at the headwaters of the Shirpuno River. One person will be singing and as soon as he or she stops, from across the river another will begin, and so forth—through the entire night and the day, there will always be someone singing, elders and youth alike. Waorani songs are like the flame in the temple of Jerusalem that is always kept alight.

Mengatue, a most proper elder Waorani, said, "My song is like a flame that lights up the darkness. As the light arises, the darkness recedes, and all negativity is dispersed."[6]

Here is one of Mengatue's songs, which he used to merge with nature, to be able to move undetected by the animals or anyone, and thus hone his skills as a hunter (a necessary trait for survival in the deep-forest Waorani way of life) and as a warrior (in the days of old the Waorani valiantly defended their land against outside intruders):

> *Bogima ñugao I'ñyey'ñyey*
> *Ñugao I'ñyey'ñyey*

> As the low-hanging mist moves unperceived through the valley
> I move unperceived through the valley

Don Casimiro's Grandfather's Rainbow Serpent Song

Don Casimiro Mamallacta is a Kichwa traditional elder from Archidona in Napo Province, with whom I spent considerable time between 1990 and 1994 when I volunteered on a project to demarcate Napo-Galeras National Park. At the Pusuno River, don Casimiro shared with me one of his grandfather's songs. After meditating on its significance I was able to interpret the song's meaning. When I realized the interpretation I enthusiastically returned to don Casimiro's house to share my discovery and he agreed, smiling and nodding. Here are the words of the song in its original Kichwa, together with my English translation, followed by my interpretation of its meaning and essential message.

Amarun Quillchic Taquina
Rainbow Serpent Song (Song of the Rainbow Serpent)

Amarun anguilluska mandas, quishpi huahua mari ani ri
Puric runa mari ani ri, hua hua hua hua hua hua hua

The boa almost got me but I escaped, because a child I am,
   because I am a walking man.

Ima mandas quishpishaliai ri? Mana imas ranguichu.
Puric runa mari ani ri, la la la la la la la.
What is it that you can do? There is nothing that you can do.
   Because I am a walking man.

Canba chupa aitabis, mana imas ranguichu.
On your boa's tail I step, there is nothing that you can do.

Tukuiy llakta puripi, mana imas ranguichu.
Through every town I have walked, there is nothing that
   you can do.

Virdi virdi quillchic ñami rikushun, jatun yaku rikushun.
Green green rainbow is appearing, big river is appearing.

Rumibimi tiarijun, cantashami shayajun.
On a rock I sit, standing I sing.

Chiri chiri chiri chi chiri chiri chiri chi.
It's cold, cold, cold, cold, cold, cold.

Interpretation

The coils or impediments of the boa represent the vices, inertia, lassitude, jealousy, and different forms of corruption that have always
plagued humanity. Such traits lead to stagnancy in the flow of one's
inner energies. Though these negativities have brought much despair,
they have also been the impetus for the great cause of spiritual development. Spiritual development allows us to escape the boa through
upholding the virtues of a child, including innocence, awe, genuine
interest in life, and a pure heart.

But this alone will not suffice, as the innocence and trust of a child
must be coupled with the wisdom of an adult, which is gathered
through the accumulation of experiences, represented by the walking

man. "Walking" in this song has two meanings: one, the balancing of both sides of one's being—female attributes and male attributes (which can also be seen as one's spiritual tendencies and one's physical way of going about things) that is accomplished through the act of walking and living an active life; and two, the actual experiences gathered via journeying and viewing the land, seeing different cities, and meeting and learning from a diverse array of people. Through coupling the heavenly intuitive virtues of a child and the attained earthly experience of an adult, one can even "step on the boa's tail" and remain unharmed. Stepping on the boa's tail means that one does not have to be perfect in everything, nor does one have to attempt to achieve total purity—it is possible to brush up against malignant influences and not be ruined by them. This metaphor can also be taken on a more practical level to mean the strengthening of one's immune system.

The mention of "every town" reinforces the notion of the accumulation of wisdom, and the idea of traveling to distant places shows that one must stay interested in what there is to learn from various locales and cultures. It means to keep one's mind open and receptive to learning new things, not confined to a provincial, limited perspective.

The green rainbow represents wisdom and balance, because green is the central color of the rainbow, found in the middle of the visible rays of light as they reach toward infrared on one end of the spectrum and ultraviolet on the other. The river symbolizes the truth of one's inner life and physical health. It shows the importance of not holding on to opinionated beliefs, grudges, or resentments—to stay flowing like the river as a means of remaining present, pure, and close to spirit.

"On a rock I sit" is the gathering together and affirmation of this wisdom within one's whole life being; while "standing I sing" portrays the bringing forth of this wisdom into the world through serving one's community and being helpful and good-natured. "Sitting" in the Kichwa tradition and worldview represents the reception and confirmation of spiritual power inside one's body, while "standing" is the assertion of authority and the sharing of personal strength. This can be seen in Kichwa meetings, where the person talking will always stand in order to transmit the message, and those listening will sit in order to receive and absorb it.

Hua hua hua hua hua hua hua: This sound is said by Taita Casimiro to represent the pure joy of an innocent child coupled with the experience of the wise adult. It could also be that *La la la la la la la* is a type of affirmation of the favorable uses of the spiritual science to clear one's understanding. *Chiri chiri chiri chi chiri chiri chiri chi* means that it is cold sometimes (*chiri* means "cold" in Kichwa). By repeating this sound one surrenders false ideologies and peels away all preconceptions in order to understand the frank, unadorned reality of life. Withstanding the cold is seen as a means toward obtaining power, true strength, wisdom, and happiness.

Such songs are called *taquina* among the Kichwa speakers in Ecuador. Other songs used for healing and calling the spirits—those sung during the ceremonies—are called more specifically *ayawaska taquina*.

The Most Sacred Possession of the Healer

To shed greater light on the significance of the icaros, taquina, or hë'hë'ñé, I offer the following story from my interviews with Amazonian sage don Pablo Amaringo. He once said to me, "An icaro is the most sacred possession of the healer." When asked more about them, he related the following story.[7]

During an ayahuasca ceremony before Pablo became a healer, he was lying down, not feeling well from the effects of the brew that were beginning to come on. "*Allí viene Altos Cielos,*" a voice said. ("Here comes High Heaven.") Pablo quickly sat up in a good posture. He saw a gorgeous woman descending from above, with crown and necklaces. Her dress was made of all flowers, many types and colors wonderfully and elaborately woven together. From below rose up many more women singing beautifully, all ceremonially dressed. One carried a small harp that she played. Pablo used all his calm to observe the phenomena taking place. He heard each note clearly. Each word of the song was audible to him.

And he most suddenly found himself in the state of ecstasy. The women surrounded him. Flowers were falling from the sky like a gentle rain, and soon the falling flowers turned to rain. At that moment all the people in the ceremony burst into tears. Everyone wept, and amazingly, everyone saw the same vision! It was her power. Soon everyone felt really cold. Shortly afterward everyone started to laugh, and then to sing with great joy. And that was how don Pablo received the icaro of Alto Cielos, and understood that an icaro is not a human invention but a gift from the divine.

Another healing icaro sung by don Pablo as part of his spiritual practice was called "Pahuahuan." This is an icaro of the mountains, sung so that the spirits of the mountains do you no harm. In addition, when you feel trapped or if someone else is stuck in an emotional bond, in a depression or sadness, this song is used and the spirits of the mountains come to assist you. Some of the words translated to English are as follows:

> *High Heaven,*
> *Dark clouds, they are leaving*
> *Far from here*

Another of don Pablo's icaros was sung to fortify his energy in order to heal and to help strengthen the spirit of the patient. It is the song of Captain Manuel Huaya and his *Aceropunta* ("Steel Point"), also known as *Supai Lancha* ("Spirit Launch") or *Barco Fantasma* ("Phantom Boat"). These various names all refer to a visionary vessel that is seen by ayahuasqueros, and by *rivereños,* the people who live along the river banks.[8]

> *Acero punta vaporninchi*
> *Acero punta vaporninchi*
> *Shamui rimun paicayari*
> *Mundo mundo tucuimanda*
> *Shamui rimun paicayari*
> *Shamui rimun paicayari*

As Pablo interpreted the song for me, I took notes. He said, "The Aceropunta moves emitting a vapor, it has force and energy; like a boa it has supernatural force, it uses the magnetism of a boa to move itself. Come to this place where we are gathered so we may see you, as you travel the world around. Come to this place where we are gathered now."

This is a long song, and these are just a few phrases of it. The song depicts the Aceropunta's smoking chimney and Manuel Huaya, the captain of this vessel, whose belt buckle is a crab and the belt a *puka-puka-naka-naka* (an uncommon red poisonous snake).

Once Pablo Amaringo heard an elder healer sing the Aceropunta song in order to heal a young man who had been bitten by a poisonous snake. Pablo was impressed with how the old man through the song alone effectively healed the snakebite. Not long after, Pablo and others saw that under the elder's house there were many kinds of snakes. The elder sang a different song to make them go away and they did! It was a fine song that Pablo was never able to repeat. How long, Pablo wondered, had it taken this elder to learn this song, to refine his science through dieting and fasting to such a place where through song he could realize these spiritual achievements?[9]

Don Solon's Legendary Healing Icaros

In Iquitos, Peru, I had the good fortune to meet don Solon Tello (1918–2010), a legendary ayahuasquero from this area. He was loved and appreciated by all who knew him and called *el Caballero de la Ayahuasca*, "the Gentleman of the Ayahuasca." I was able to participate in his healing ceremonies in 1997. I detail his great example in the "Lineage Holders" chapter.

Singing, don Solon Tello prepared the medicine for us to drink. I faintly made out some of the Spanish words interwoven with the Lamista dialect of the Kichwa shamans he had trained among. I found the icaros of this elder healer of the urban ayahuasquero plant-medicine tradition in Iquitos to be exceptionally captivating. His songs were simple, humble, and profound.

Don Solon allowed me to realize how language as we normally conceptualize it is irrelevant to this medicine science and to the divine spirits that support the healers. What matters is the ability to unify with the higher-energy realities that are beyond language, and to fuse this intention into the present moment. We are born into a cultural circumstance where language is used to communicate, to transmit concepts and exchange information with one another. The energetic reality made evident through the effects of the medicine, however, allows one to understand how the healer uses vastly diverse techniques that regular language knows nothing about. Words are stretched far and wide, then they are pushed closely together; the healer uses them to try to meet the demands of the circumstances. To communicate the language of spirits, regular words are transformed to become carriers of designs, messengers of prayers.

Below I reproduce a short portion of one of his icaros. This icaro I could understand because it was mostly in Spanish, in an idiom that had been made more sensitive, brought closer to spirit, by the medicine.

So-pla-ri-ngi-So-pla-ri-ngi	*Blowing, blowing*
Me-di-ci-na-So-pla-ringi	*Medicine, blowing*
Cui-de-nos-dios-ci-to-lindo-tu-hijos	*God, care for us, your children*
Cui-de-nos-ma-dre-ci-ta-tu-hijos	*Mother, care for us, your children*
Ilu-mi-ne-nues-tro-ca-mi-no-lin-do	*Illuminate our path*
Esta-mos-en-mi-ca-si-ta-su-ca-sa	*Here we are in my humble abode, your home*
Me-di-ci-na-me-di-ci-na	*Medicine, great medicine*

It seems simple, but each Spanish word means much more when infused with life brought forth by the medicine. For example, *soplaringi* refers not only to blowing but also to "vital breath," to be filled and made new again; to be blown on means to receive vitality and be filled with the natural power of life.

Elements of the Experience ❈ 97

"Spirits read not your lips but rather your intentions, and the vibrations of your heart," said don Solon once as we sat talking and smoking the strong native tobacco after a ceremony.

Glimpses into the Songs of the Always-New Ones

August 2006, Secoya territory: Agustin Payaguaje, or as friends call him, "Tintin," feebly arose for a second round of yagé, drank, and retreated to his hammock. He was still weak after having been lost in the forest for four full days, and we were all tired from the long days of searching for him.

Fifteen minutes later he got up and asked for a full gourd. His friend Fragrant Medicine Bark—Cesareo Piaguaje—filled a gourd to the rim for him to drink. He began to blow and cure the brew. I'll never forget this moment. The intensity of the song, the earnestness of his prayer into the yagé, were like none I had ever heard.

Tintin drank the gourd passed from the master's hand. He drank and drank and drank and drank . . . and drank. I had only taken a few sips as my own dose earlier; the brew was evidently strong and I was barely holding on. It took all my might to stay still, which thankfully I did, as I did not want to be the one to interrupt such a moment. I was already so woozy that just hearing each of his gulps go down, one at a time, made me feel more and more delirious. With each gulp that coursed down his throat, I myself felt the yagé come on stronger and stronger inside me, and by the time he finally had slurped down the entire gourd, I was curled up in my hammock shivering.

Shortly afterward, Tintin began singing, and that soon led into a heavier chanting, then a moaning, then a howling—bursting open the stillness of the night with a fury, as if he were cutting his way through tangles of vines, incessantly focused on discovery and transformation. He was discovering what was holding him back and transmuting it. He grabbed the bottle of yagé and gulped down even more. This was serious work and he needed to be fully engulfed in the inebriation to accomplish it. Sweating, he sang, howling into the canopy of the screaming bird-filled night. The lodge was small and the participants of the ceremony were huddled close together. I thought, 'For sure this guy is going to go running shrieking into the woods,' but he only stumbled onto the patio and pranced around like a capering jaguar, skipping back and forth from one end of the patio to the other, then returned to the lodge.

Back in his hammock he chirped and let out other noises impossible to describe, other than to say they sounded like what one would expect a whirling goblin to sound like. There were whistling sounds like high-pitched flutes emitting piercing shrills, and all the time blowing, and more blowing, until after a while he eventually returned to a rhythmic melody, and the intensity waned. The long melancholy moaning glided into an *ooo*ing, a long and persistent *ooo ooo ooo*ing, and this went on for a while. Mesmerized, I wondered what on earth was happening.

All the while, seeming as though it came up from behind him, the sound of soft blowing could be heard. Through the blowing the negativity was being released, and it was if he were inviting it intimately near, to recognize and allow it to surface, and thus he released what was no longer needed. It was as if he were pulling out a grim complexity from deep within himself or the surrounding environment.

It seemed as if through the chanting, the *ooo*ing, and melodic and vocal trance-inducing intonations he was unraveling an old, limiting, seriously negative pattern. Through his focused intent this thing or energy disappeared into itself, vanishing into the void. There was some sort of snapping sound, and his song shifted; he did more blowing and singing, blowing and singing, until he finally succeeded in thoroughly blowing out the goblin he had just crunched in his newly re-established diamond body. With complete triumph he sang, "Haaaaaaaaaaaaaaahahahahahahahaaaaaaa," which reverberated throughout the hut, verifying that he was healed.

He sang, "Hahahahaaaahaaaahaaaaa, mea'sooo measooo so so so . . . wiña'so so so so so. . . ."

Soon he arose to stand next to his hammock, wet and smelling all fresh from the green leaves he had tucked into his armbands while he was out prancing around the patio. He stood there, swaying back and forth. Cesareo passed him the matipë, the ceremonial scepter, and the leafy rattle called the *hookasayepë* made from a tied cluster of mamecocó *(Pariana radiciflora)*, which is a broad-leafed grass. He sang rhythmically, echoing ancient voices. Soft crowded faint notes filled the room, interlaced with abundant blowing, soft notes and blowing, soft notes and blowing—the ship was on course again and it seemed as though he were unfurling the scrolls of this time-honored healing method for all present to see.

Rhythmically dancing back and forth, back and forth, lifted by the energies of the heavenly people, Tintin was restored. He had burst through and was now healed, his original energetic body fully reintegrated and recuperated with the energy of the divine immortals.

The drunkenness soon passed. It had reached a climax for all of us and almost as suddenly as it arrived it faded away. After this a deep peace prevailed. I touched the pure calm of the good way of life. All the participants of the ceremony felt the good energy, the positive transformation that occurred in us all, and everyone was satisfied knowing that the healing had been effective, especially for Tintin.

As the new morning advanced, participants lay silent and still in their hammocks, gently swaying, the copal incense burning softly, thin wisps of aromatic smoke rising from the embers of the fire.

Later that day, Cesareo expressed satisfaction with the powerful ceremony, during which, he said, his and Tintin's spirits had traveled to the realms of the Jaicuntipai, the spirits of Napo-Galeras.[10] There Cesareo thought, "I will see if I can arrange a marriage for him." Cesareo was with his spiritual wife and children and was just about to tell her of his plan when he noticed that over there, in a different place, Tintin had already married long ago and even had a son. Cesareo's wife knew what he was thinking and laughed at him—"You didn't know?" When Tintin sang his high-pitched whistling notes in the night, this was due to the arrival of his spiritual son, who had found him again thanks to the strong, properly cured yagé.

Tintin had lost contact with his powers and now had regained them.

The times had been changing. He had attempted to follow the way of the Evangelicals for many years and stopped drinking yagé. But he was obliged to begin again after having been spiritually damaged. Prior to this healing, Tintin had suffered for several difficult years. He would get lost in the forest, lose his belongings. . . . His wife had died from a snakebite, and he had lost both his children as well—his son drowned in the river, drunk on *guanchaca,* sugarcane moonshine brought in by the colonists.

Now Tintin was fine again and at peace with himself after this healing that he had accomplished with the assistance of his spirit son. Tintin later shared with me his ceremonial yagé name, which he had almost forgotten. It is Këhna'curipiarazá, "Golden Sky-metal Bird." Today he is among the last living lineage holders of the Secoya yagé tradition.

Infusing Water with Sacred Healing Energy

Infusing water with fragrant plants and praying over it to bless it with healing power is a widespread practice, probably pan-Amazonian if not global. This water is then sprinkled to cleanse spaces, or drunk to bring healing energy to a person, or employed in a multitude of other ways.

Among the Secoya, a rhythmic singsong chant is often sung at dawn after a ceremony for healing water. Once I had the opportunity to jot some of the words in my notebook, and I reproduce them below. These songs, known as ocoraca jujuyë, "preparing healing water," may be chanted for up to an hour in order to charge water containing the fragrant herb ñumi. The arrangement of soft crowded notes culminates in the master reciting sagas of celestial beings and their eternal love for humanity; their energy, of which just one little drop can bring forth countless healings; and the way they descend to the edge of the house, to see, to watch, to witness the cure, to charge the medicine so it may be effective. The water absorbs the energetic emanations of the chant so that when a patient drinks it, this energy as well as the plant energy and molecules enter his or her body and infuse it with the memory of intact health and positive energy, replacing the stagnant negative designs that are causing persistent illness. This historical application of song foreshadows the now-famous work of Japanese researcher Masaru Emoto,[11] who experimented with the transmission of intentions to water. When water infused with love and good intentions is drunk, it can be used to transform the energetic state of being.

Here is a segment of Tintin's ocoraca jujuyë:

> *Wiñapi ocopí*
> *Payo tututeh*
> *Sá wiña sásá*
> *Toyá wiña maapí*
> *Heh heh heh hee, heeeeee. . . . .*

Each Secoya word is a world of meaning, especially words such as these that are not used in everyday speech and pertain to the songs of yagé. With the help of Miguel Payaguaje, Tintin's nephew, I was able to acquire the following interpretation. *Wiñapi* is to become new. *Ocopí* relates to water that is healed through infusing it with charged sacred intentions. *Payo tututeh* means filling the liquid with supreme spiritual strength that will affect the physical reality. *Sá wiña sásá* says that the energy of the shaman is making something powerful, transforming the old into the new, infusing something with the ability to transform and renew itself. *Toyá wiña maapí* refers to trail of the celestial designs that is always new. *Heh heh heh hee* is a powerful affirmation that strengthens every level of life and wards away negative energies. It confirms and ensures one's intention that the sacred words come true, and that the spirits will look favorably upon one's acts.

My English rendering and summary of the meaning of the song goes like this: "Infusing into the water the designs of the everlasting always-new ones, may their energy charge this water, may the patient that drinks this water be made new, be made fresh, like the always-new ones of Heaven; may these be the designs that fill this water, and may the people walk this complete path of renewal."

The Secoya also have invocations used to ward off negative spirits.

These are the watí ujá mentioned above. They can be sung onto a piece of wood like a twig or thin branch, which is then tossed to where the negative spirits are, making them recede with their unruly, mischievous, life-threatening plots.

The Language of the Celestial Realms

A Secoya legend tells of an ancient yagé drinker named Quequero who died a sudden death and used his powers to take the souls of his wife and son with him to the next world, to the house of Repao, the wife of Ñañë, our creator. Quequero had fallen into sorcery, while his wife and son were very pure-hearted and good people.

This legend illustrates that song is the language of the celestial beings, and for this reason I share it here. It is believed that when a traditional Secoya dies, their soul travels to the house of Repao. Not all human souls can travel there because many are too heavy to find the way; only those who have lived according to the traditional standards, and drinkers of yagé who are versed in soul travel, find their way to Repao's house. Quequero was a seasoned drinker of yagé, and for this reason was able to navigate the next world after his death, and bring his wife and son, although they were not even dead. But the evil deeds he had committed during life would not permit him to be sent to live a life of abundance and unlimited freedom among the good ancestors along the shores of the heavenly river.

Inside Repao's lodge is a hammock where the souls of the deceased are laid to be judged. Every action they took and every thought they had during life are visible on them. A swarm of hummingbirds, whose nest is above the door, descends onto each soul to determine the caliber of virtue by which the person lived on the Earth.

Quequero's wife took one of Repao's clay pots to fetch water from the river. When she was walking back up the hill on the path to Repao's house, she saw the house get swallowed up in dark clouds. At the same time, the path before her closed up, blocked by spiny vines. At that moment the hummingbirds had read Quequero's soul and found that he had practiced sorcery and killed people. His soul needed to be sent to the other side of the heavenly river to suffer and purify itself. Startled by the clouds and the spiny vines, his wife dropped the clay pot holding the water. When it hit the ground and broke, it transformed into a big anaconda that slowly slithered off. Soon the clouds lifted, the vines receded, and the house again appeared atop the hill.

Repao did not understand how the woman and her son arrived there since they were still alive in the mortal world and not meant to be at her house. Moved by the woman's nobility, grace, and goodness, Repao arranged to send them back to their home on the Earth. Repao sent two Wiñapai, each transformed into a white king vulture, a *pëpërí*, to scout out the route back to Earth. Upon arriving on the Earth, one of pëpërí-Wiñapai became ensnared in a hunting trap, then yanked itself free. When it returned with the injury to the house in heaven, Repao asked the woman if she knew how to heal this type of wound.

To the immortals, who perceive things differently, it seemed as though the vulture had incurred a snakebite, though the mortal woman could see that it was actually a rope wrapped tightly around its ankle. She retrieved a sewing needle she held tucked in her shawl and began loosening the knot. To the immortals it seemed that she was singing a song—her hand swayed rhythmically back and forth as she loosened the knot. For people who sing among themselves to communicate, this was a beautiful song.

When the knot was loosened, the immortals were very happy with her. Repao gave her the *Matiyai*, the magic scepter named Heaven Jaguar, advising her not to overuse it, not to show it to anyone, and always to share with others the abundance it brought. Then Repao placed her and her son each on the back of one of the white king vulture spirits, who took them home, spiraling downward through the clouds.

With the Matiyai they could point to a patch of forest and it would transform into a garden, or to some game animal and it would fall dead. The woman and her son lived well in a remote part of the forest. Other Secoya were impressed by how the two of them were able to always have food and a nice garden. Eventually they got the son drunk and he showed them the Matiyai, which was stored in a clay pot covered by a leaf. The following morning there was a hole in the pot, and they saw a big jaguar leaping up through the sky. The scepter truly was a "heaven jaguar." Later scepters built after the model of the Matiyai were dubbed *matipë,* "heaven rising."[12]

SEEING THE SONG

Fragrant Medicine Bark blows on the gourd of yagé. A glistening blue star alights on its surface. Intricate patterns coalesce. Delicate designs make the brew potent. It is as if the song does more than create the designs that appear—it also creates a space in which they *can* appear. Like a harbor protects boats, a curtain shields a place from being seen, the song gives the eternal designs an opportunity—a temporary space in linear time—to appear and become known to us. Like light pushing through darkness, like bubbles rising through water, the songs of yagé force their way upward, creating a space where infinite energy can incarnate in the limited world.

In the small area in front of the master's lips, which are rhythmically moving above the gourd of yagé, a song is flowing from the deepest recess of his memory where he unites with the immortal realms. The blue star shimmers inside the brew, quivering rays of light energetically filling the liquid. Fluffs of the purple and white cotton of the *toyá ma'a,* the designs trail, begin to rise above a hillside of golden green swaying grasses . . . in a sunlit prairie . . . where summer winds gently blow. All spirits are rising toward omniscience, toward a sublime unification with the whole. Auras bend upward and back and around, emanating circular colors, extending out like the translucent wings of a celestial bird, white and speckled with the cobalt-blue darkness of the star-lit night. The star in the cup. . . . Can words ever describe such a mysterious phenomenon? They can only guide the mind closer to fathoming what is made a reality through the traditional drinking of yagé.

And the *yagé toyá* is much more than enigmatic imagery. One could reckon it is the atmosphere of spirits and supernatural beings, the aura of the vast array of energetic emanations that comprise creation. Wordlessly, they impart original instructions that can connect us to spirit, pushing our entire being toward physical and spiritual sublimation, inspiring integration with the higher universal energy realms, and thus transforming heavy, stagnant energy patterns into light, freely flowing patterns of a good and healthy life.

Yagé Toyá: Designs of the Visionary Realms

"The *huairamama* arrives with great whirlwind and energy from outer space, which you can see as the multicolored waves to its side. This whirlwind uncovers the pot of ayahuasca, and the spirits and muses appear in the flames to meet the arrival of *a'tun supai lancha* [great spirit boat]. They hold musical instruments from which blissful transcendent melodies emerge, both in sound and vision."
—Pablo Amaringo, *Ayahuasca Visions*[13]

Yagé toyá—"yagé designs" or "visual patterning revealed by the yagé"—are a phenomenon of the world of yagé, appearing to people under its influence. There are many kinds of designs that can be generally called yagé toyá, some easier to see than others. One must follow certain methods of training and discipline in order to experience and acquire the more refined medicine designs. This learning is at the heart of the mystical science. The visions revealed by the yagé toyá, including the multiple worlds and countless beings, can only be perceived by those who have learned how to pierce through the veil that separates us from the fullness of spirit. Then at that stage descriptions are no longer necessary. If words cannot come close to describing even a single vision, how would they ever approach such an immense topic as this? And while all that is there to be seen is as close as the tip of your nose, preserved perfectly for eternity, it is simultaneously as distant as the Southern Cross.

All the beings, deities, and elemental powers of the universe have their own yagé toyá. The highest and most fortuitous is that from the realms of the Wiñapai. Also of great benefit to learn about is the *Jujupai toyá*, the patterns of the doctor people. When they enter a patient they quickly unwind, swirling through the body with a thousand and one ways to apply themselves to constrictions, imbalances, and impurities. Immediately they bring the patient much closer to his or her original state of health and well-being. A master can direct these energetic emanations to enter the body of a student so he or she may learn, or into a patient for healing and restoration of personal balance and wholeness. The Jujupai toyá will not permit any distortion of the healthy energy patterns of life in their presence. Inside the human body they recognize immediately what is not a design of good health and work diligently to rectify it, until their limited energy allotment fades and they depart like a multitude of little people who, upon hearing the whistle calling them to return, drop what they are doing and leave running. A few higher-energy stragglers, concentrating on their work, jump off last, running behind the others in utter despair that they will be left to evaporate alone, since the yagé toyá departs almost as swiftly as it arrives.

A vibrant cascade of phosphorescent yellow beads bounces across the table and rolls across the floor. The beads are scintillating and ungraspable, jumping like popcorn, slipping through the fingers of the students and elders alike who, although still in their hammocks, in their visions see themselves in laughing drunken chase, crawling on all fours after them. Rolling off in all directions, the beads vanish back to the void from which they came. Words can be used, yes, but they can only guide one's mind a little closer toward the many types of pure non-verbalized energies that comprise the infinite and utterly profound universe that we are a flesh-and-bones part of.

Seeing the variations of the yagé toyá can only take place through experience and practice, although one can talk all day and night about the different forms they take—such as the *Jaicuntipai toyá* that assemble themselves as intricately woven beaded medicine patterns in tones of royal purple and emerald green, earthen brown and opaque white, cobalt blue and pearlescent pink. Being that spirit is the thread that holds the energetic configuration temporarily together, the designs can be seen quivering as if breathing.

To see these realms, one must drink strong yagé with the elders and the more experienced students who enjoy laughter and are firm in their virtue. After more and more ceremonies, the yagé toyá begins to accumulate in one's body. Then one is meeting yagé toyá halfway, and the yagé toyá in turn approaches, revealing itself even more, entering and engulfing the body of the student and filling him or her with its supreme and sublime energy. When that happens the yagé grips one without pity and it's necessary to use all one's spiritual and physical strength to stay still and quiet. Varied patternings of the yagé toyá include molecular shapes, fractals, tunnels, exploding chrysanthemums, saturated swirling colors, and much more among the wisps and onslaughts of "visual language" (as the shamanologist Terence McKenna dubbed it) that one perceives. The toyá can bring one to dreamlike experiences such as turning into an animal, a plant, or a rock in a river. It might lead to the vision that someone is placing beaded necklaces and flower leis on you, or that you are dancing with multitudes of celestial people. The most traditional destination or goal according to our Secoya elders is to meet with any of the legions of divine immortals, who must be called and invited sincerely to join the ceremony. What is important is to know where one is coming from and where one is going in order to keep to a good path while always negotiating to see more of this resplendent reality, a negotiation that happens through one's commitment and desire to learn. Note that traditionally as well as today, this can be an expensive education in addition to a demanding curriculum. One must not only devote great care to the dieta but also provide significant payment—monetary and/or service work—to the master and helpers.

The master drinkers of yagé who embody the yagé toyá can maneuver in these sacred realms and enjoy incomparably exquisite visionary experiences, such as heavenly banquets. The multiple dishes—among them, ripe fruit, smoked fish, and meats—simply appear on the table.

Afterwards, the unwashed dishes and serving bowls just vanish and the table is spotless and clean.

The elders attest to the appearance of the toyá ma'a, the designs path that manifests before them and allows them to visit the immortal realms. On many occasions during the years I lived at don Cesareo's home (1995–2000), he shared tales of his experiences among the Jaicuntipai. On one such occasion he spoke about having visited the abode of the Jaicuntipai where his spiritual wife resides. She did not want him to return and took away the toyá ma'a. He pleaded with her to return it. She pleaded with him to stay. He explained that he would love to but he had obligations: his earthly family needed him. In sympathy and consideration for them, she returned the toyá ma'a, along which he was able to get back to his earthly home. He refrained from drinking yagé for a while after that and only hesitantly approached it later. Now his spiritual wife never removes the designs path, since she knows this way he will return more regularly. When he sings, she follows the same designs trail to the ceremony, and sitting inside his body she sings and heals people. When she arrives, his voice becomes much finer.

The elder yagé drinkers have seen so much. As holographic emanations of the spirit world made manifest to us, the yagé toyá sometimes cover the master like a cloak. During the ceremonies it's possible to actually see the master engulfed in designs that flow over his body in rich saturated arrays as if they were a layer on top of his tunic. The yagé drinkers' cloak, called among the Secoya the *toyákä*, is a profound sight.[14] As there are many kinds of yagé toyá, there are many types of toyákä, as illustrated by the powerful and bizarre story of Yai Yoí (Jaguar Grunge)[15] and the *yai toyákä*, the jaguar designs cloak that represents merging with and having the power of the primal energies of the Earth. The *Wiñapai toyákä*—the Always-new-people designs cloak representing the freely flowing energies of the celestial spheres—is the ultimate symbol of spiritual authority. The elders attest that its glory is beyond description; it makes the vastness of the star-filled sky seem close at hand, clarifying all the normally hidden wonders in the infinity of the universe.

The energy designs and patterns of yagé stem from antiquity or maybe even the dawn of creation, yet they are always fresh and new like a spring morning's blossoming buds covered with dew, or the sounds of songbirds in the garden, or the gushing of clear pure water from a spring. The visionary realms revealed by the medicine spring forth from countless possibilities, and the images one's mind brings up when it touches these energies are not only diverse but usually strange beyond language.

When it comes to revealing the visionary world of ayahuasca, no one can speak more eloquently or paint more revealingly of this incredible topic than could don Pablo Amaringo. Once while I was admiring his art, he said to me, "I am just one man and look at what I have seen. Who can record the countless visions seen by the many elders and spiritually developed maestros of the many great Amazonian traditions?"[16]

The yagé toyá cannot be corrupted or manipulated. It can only be released by a skilled shaman and allowed to do its work for the short time it has available in this three-dimensional realm. To obtain the celestial visions of the yagé toyá is the deepest desire of all lower energetic entities (including us) because it is a path to our evolution and spiritual salvation. Once individuals become aware of the existence of the phenomena of the Wiñapai toyá, they change. In this light we can say the yagé toyá is an impetus for evolution.

Collective Visions

I touched on the phenomenon of collective visions in the opening chapter on indigenous science because this is one of the ways in which "proof" of the spirit world is obtained by each person for him- or herself. This happens when two or more people experience the same vision. This can take place during a single ceremony, or when the shaman sets an intention for a particular thing to occur and the participants share a common vision, or over a career or regimen of multiple ceremonies. All students of the tradition seek to see the same visions that their predecessors did, and in this way they verify the reality of these realms that exist in a dimension beyond the limitations of space and time. As more and more people share the same or similar experiences, the details of the visions become common knowledge—cultural artifacts. Seeing these common visions is a confirmation of one's spiritual progress, and though the visions are transient, the energy that one touches when experiencing them is not. This energy deeply nurtures every cell in the body and gives great strength to work daily in a diligent and dedicated manner. This spiritually infused energy helps one to stay focused in a world full of distractions.

Among the great collective visions from the tradition of the Secoya is that of the red celestial sky-metal canoes, the *makëhna yowë,* and the white ones, *pokëhna yowë.* Reinaldo Lucitante shared with me his vision of a celestial canoe that he saw once when drinking yagé with Fernando Payaguaje at the lagoons of Cuyabeno. Many crowned masters waved from its deck as it passed by in billowing red energy clouds. Other collective visions include the Matëmo Cou, the Sky Turtle, who lays her papaya-size eggs on the shores of the Matëmo Tsiaya, the Sky River. The Toyá Uncucui, the Designs Boa, is an incredible reality of the world of yagé. From its mouth scintillating showers of sparkling light engulf the drinkers, bringing on even more spectacular visions of the celestial realms. This is one of the first serious visions the student receives, after which it becomes possible to begin to see the various legions of Wiñapai such as the Cancopai, who are the shimmering cicada people that drinkers strive to see during the celestial summer when the sounds of myriad insects fill the night air.

As discussed in Chapter 1 in terms of a spiritual education, Cesareo and other elders share that after one has had sufficient celestial visions, one must see the terrestrial visions. One must meet the Demon King, Pai'joyowatí, and other deities of the Earth—primal energies such as Wanteanco, the Jaguar Mother, who transforms throughout the year, young, attractive, and docile during the summer months and an ornery old hag during the rainy months. Oco Wanteanco, sister of the Jaguar Mother, lives in the water and has underground tunnels through which she travels from one river system to another. She's the mother of the water jaguars, as her sister is mother of the terrestrial jaguars. We've already met the Camiyai (Crab Jaguar), Menkoyiyi (Electric-eel Water-dragon), and Añapëquë (Snake Black-caiman), elemental powers of the Earth. Then there are different types of Watí or earth spirits such as the Curiwaripai, the spirits of different kinds of plants, and the Mawahopai, the morpho butterfly people. Unpredictable spirits with volatile tendencies, Watí can help a healer do good and accomplish difficult cures, or aid the evil plans of sorcerers. Terrestrial spirits often are tricksters, which is why in traditional Secoya yagé drinking they are met only after one has established relationships with the Wiñapai.

Graduation occurs when one is crowned by the celestial spirits, confirming that one's virtues have reached a certain level. There are many levels of graduation that allow the adept to see and know even more, and to further interact with the spirit worlds and powers of the universe. Elders speak of celestial beings who wear four crowns, implying that even among the celestial spirits there is a process of evolution taking place. To the student aspiring to graduate, and to the experienced yagé drinker pursuing further graduations, each crown one receives, each necklace given by the celestial spirits confirms another level of graduation. These are only some of the most basic concepts that illustrate the tremendous body of collective visions known to the Secoya people as part of their spiritual science.

A VALUABLE CURE LEARNED FROM A YAGÉ VISION

During a graduation he underwent with thickly prepared pejí (*Brugmansia suaveolens*), Fragrant Medicine Bark, don Cesareo, learned a song to help women who are having difficulty conceiving a child. A middle-aged couple that owns a small tourist lodge upriver from the Secoya village of Sehuaya was unable to conceive. They now have three children thanks to this unique healing tactic that Fragrant Medicine Bark acquired directly from the spirits. The cure is simple: a flower from a cultivated cotton plant is placed in water and softy chanted over for thirty minutes or more. The water is drunk by the woman, and the couple is instructed to wait until seven days after her next menstruation to attempt conception. While this cure is simple and effective, it took tremendous effort on behalf of the healer to attain this spiritual achievement that now has become yet another tool for him to uphold the culture of service.

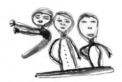

A Word of Caution about Revealing One's Visions

Note that if you are to reveal your visions, you should do it with purpose, not simply to brag or tell stories. They should not be spoken about prematurely or inadequately. This was a precaution I wanted to know more about, so several elders patiently explained that it is okay to speak about the visions to friends of confidence, the morning after or during the ceremony. Afterwards, though, it's best to just keep quiet. There are two principal reasons why. The first is in order to avoid dissipating the energy transmission that is specifically for the person who received the vision—an enrichment from the origin of the universe, in response to one's devotion and spiritual cultivation. (The same holds true for powerful dreams.)

The second reason is that many people do not have the dedication to follow the correct way of life. But deep inside everybody wants to have this intimate an association with spirit. They want it but are not prepared to do the work. For this reason it is risky to share one's visions with people who are not at the same level or who do not share the same good energy. The person who divulges a vision to ordinary people runs the risk of arousing their jealousy, resentment and/or ridicule, and this in turn leads to enmity, something that no sincere follower of the medicine path wants. Thus the elders counsel that unless there is a specific reason for divulging one's experiences, you should keep quiet about them.

When the energy of the vision is allowed to grow within, the adept can use it to gain power and strength for healing. One can reconnect with this energy in any present moment. Dreams have the same weight and can be used in the same way. For example, while accomplishing a healing, one recalls a powerful dream or vision and by doing so touches again that very same energy, which helps carry out the healing. Think about what has more value: sharing an amusing tale and running the risk of dissipating one's personal energy, or sharing the results of the vision by manifesting its energy in the world in a practical and beneficial way.

Dreams and visions are secret tools to awaken your personal power in order to help you be more effective in enacting service and accomplishing healing work and solidarity. There is then no need to speak about the visions seen because you are sharing your life energy with the world. This does not mean that the elders don't talk about their visions—they love to talk about them, but usually only years afterward, when they have merged with these energies and are past the stage where they run the risk of dissipating the precious spiritual gift.

The Ceremony of Yagé

"In the past, when ceremonies were led according to the ancient customs, and the medicine was well cared for, during the ceremony the ayahuasca was always kept in a medium-sized open clay pot. It was important to leave the pot open so that the energy of the medicine could rise and fill the room where the ceremony was being held. The master would serve each person a small gourd. He would blow over the medicine and serve it from the side on which he blew. He would establish the *arcanas* [the protection] for the group, and then call the *mareación* [the reverie of inebriation and visions], that when it comes is a splendid thing."

—Pablo Amaringo[17]

All sessions of drinking yagé (or ayahuasca) are ceremonies, and all aspire to learning, integration, and healing in some form. In a specific healing context, for which a person might seek shamanic assistance, the medicine will be cooked and all will fast during the day prior to the night-time ceremony. The patient(s) will often but not always partake of the thick and bitter drink as part of the treatment.

The carefully prepared and well-refined brew is brought from its cooking or storage site to the master's side after sunset. In order to avoid dispersing the pinta, the cooks do not shake anyone's hand or walk around the room. As in the cooking process (detailed in the next chapter), the path along which the medicine is carried is always respected by recognizing it and not crossing over it. This is because the yagé toyá must make its way from where the yagé was cooked to where it is now being served. Once the toyá has arrived and the drinkers are engulfed in visions, then if someone walks across the trail nothing occurs, but if this happens at the onset of the ceremony the yagé toyá arrives to the location where the trail has been walked across and becomes confused; the toyá does not know which way to go and so it returns. The master can call it and it may eventually come much later in the night, but it is much more work and the participants feel primarily stewed and drunk rather than engulfed in enigmatic visionary experiences.

Initially the master serves out just a few sips. The master drinks first then the cooks, followed by the rest of the people participating. In a traditional Secoya yagé ceremony the women always sit on one side of the lodge and the men on the other. Usually there will be several gourds, one for the men, another for the women, one to scoop the brew out of the pot with, and another large gourd for water used to rinse the mouth of the medicine's bitter flavor. If many people are participating in the ceremony, the inner circle of traditional elders, cooks, and the ceremonial guide will often drink from a separate gourd. A man whose wife is pregnant must not drink from the same gourd as the others. He can drink but he must use his own gourd—this is to ensure that the developing fetus won't get dizzy in the womb. Also, this man must only tie up his own hammock and tie it up slowly. If he helps too many others tie their hammocks, it is believed that the umbilical cord will wrap around the baby's neck and cause complications at birth.

While waiting for the medicine to take effect, the elders often will be talking about past yagé ceremonies, relating with great detail descriptions of visions and experiences and discussing the vast array of subjects that constitute the ancient body of wisdom and cultural heritage of the people. I recall one night drinking yagé among a group of Secoya elders when they remained entranced in animated dialogue for hours. Eventually curiosity got the better of me and I overcame my reservations to interrupt and ask what they were talking about, my knowledge of their language being minimal. I wanted so badly to know, even to get just a hint. One kind elder, laughing, said, "Ahh, yes, he's talking about the time he was swallowed by the Toyá Uncucui [the Designs Boa]. He was squeezed through its stomach. He wanted to scream but held on tight, holding good silence, and when he came out its ass there was a loud slapping sound. He suddenly went flying at top speed off into the universe. How he got back, he doesn't even know." Bursting out in laughter they continued on with their animated conversation.

Usually after an hour or two a larger gourd will be served and the intentions shift to meditation and deep concentration. The master blows on the medicine in order to awaken the yagé toyá or pinta, and the participants and masters alike all enter into a deep and solemn trance, where often call-and-response chanting goes on among the ceremony's leaders and the participants who are drinking yagé. In order to not lose the trance and to keep the designs flowing, the master of the ceremony, holding the matipë made of erect tail feathers of the scarlet macaw and tied with colorful tassels and fluffy feathers, will chant and sing until sunrise, drinking copious amounts of yagé throughout the night to call forth and maintain the connection with the auspicious spirits.

The echoing tonal vibrations emitted from the master's throat, invocations of the celestial realms, help bring all the drinkers closer to a group vision, where any part of the ancestral cosmology might come to life, to each in his or her own way, as each ceremonial participant lets the medicine do its work.

When everything is aligned, the master sings wonderfully right from the start. The entire night his body is light, he feels no pain, and the most exquisite of all energies flow uninhibitedly for the other drinkers to witness and absorb. The master communes with the Jaicuntipai and other Wiñapai who visit during the ceremony. The Jujupai, the doctor people, usually arrive later in the night to help with the necessary healing. Countless other profound adventures will have been experienced by the coming of dawn. If a complex cure must be undertaken, the master will call the Demon King himself, Pai'joyowatí, whose chest is like a mirror, reflecting and making visible the root cause of all illness. Once the illness is identified, the Demon King summons the lower-level earth spirits or Watí responsible for having caused the illness. The Watí are instructed to remove the damage. They remove the root cause of the disease on a spiritual level. Then the Jujupai seal the patient's energetic body. Starting the next day, the patient will follow a diet and recuperate. Perhaps plant spirits like the Curiwaripai will recommend particular medicinal herbs. This I am told by my friends the Secoya elders, who know these realms.

As the sun rises, villagers come to be healed. Women and children receive herbal water that has been cured by the master(s), chanted over for hours, arranged as a catalyst for the yagé tutu (power or strength) to reach the deep recesses of body and soul. The patients sit one by one on a low stool before the master, who heals chanting softly, rhythmically. The green leaf fan and the red macaw feathers of the matïpe tremble to the rhythm of his chant, as mothers and children are healed in the crisp morning air filled with birdcalls. Everyone in the house drinks a few sips of this same aromatic water in order to allow the yagé tutu to pass, and in order to live on into another day, again made new.

All the overnight participants stay quiet and still until just after dawn. When the master passes the matipë to an assistant, who lays it carefully down, the ceremony is over. After the ceremony the patients leave and the elders rest, swaying gently in their hammocks, until the effects have fully passed, which, depending on how much they had drunk, can be up until midday or that afternoon.

Chapter 6, "The Celestial Summer of Cicadas," explains further aspects of the Secoya yagé ceremony, which is among the original, ancient, and celestially ordained heritages of humanity.

Cultivating the Sacred Within

Have no doubt, the drinking of yagé is much more than a psychedelic experience created by particular chemical combinations. In contrast to the Western use of recreational drugs for entertainment or maybe insight, the ceremony of yagé in a traditional context—for example, as practiced among the Tukanoan-speaking people of northwestern equatorial Amazonia—is at the living heart of the people's traditional way of life. It touches upon every aspect of their cultural and spiritual development and worldviews; and it is used with a sacred intent to maintain their connection with mythic ancestors and the heavenly immortal medicine islands. These tribal traditions are refreshed and reconfirmed through the drinking of the yagé, thus allowing for continuation of the celestial energy patterns among the people of the Earth. In this way yagé serves as the very essence of the divine immortals themselves and is the source of universal integration, knowledge, and deep spiritual communion. The elders attest to having witnessed the most fantastic celestial phenomena, visions of colossal beauty in rich, all-engulfing, saturated tones. The fluffy and ultraclean medicine people of yagé reconcile all gaps between our inner and outer harmony. To see them only once positively marks one's life forever.

The inebriation is used ceremonially to transcend the physical realms in order to experience, to know and to see, the supernatural and eternal realms. In a well-guided and successful ceremony all the participants receive a renewed perspective on life and will be realigned and reintegrated with an original way of being. The participants and master alike are left with a refreshed understanding of the path of spiritual self-development, and of the calming, gentle, and rhythmical motions that align one with a life of happiness and fulfillment. As participants see clearly the path to an integral salvation it deeply benefits one's self, family, community, and all species alike. Even if one never drinks the medicine again, to have been touched by this energy only once can potentially provide the jumpstart to joyously follow a lifetime of spiritual cultivation and service.

Upon receiving the energy one must allow it to grow from within. The methods for allowing this energy to accumulate within oneself, the ways of transmitting this energy, and its appropriate uses and expressions in the world are the branches of the ancient mystical science. What at first seems elusive and mysterious eventually becomes self-evident, and then it becomes a matter of how one lives and the perspective adopted.

To conclude this section I leave you with the following thought. There is a Secoya saying regarding the drinking of yagé—in essence it is this: "If you want to drink, it is a personal choice. No one should tell you to drink or not to drink." Among the Secoya for this reason you will never be invited to drink yagé. They may tell people that they are drinking on a certain night and make the ceremony known. Then if others want to come they will go through all the efforts necessary to come. The Secoya adamantly insist that no one can coerce or invite anyone to want to drink yagé. The decision is something that each person takes one hundred percent responsibility for. Oddly enough, this saying has something to do with the tentative notion that if you become a sorcerer and start damaging people, it is your own fault.

When someone wants to drink yagé they will travel a long distance and no obstacle will seem too large to overcome. In days of old when the Secoya wanted to drink yagé and they heard there were ceremonies taking place, they would walk barefoot for hours through the night with only the dim light of a copal torch to illuminate the winding path through the thick bush, to the ceremonial house of yagé.

La Dieta: For Purification and Spiritual Mastery

The core process of mastering or even approaching the mysteries of traditional Amazonian medicine is submission to a "self-challenge program." Known throughout the Amazon and the world now by the Spanish term *dieta,* this process varies greatly because the use of plants, especially sacred ones, is deeply culture-bound.

To take on a dieta ("diet" in English, but without the emphasis on weight loss) is much more than simply restraining from certain foods. A dieta is a way to concentrate, refine, and purify personal energies—to achieve mastery over all actions, thoughts, and words, to refine one's life essence until it becomes piercing and true. Like this one becomes worthy of meeting divine beings and obtaining allies from the spiritual realms. While a dieta can be viewed somewhat as a health regime in that abstaining from certain foods, activities, and emotions is a way to improve health, in the framework of traditional Amazonian medicine adhering to a dieta primarily carries the goal of preparing oneself to commune with spiritual energies (plant and tree spirits, mountain spirits, elemental forces and powers of nature, supernatural beings, divine immortals, mytho-historical ancestors, and ancient spirits and deities from many realms and lineages). Vitality, happiness, and good health become some of the side effects experienced during a successful dieta as body, mind, and spirit are integrated. In this regard the dieta is also a form of preventive medicine. The essence of an appropriate dieta is to learn to use less resources and make less of an impact on Mother Earth, to walk lightly and gain the energy to do so. At advanced levels the goal of these dietas is to gain the necessary energy to "carry the weight of the world on one's shoulders" but in such a manner that it is "light as a feather."

Traditional Amazonian medicine encourages everyone to be independent, to follow a disciplined health regime, to be virtuous and align oneself with universal law. Among the Waorani, for example, by the age of eleven each individual has already reached self-sufficiency. Virtuous fulfillment through selfless service is well recognized as the fastest way of attracting celestial spirits. The core and upshot of many spiritual practices, this means not being a burden on anyone and caring for self and family, giving more than one receives, living appropriately, eating clean and wholesome foods in moderation, exercising sufficiently, being optimistic and enjoying laughter, and learning to adhere ever more closely to the social and cosmological order of things. Such a personal program is far beyond abstaining from certain foods, or drinking certain medicinal plants, though these are elements of it and ways of obtaining results. A real dieta is in essence the great path of spiritual development that must be seen as the true progress of humanity.

Dietas tend to be more stringent during periods of training and initiation, as well as new levels of learning, while shorter dietas or less limiting guidelines are followed for energetic maintenance.

There are various methods of training, and distinct traditions and disciplines are followed to obtain the spiritual energy that gives access to celestial visions and knowledge. All require the student to abstain from indulgences and to live a life in utmost moderation. The point of all the different practices is to be able to concentrate one's energy in the supreme high-vibration channels of life, until it can become discerning enough to "see" and "know" the truth of things, and to experience the astonishing beauty of the normally unseen realms. Then one meets the toyá—the designs and visual language of reality's foundations, highest levels, and infinite diversity and magnificence. The toyá in turn approaches because the spirits take notice when one gives of oneself in the process of dieta.

There is also the concept of a trade—something given (to spirit) so that something can be received (by the student). One gives of oneself because abstaining from things that one likes is a form of giving. Each individual knows what is a sacrifice for him or her personally, in addition to the usual abstentions.

By following a dieta, one's personal energy is refined daily to become stronger, more upright, shining and active. The dieta and its duration are sustained in different ways, depending on the tradition and the instructions of the master. In order to gather the heavenly toyá or pinta (Spanish for "colorful patterning"), one must abstain from sexual activity, from all fermented beverages, and from certain edibles such as fried and oily foods, canned foods, pork, onions, salt, sugar, red-hot chili peppers, and other spices. Some students refrain from bathing, drinking, or touching plain water. One must maintain a calm and tranquil demeanor yet be always ready to lend a hand, overcoming inner inertia, apathy, and listlessness through a good daily work ethic, spiritual concentration, and sincere approach to life.

One method of concentrating energy is to devote oneself to helping others, passing up not a single opportunity to serve, and seeing that each opportunity to help someone is truly a precious gift, directly from the Great Spirit. The objective is to practice multiple random acts of kindness every day and to give one's life energy selflessly.

On an internal level the student must be present and hard-working, as well as alert in his dreams—he must be aware not to take something offered in a dream—and it is necessary to learn how to be spiritually centered by rejecting the majority of what is seen in visions in order to avoid spiritual pitfalls. Having gained an initial insight, they must cultivate themselves beyond the level of premature desires for obtainment, letting go of attachments and following the guidance given by one's maestro, as well as the wordless teachings of the medicine and the divine spirits.

Once the initial "threads" of the heavenly energies have been obtained, the student must keep "rolling the ball in," so to say. This represents gathering and refining the spiritual energy designs, which must be accumulated with care since the threads are thin and fragile. As these designs grow in strength within the body of the student, though they may seem non-existent they are always ready to assist the individual on his or her spiritual voyage or life path of service, providing daily fulfillment and joy. Acquiring these designs was once at the root of the basic education system of the people and was their main interest, a self-challenge program dedicated to aiding one on every level of life. In the days when these traditions reigned this was considered to be the foundation for spiritual salvation as well as a successful mortal existence.

Don Pablo's Rigorous Dieta

"To become a sage is a very serious thing," said don Pablo Amaringo when we became friends in 1994. It does not come easy and this is why today we have many false sages.

Don Pablo told me about the dieta that he followed for an entire year. Later he underwent similar dietas for shorter periods of time. He said it was the basic program for becoming a vegetalista (a healer who uses plants). For our purposes of illustration it serves as a good sample dieta. Don Pablo had drunk ayahuasca on many occasions prior, but it was only after he recovered from a serious illness that he realized the true value of this path. After several years of indecisiveness he finally made the solid decision to become a vegetalista. Following some personal hardship, he wanted to heal and strengthen himself, and he was ready to accept the responsibility of committing to the training with his teacher, don Pascual Pichiri. It was the year 1969, Pablo was thirty-one years old, and he was sincere and determined to learn.

Pablo ate only twice a day, at ten in the morning and three in the afternoon. His meal consisted of one sardine and one straight plantain. He would eat these food items from one end to the other without breaking or cutting them into pieces. The fish he ate from head to tail. Not breaking the food items ensures that the spiritual energy being cultivating will also be unbroken—that it will act like a continuum, a circle, a continually whirling energy loop. In other words, the dieta will serve its purpose of allowing one to obtain a "whole," "complete," or "integral" energy. Along these lines, it is also important that all leftovers, fish scales, bones, and plantain peels be buried in a hole where the ants will not carry any pieces away, again ensuring that one will not lose any of the energy being accumulated.

In order to prepare fish for his diet, don Pablo dried them on a smoking rack placed over a bed of hot coals. It was imperative that no parts fall onto the ashes. Nor could any ashes float up and touch the food. Observing this separation was intended to help him differentiate the vast and distinct pure energies, so that the ayahuasca visions would be unequivocal, the energies perceived clearly and not chaotically. For this purpose he used certain kinds of firewood that would, when reduced to embers, hold consistent heat but release no rising ashes.

Sometimes he would catch other types of fish. The ones necessary for his dieta were fish with small mouths that are primarily fruit eaters; these are small and silver-colored, and have scales. Any fish that meets this description will work for a dieta, and there are many kinds.

In addition to eliminating certain foods, many aspirants avoid hot and cold foods. Pablo was instructed to eat only room-temperature foods in order to adhere to a middle-of-the-road approach to daily life. It was equally important to refrain from expressing intense emotions of anger or sorrow, or getting caught up in emotional conflicts of any kind. Avoiding strong-smelling odors and perfumes and abstaining completely from sexual or intimate encounters were necessary aspects of Pablo's dieta. He was for the most part to avoid people altogether and be especially wary of whose hand he shook. Some people can absorb the energy of others, making them weak and sick, then one has to start over again. Other people can pass their negative energy to you, and you absorb it like a sponge. After a certain period of following the dieta, your energy seals within and you becomes strong. You can then live again among people without so much precaution.

Don Pablo said that he couldn't eat just any kind of banana—only a certain kind of plantain that grows straight, not bent. Most plantains grow in a curved shape, but the dieta required the straight ones, for if you eat a curved plantain your diet and energy become "bent." This implies that the spiritual energy being cultivating is weakened; maybe there are stress points in the energy circulation. The energy is interfered with, stunted and rendered non-effective. Eating straight plantains to ensure that one's energy will grow straight is an act that symbolizes a truthful and uncorrupted way of life.

Pablo was instructed to avoid prolonged exposure to direct midday sun, so he lived in the shade of his hut in a remote jungle garden. And he could drink no plain fresh water, only *chapo verde* (green plantain mashed in water) or *shibe* (also known as *farina remojada*). This is a popular food of Amazonian Peru, like a kind of granola made from yuca tubers *(Manihot esculenta)* soaked in water, ground, then dry-toasted over hot coals in a large pan.

According to don Pablo, when undergoing a dieta you must not sleep during the day. You can sleep from three in the morning to just after sunrise, at seven in the morning. You have to stay awake! You have to stay alert! From nine in the evening to three o'clock in morning is when the spirits come to teach in accordance with Earth's electromagnetic sphere. In a traditional setting, after nine in the evening a shaman's wife will not speak to anyone. At that hour she is quiet in order to not interfere with the arrival of the spirits.

After some time of following the dieta—and this can vary from person to person, but it ranges from one month to a year—one begins to see the most exquisite visions, then it becomes part of one's life and such visions are no longer difficult to attain. Don Pablo said, "One must be sincere with oneself and not afraid to do things correctly, then you will know when to stop the dieta. If you are studying with a master he will help guide you on this process. If you are studying alone you will know in the quietude of your self-reflections, so strive daily to be in touch with your authentic inner voice."

When I asked him to elaborate on the "authentic inner voice," he replied solemnly, "You hear it when you are alone, when you are still and calm."

Like a pillar holds the roof securely above the floor of a house, the developed spiritual person upholding the dieta becomes a pillar between Heaven and Earth (the pillar symbolizing one's body). The folk saying of old, "To see God in Heaven you must see God on Earth," becomes a living truth, and everywhere you look you see God. In other words, you recognize the non-separable unity of all creation, and realize that this unity of all animate and non-animate objects is the one living God. Upon recognizing this, you naturally awaken to the culture of service, for everyone you see is God—and yourself! The dieta gives strength and conviction to life and helps the practitioner not get depressed at the state of the world, or self-absorbed in his or her own petty desires. This is why the healer must accomplish many types of dietas and practice multiple acts of self-denial, so that he or she can gain the spiritual strength necessary to sustain a positive, optimistic, and non-discriminatory approach to life—the same that for the most part keeps you smiling. This stance goes everywhere you go and becomes part of a well-rounded and stable personality. This is the greatest secret of all the ancient masters, worldwide.

Another Type of Dieta: Don Solon's Method

Don Solon in his time of initiation had undergone extensive dieting for much longer periods, holding firm to the dieta for up to a year (similar to don Pablo's experience described above). Once don Solon was initiated and had gained his powers, he would regularly (at least once a month) hold shorter five-day, seven-day, or nine-day dietas in order to keep his spiritual energy "close," as he would say. During this time he would also drink medicinal plants for strength and to learn their qualities. When he went back to regular life, he continued to monitor the food he ate, preferring wholesome natural foods, and holding to moderation in all his doings. But he would not be so severe—he would sleep with his wife and share the food his family was eating. Except of course when he planned to drink *la purga* (ayahuasca) in the evening, he would fast the entire day.

Most notable about don Solon's method was the unique way in which he ended the dieta. He would take a lemon, cut it in half, rub some hot chili pepper on it, and then sprinkle on a little salt. He squeezed the juice of the lemon into his mouth and swallowed it slowly. Two hours later he would quietly leave the area where he was dieting and return to regular daily life.

Zasina of the Kichwa of Napo Province

In Ecuador the concept of dieta takes on different forms. The Kichwa people call it *sassy* or *zasina,* terms that unfold into a university of meaning that relates to the methods of gathering and refining one's personal energy through a process of abstinence over a given period of time.

The classic zasina will involve abstinence from *kachi* (salt), *uchu* (chili peppers), *wira* (oily foods), *cuchi* (pork), and hot and cold foods (one eats at room temperature), as well as plain water, drinking only *mazamora,* green banana boiled and mashed in water. The zasina includes sexual abstinence, and the person must sleep in a separate bed from his or her significant other during the dieting process.

In traditional Kichwa culture the zasina touches upon every type of energy-cultivating discipline and many facets of daily life. For example, the cured strong black tobacco called *taucumasu* is prepared in a very special way. From the time it is planted until the time it is harvested one follows a dieta, and every aspect of the cultivation of *taucu (Nicotiana tabacum)*[18] is accomplished with zasina. When the seeds are sown, the zasina is to hold one's breath and not look. Then when one returns to weed the taucu patch, another method of zasina. Like this these tobacco logs come out very strong and can be used to cure many types of ailments, including skin problems and snakebite as well as spiritual imbalances such as fright and discomfort, making it especially helpful for soothing crying babies.

Kutipa is the term for when the zasina is not followed correctly. A series of illnesses can arise, especially if one breaks the zasina after being granted powers or energies by one's master teacher. Such illnesses can only be healed by a good ayahuasquero. This is one of the reasons many youth are afraid to learn. They fear the kutipa, the consequences of breaking the diet, and the illness it brings and the difficulty and suffering inherent in the arduous process of healing oneself afterward. If you are *not* training as a disciple or undergoing an initiation program with a master, then a basic dieta can be followed to gain strength and spiritual integration as long as you feel it is beneficial; and when it is over, you don't run the risk of instigating kutipa.

The Secoya Method—Spiritual Control and Self-Restraint

Secoya traditional elder and healer Cesareo Piaguaje shared with me the following, which I transcribed from a journal entry I made at his home along the Aguarico River in August 1996. In his youth, when he was studying the spiritual science with his grandfather, he spent four years in the wilderness fasting with his grandfather and three other students. They devoted themselves to growing some basic crops like yuca and plantain, as well as yagé and the admixture plant yagé ocó, and they drank copious amounts of yagé there in the solitude of their wilderness glade. They would drink for three nights and rest for two nights, and like this they lived for four full years, dedicated solely to the drinking of yagé. On some occasions when the energies were supreme they were not even hungry and would go up to four months without eating any kind of food, only drinking yagé that Cesareo calls *"gran alimento"* in Spanish, meaning "great food." When they wanted to eat they made *aun,* called *casave* in Spanish, which are large tortillas of grated and then squeezed yuca tubers. When the yuca is spread onto a clay pan it is like flour, and when lightly cooked it produces one of the most important foods of the Secoya people. Young Cesareo and his companions would also catch small fish and forest doves, the meat of which were dried on the smoking rack and eaten dry, and they ate green plantains carefully dried over the embers. This is all they ate! When I asked him what he saw, he replied, "Everything!" It was during those years, he went on to say, that he learned how to heal.

It is important to note that among the Secoya the most fundamental part of a dieta is living a virtuous life. This is why when the first missionaries arrived many agreed that the Indians were the true Christians! A virtuous life entails moderation in all measures; it also means taking things casually and not overreacting, and not being impulsive but rather deeply observing. Additional guidelines when learning the sacred science and acquiring the toyá (the energetic emanations of the yagé) include avoiding direct sunlight, bathing only from a bucket on the land (not swimming in the river), avoiding all alcoholic or fermented beverages, abstaining from sexual activity, and most specifically not receiving any food prepared by a menstruating or pregnant woman. The student must be service-oriented and work to eliminate lassitude from his or her body. While there is no prerequisite to do anything good, it is absolutely necessary to do nothing wrong, and being lazy is considered one of the greatest setbacks in learning the science. Students are expected to have a strong work ethic and to devote long hours to this. They are not allowed to lounge in their hammocks during the day or sleep after a short rest period that is customarily taken after lunch. One should sit up, not lie down. Students dedicate themselves to any of the vast areas necessary for sustaining jungle life, such as clearing space for gardens, planting and weeding them, hunting or fishing and preparing food, making or repairing canoes, washing one's clothes, making arts and crafts, or anything that keeps them active and in a state of contemplative meditation that encourages a focus on unifying mind and body—that is, spirit and matter.

To help eliminate laziness and to cleanse the body, the Secoya utilize a "sunrise renewal ceremony"—what they call *tzí'tzó'huajëye,* glossed as "renewal through bringing something in that comes quickly out"—in which powerful alkaline-rich medicinal plants that are emetics (they encourage vomiting) are blown on ("cured" or spiritually infused with one's breath and intention) by the elder who has no laziness and then consumed by students in large gourds at three in the morning. Cleansing plant substances with deep-acting healing qualities used for the sunrise renewal include the rasped and boiled blood-red root bark of the understory vine *mañapë (Callichlamys latifolia);* the peeled and soaked bark of the young *monsë* tree *(Cedrelinga caeteniformis);* the split and soaked heart of the *wi'gonzá,* the bamboo palm *(Oenocarpus mapora),* said to open the throat so one can sing; and the finely sliced inner seed of the *cantsé* tree *(Grias neuberthii),* believed to be a cure for any lung ailment. Other vomitives include *yoco (Paullinia yoco)* and the fragrant rasped bark of the *sensé'bëquë'sonquë'ó (Myroxylon balsamum);* the latter is also good for cleansing the lungs. The powerful ibogaine-containing *pai'su'u'witó,* known by the Kichwa as *tzicta*

(*Tabernaemontana sananho*),[19] is an emetic used to heal the body of laziness. Then there is the infamous "snake-head soup," as don Cesareo jovially calls it, consisting of the leaves of the yagé plant and the admixture yagé ocó, boiled for two hours in a large pot (also called *yagé hao*). There are other purgatives but these are the most prominent. Each has its specific preparation.

At the early hours of dawn the elder and students arise, and the elder uses his gourd to tap lightly on the large pot and then serve up the contents. Everyone is drinking and vomiting, drinking and vomiting until after sunrise. This cleans out the "cream" or "cheese" found at the bottom of the gut that is considered to be the source of laziness. When this is removed, one's natural energy returns and begins to grow daily. At sunrise one is instructed to clear the weeds from the patio. This is always done barefoot and in a squatting position, so that the negative energy of laziness can leave through the soles of one's feet and be absorbed back into the ground. As one goes about working in silence, the positive energy of the Earth enters one's body and strengthens it.

As a prerequisite to meeting the celestial spirits and the doctor people, the aspirant must not be stuck at the level of general sexual desires. Celibacy is obligatory at the beginning of the spiritual path as a means of strengthening the body, obtaining energy, overcoming illness, and infusing spirit into matter. The sexual energy is raised and transformed into physical vitality through a solid work ethic. This is why the Secoya highly recommend a strong work ethic as a precursor to learning the sacred culture of yagé, and it is believed that lassitude is the greatest obstacle to learning. The physical energy then merges with spiritual energy, and the higher the vibration of energy in one's body, the higher the energy one can connect with on a spiritual level. One must devote a significant portion of each day to being active, useful, and serving or helping others. One must maintain daily hygiene and keep a clean house, not accumulating anything extra and living the simplest life possible.

The objective is to allow the sexual energy to vaporize and rise up in the body to make one vigorous and strong. In the case of married couples, the Secoya abstain from sexual intimacy for at least a week before the customary annual drinking month of the celestial summer. They will also refrain from sexual activity afterwards until they feel that the energy of the yagé has completely dissipated from their bodies (a minimum of one week).

Living with integrity is not only a prerequisite for a successful dieta, it is an essential part of spiritual growth and true spiritual progress. In essence this means to act with integrity in all one's doings and see that one's actions cause no more confusion, to oneself or others. Nonetheless it is important to mention that a moral person will not necessarily be a spiritually achieved person, but a spiritually achieved person will always be a moral and integral person. Being moral and living an upright life of integrity is a definitive part of being a Secoya, one of "God's Multicolored People."

In the section on "Natural Celibacy" in contemporary Taoist master Ni Hua-Ching's *Workbook for Spiritual Development of All People*, we find the following applicable passage: "If you are to fully enjoy or exercise the value of something, then some difficulty must be overcome, or some price needs to be paid. This is the world, this is human life, practically speaking. Family life provides the source of manpower, and the harness of that choice is no lighter than that of celibacy." Master Ni continues on the next page, "People of self-delivery, if inspired, try to discover the profound secret of being absolute, which is where true freedom lies. An absolute being can light up the meaning of all worded and wordless teachings, of all ancient great minds, in one instant. He shall breathe the breath of all enlightened ones. He dissolves his mind in the ocean of wisdom. He shall reside in all the enlightened realms."[20]

Living among the Secoya between 1995 and 2000 and having the good fortune of participating in many ceremonies with the elders, I was able to see that to the Secoya, dieta involves living an upright, moral, and absolute life. This is clearly synonymous with spiritual development, which is a necessity for awakening to the larger truths of our world and this universe. And clearly such a goal is the ultimate purpose of traditional Secoya yagé drinking.

The Dieta of the Highland Puruwa Kichwa People

In the central highlands of Ecuador, in the mountain province of Chimborazo, we find a stronghold of Kichwa culture and tradition among the Puruwa people. The high Andes and the people there are as different as the mountain environment is to the rainforest, yet both the Kichwa and Secoya (the latter a lower-elevation rainforest tribe) greatly value upholding the culture of service as a means of building spiritual strength. Among the Puruwa Kichwa it is wholeheartedly believed that everyone intent on being a virtuous example to others should practice some years of selfless devotion to the path of community service. One takes each day as an opportunity to engage in service and solidarity, always ready to rise to the occasion and be of service or support when needed. Sustaining this approach to life is considered a form of dieting for the accumulation of spiritual energy, and it is no doubt one of the safest and most satisfying methods. A confirmation comes from an entirely different culture across the ocean, again in the work of Master Ni: "If one wishes to increase the number of his body spirits and his spiritual strength, the easiest and simplest way is through selfless, virtuous service."[21]

I also like this quote from a native American, Essie Parrish, the great California Pomo Indian shaman: "'Be careful on the journey,' they said, 'the journey to heaven,' they warned me. And so I went . . . Then when I entered into the place, I knew: if you enter heaven you might have to work."[22]

Gaining Paju: The Power to More Effectively Use Certain Plants

The Kichwa people ascribe importance to *paju*, which can be translated as "a power." Viewed as a spiritual ability, paju is something that can be obtained from a yachac, a person of wisdom, a.k.a. medicine man/woman, usually someone who is versed in the drinking of ayahuasca and has undergone zasina (dieta) as a means of gaining spiritual powers and strength. Paju is a power related specifically to enhancing the use of certain medicinal plants, such as taucu (tobacco, *Nicotiana tabacum*), *chiriguayusa (Brunfelsia grandiflora)*, and *tzicta (Tabernaemontana sananho)*. Someone who has a paju can use these plants with greater efficacy and thereby heal a wider array of illness and more complex ailments than someone who does not have the paju. Of course, anyone may use a given plant to heal simple ailments. For example, anyone can heat some of the strong black taucumasu (tobacco log) with water and use this liquid topically to alleviate a minor skin rash, but only someone who has received the paju of the tobacco (by undergoing a zasina with the tobacco and receiving the paju from an elder who has it) will be able to efficiently heal stubborn skin rashes or fungal infections. It is as if the potency of the plant medicine is enhanced as it becomes a vessel for the synergistic transmission of the healer's positive energy.

In 1996 I was with don Cesareo in the Secoya homelands on the Peruvian-Ecuadorian border region. He showed me a plant called *pë'mëtó*, "caiman's tobacco,"[23] used for helping someone regrow their teeth. Naturally this aroused my interest and I questioned him further. A skilled drinker of yagé can cure a water of those leaves, he explained—and not just anyone, but someone highly skilled in this science and possessing the necessary paju. (Actually, the Paicoca term is *juju.*) Cesareo has seen this take place. It is amazing what skills the drinkers of yagé have been able to obtain through their perseverance and devotion.

Some plants cannot even be touched unless the person has the paju to do so, such as the rare and barely known plants called *pishkuri,* "bird-wealth," and *pumallullu,* "mountain lion-sprout." (They may be the same plant.) Such mysterious flora are believed to have been obtained in ancient times from the heart of the Ingaru Supai, by a yachac who adhered strictly to a zasina. The Ingaru Supai is a spirit of the deep forest who protects the wilderness. It lives in remote rainforest areas without people, and it will defend its territory if necessary. The Ingaru Supai is believed to have a hollow chest cavity where his heart can be seen hanging. The ancient shaman while fasting was able to hide behind a tree, and when the Ingaru Supai passed the shaman grabbed its heart and ran. He put the heart in a clay pot and buried it. Where the heart decomposed a fine soil called *maiangi* formed, out of which grew these plants. It's possible that they were still used not long ago, but it seems as if now their use has faded into the past.

Among the most traditional families who protect large swaths of territory, the plants would be used in the following manner. Upon the birth of a child, a few drops of one of these plants would be placed in a baby's nose by an elder who has the paju to do so, and the child will live out his or her life. Upon death, the spirit of this person reincarnates as a puma or jaguar. I learned about this from Casimiro Mamallacta, whose family members are the long-term keepers of the western slopes of the mountain of Napo-Galeras. From his home in the outskirts of Archidona it is a stiff two-day trek to his purina tambu, the wilderness area where he accomplished many diets in his youth with his grandmother. There at the Rio Pusuno, he wandered the land, enjoying it, living lightly on the Earth with all her myriad creatures. On many of our walks there we would see fresh jaguar tracks, in the same direction we were going. Casimiro said this was his grandfather, who had been given the pumallullu upon birth. He died an old man, a man of deep wisdom, who knew these forests well; Casimiro believes that now he roams these lands as a jaguar, and it was his tracks that we would see. Knowing that his grandson was wandering the forest, he would go before us clearing the path of poisonous snakes and other types of harm, Casimiro said. And never once were we endangered on these wilderness treks. On the other hand, one of Casimiro's younger sons enjoyed the disco halls in town, the dancing and the drinking. Obviously he did not have the paju to touch these plants and thought the prohibition was a thing of the past. He touched a pumallullu plant without following the obligatory dieta. After that he began to go crazy—at the discos he would strip down completely nude and dance on the tables and bar, doing things he never did before every time he drank liquor. He joined the army and the discipline cured him. Today he is a skilled jungle guide.

Dietas with Poisonous Plants

Following are two unique types of dieta endemic to the deep-forest tribes. The first was shared with me by don Casimiro, and it is a practice no longer upheld. His grandfather, a master healer by the name of Huagrabula, and the grandfathers before him followed a dieta using the deadly toxic bark of the *huambula* tree *(Minquartia guianensis)*. *Huambula* is the Kichwa name; among the Secoya it is known as *yajisiu,* and among the Waorani, *cubacarehue.*

The huambula is one of the powerful trees held sacred by the people for many reasons. For one, its wood never rots, not even when left in the rain or planted in the ground. In the old days all traditional houses were built from the heartwood of young huambula trees found downed in the forest, knocked over in windstorms or hit by other falling trees. The people would seek only the posts ready to carry home for building the lodge. These posts would be inherited from generation to generation, and many indigenous peoples' homes today use the same posts that their ancestors did. For this reason the tree represents the continuum between generations.

The tree has several peculiar uses: for example, when its bark is pounded and placed in pools in the river, it temporarily eliminates oxygen from the water in that area. Then the fish, gasping for air, come to the surface where they can be caught. The edible fruits of the huambula are like small avocados. Once while in Galeras I was able to try these fruits. Casimiro and I mashed them in some water, and the deep rich oily green drink was indeed fortifying.

Don Casimiro told me that his grandfather would diet with the poisonous bark of the tree under the supervision of his master—first just holding the bark, then inhaling a bit. The doses would be increased little by little over time, the whole while following a diet of green bananas. Eventually the dieter would consume what would otherwise be a lethal dose! The person gains the strength of this tree; he receives its paju, its power or energy, and with this fortification a challenging life in the wilderness becomes easier on many levels. This process gave aspirants extra-special healing abilities to use in the service of their families and people.

The Waorani carry out a similar diet with their arrow poison, called *curare* or, in their language, *oomae.* This is another amazing product of the indigenous science, a most sophisticated technology that the Waorani extrapolated from an ancient myth. The grandchildren of Grandfather Creator made a new Grandfather Creator to bring around a time of peace, during which people could live happily and prosper. The Waorani needed a way to catch food more easily. They observed that snakes have fangs with poison that they use to hunt and feed themselves, and that eagles have claws for the same purpose, and so on with all the other animals. And what about the Waorani, living naked in the jungle? This deep yearning to transform allowed them to discover how to make oomae, a combination of various plants including muscle relaxants. The animal thus dies slowly as its heart relaxes to the point where it no longer works and oxygen no longer reaches the bloodstream. Oomae is not a poison; it is a muscle relaxant that is rendered ineffective by heat, so after being cooked the meat is perfectly suitable to eat.

For the dieta, the Waorani will first eat a very small dose of the tar-like black poison, gradually increasing it. Eventually they can swallow a large ball, an otherwise fatal dose, and be unharmed. They achieve special hunting abilities through this process that last many years. This is an ancient custom of the Waorani people when they are training to become hunters.

There are various methods of training, and distinct traditions and disciplines are followed to obtain the spiritual energy that gives access to celestial visions and knowledge. All require the student to abstain from indulgences and to live a life in utmost moderation. The point of all the different practices is to be able to concentrate one's energy in the supreme high-vibration channels of life, until it can become discerning enough to "see" and "know" the truth of things, and to experience the astonishing beauty of the normally unseen realms.

Cultural and societal conditioning as well as each person's own life history will affect everything one experiences and believes to be true. For this reason it is imperative to not consider all that can be seen or heard as the final truth—it is only what it is. Nor is it wise to believe all one's thoughts. To strive to understand the truth one needs to practice discernment on every level of one's being.

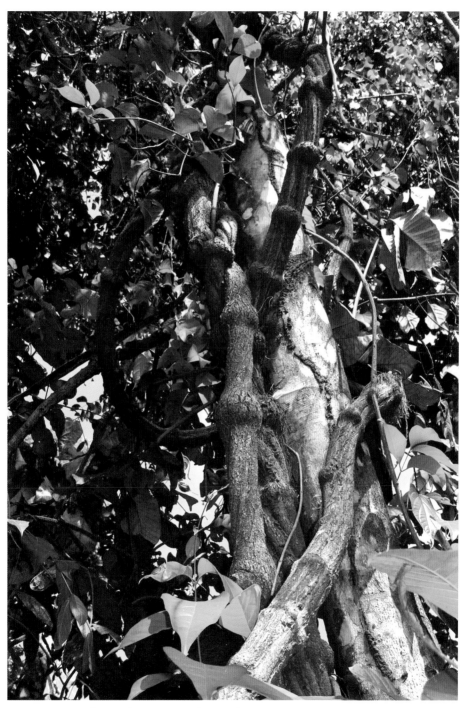

Mucutulluwaska (Kichwa), tzinca yagé (Secoya): the swollen-node variety of
Banisteriopsis caapi

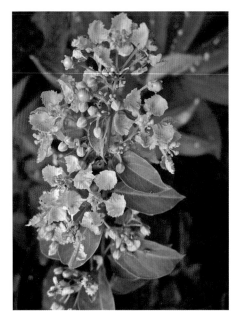
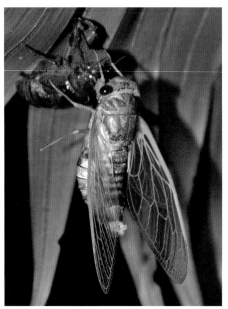

Tara yagé in flower *(B. caapi)*　　　　Newly emerged cicada (by Keith Hinman)

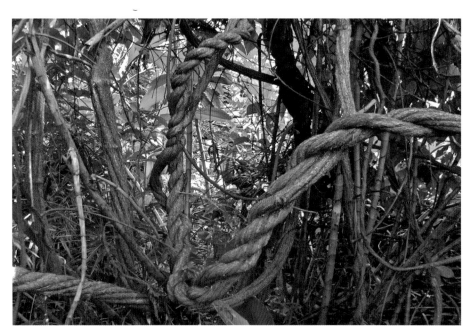

Long running vines of the sëño yagé variety

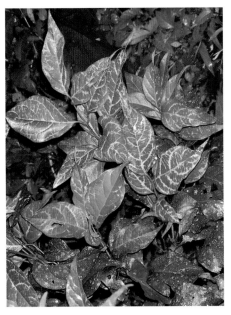

Splotched leaf variety of waiyagé *(B. caapi)*

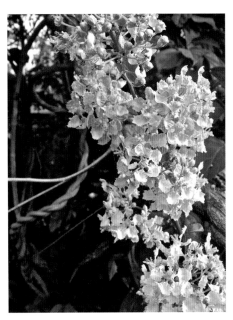

Tara yagé in full flower *(B. caapi)*

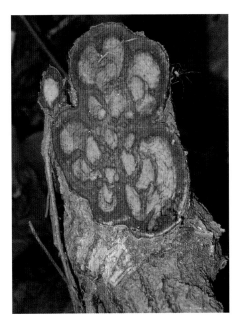

Cross-section view of tara yagé

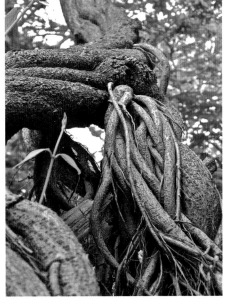

Tara yagé roots and vine

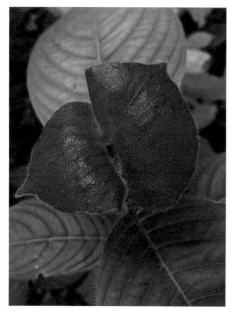

Sachawarmy, *Cephaelis tomentosa*

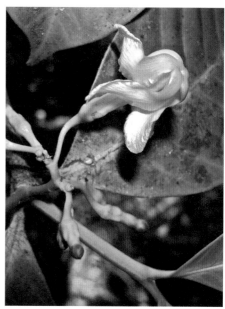

Tzicta, *Tabernaemontana sananho*

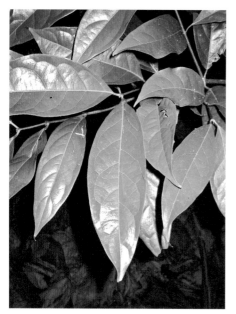

Yagé ocó, *Diplopterys cabrerana*

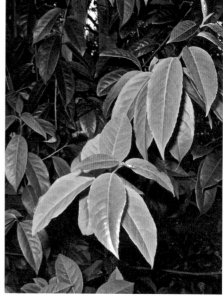

Waísamama, *Ilex guayusa*

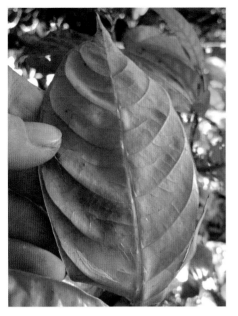
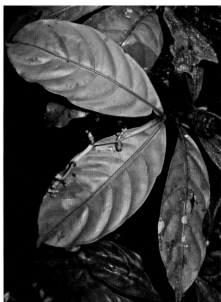

Chullachaqui panga, "leaf of the one-legged spirit," *Psychotria* sp.

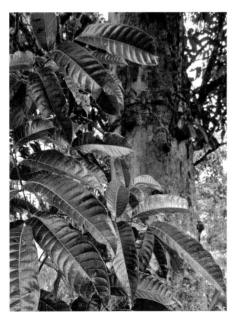
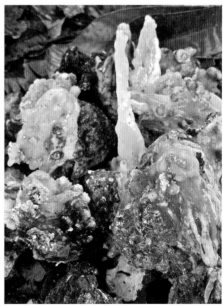

Copal, *Dacryodes peruviana*

Sacred copal resin

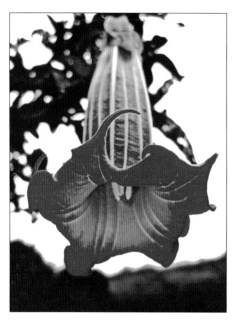

Wantú, *Brugmansia sanguinea*

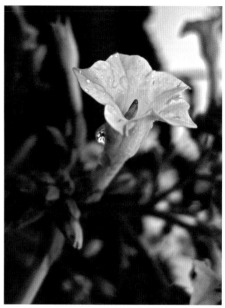

Taucu, *Nicotiana tabacum*

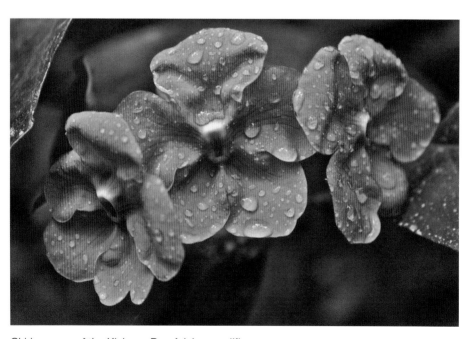

Chiriguayusa of the Kichwa, *Brunfelsia grandiflora*

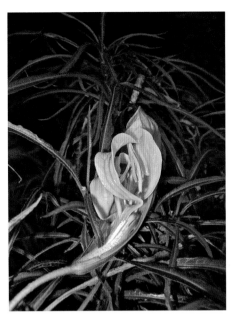
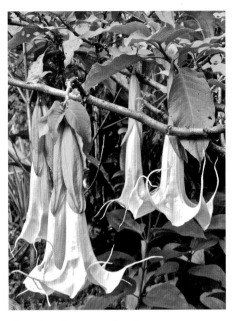

Culebra borrachera, *Methysticodendron amesianum*

Guanduc, *Brugmansia arborea*

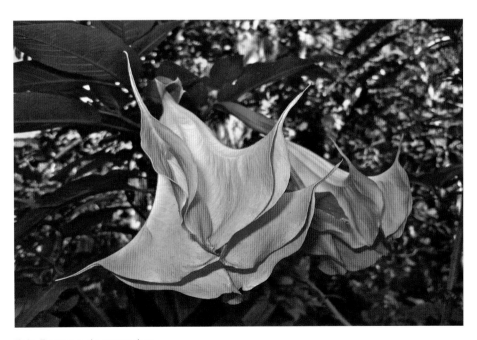

Pejí, *Brugmansia suaveolens*

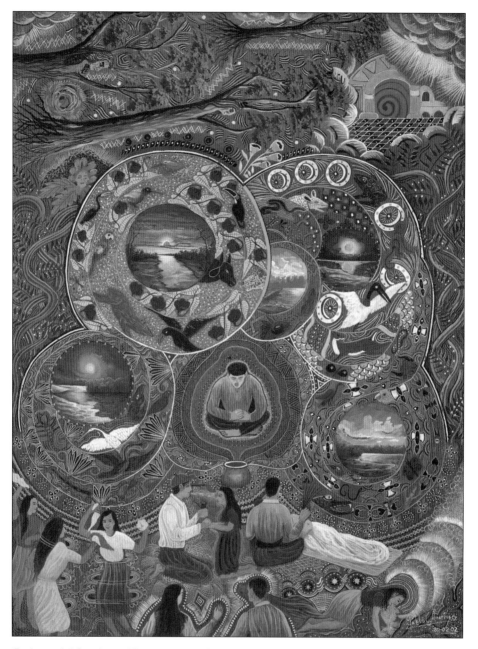

Poderes del Sumiruna, "Powers of the Sumiruna," by Pablo Amaringo, 2002

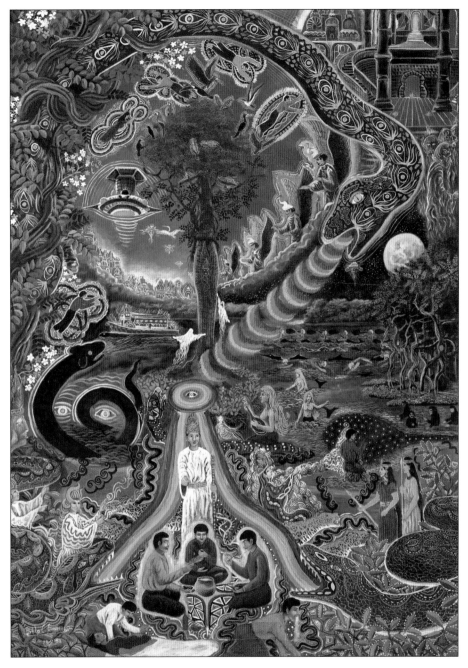

Cosmología Espiritual, "Spiritual Cosmology," by Pablo Amaringo, 2002

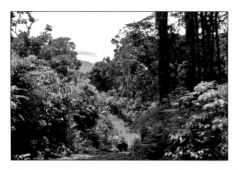 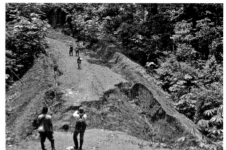

Illegal logging roads like this one threaten the Tropical Wet Forest (2010)

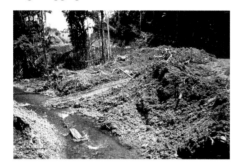 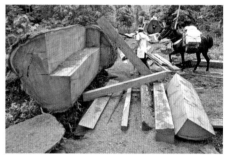

Degrading the environment and rivers at Napo-Galeras (2010)

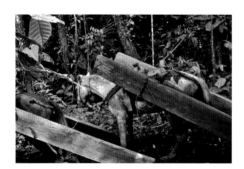 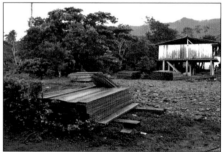

Unregulated logging like this east of Napo-Galeras is occurring all over Ecuador (2010)

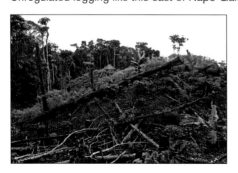 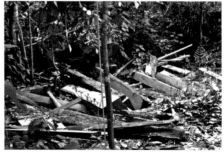

Illegal squatting and logging within Wairachina Sacha reserve, east of Napo-Galeras (2010)

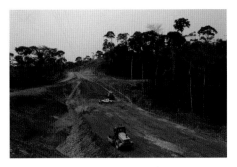 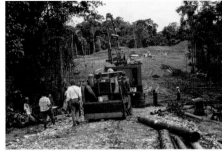

Oil roads in Waorani territory (left, 2009; right, 1994, by Murray Cooper)

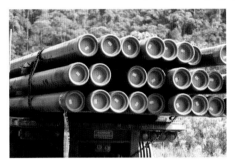 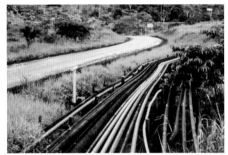

Our addiction to fossil fuels brings permanent destruction to the rainforest (2010)

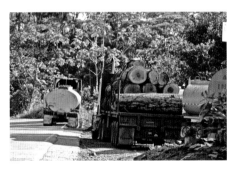 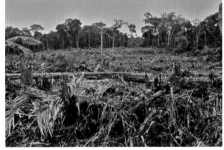

Extractivism, the plague of our era

Clearcut for oil palms, 2011
(by James Ficklin)

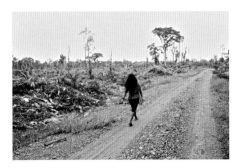 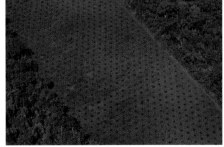

Oil palm plantations bordering Secoya territory, 2011 (by James Ficklin and Murray Cooper)

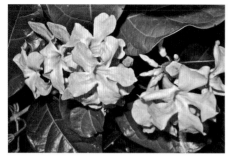

Ajuswaska, *Mansoa alliaceae*

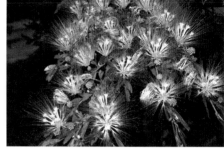

Yutzu, *Calliandra angustifolia*

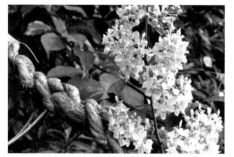

Tara yagé, *Banisteriopsis caapi*

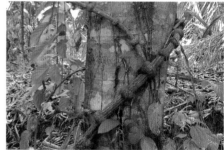

Tzinca yagé, *B. caapi* variety

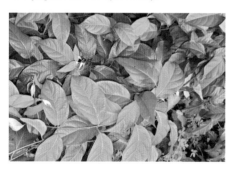

B. caapi young leaves

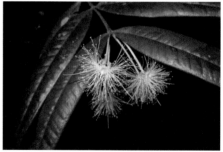

Shingi guayusa, *Calyptranthes ishoaquinicca*

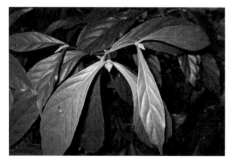

Amiruka, *Psychotria viridis*

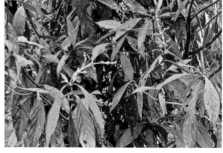

Chacruna (amiruka) in flower

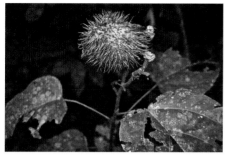

Pajumanduru, *Bixa orellana* variety

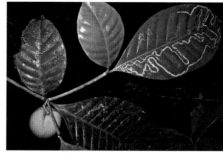

Tzicta, *Tabernaemontana sananho*

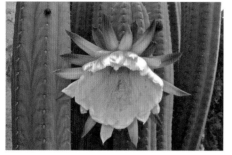

Awacolla, *Trichocereus pachanoi*

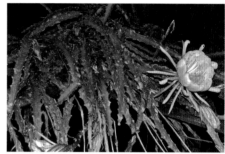

Pitajaya, *Hylocereus* sp.

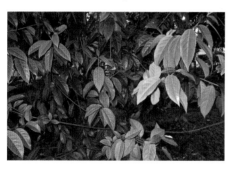

Waísamama, *Ilex guayusa*

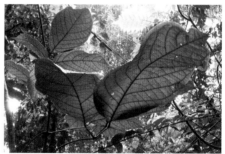

Mañapë, *Callichlamys latifolia*

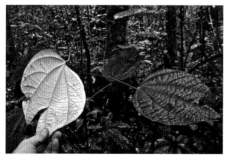

Oonta, *Curarea tecunarum*

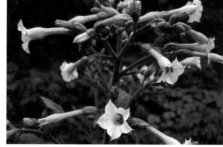

Taucu, *Nicotiana tabacum*

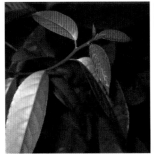
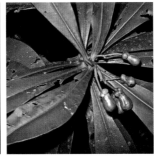
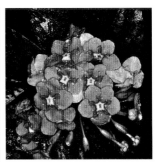

Ilex guayusa leaf shoots

Ujuangu, *Tovomita weddelliana*

Yai ujájái, *Brunfelsia chiricaspi*

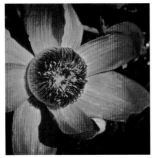
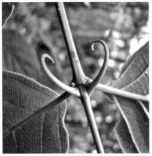
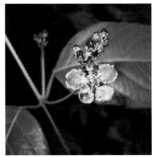

Nonginka, *Gustavia longifolia*

Uña de gato, *Uncaria guianensis*

Sense yagé, *Banisteriopsis* sp.

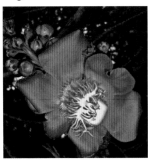
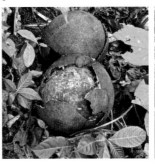

Ilushtinda muyu, *Couroupita guianensis*

Tamia yura, *Leonia crassa*

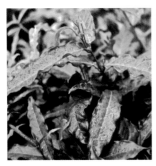
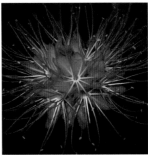
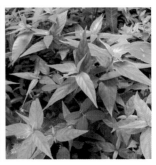

Machakui wishuk, snakebite root

Cruzcaspi, *Brownea grandiceps*

Ocomaña, *Justicia pectoralis*

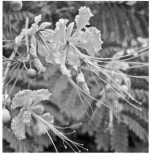

Sen, *Caesalpinia pulcherrima*

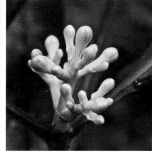

Curarina, *Potalia amara*

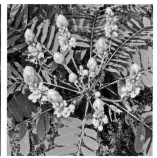

Retama, *Senna alata*

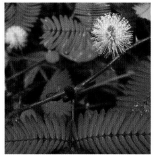

Jurema, *Mimosa hostilis*

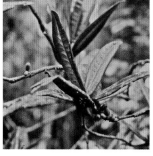

Mishqui panga, *Coussarea dulcifolia*

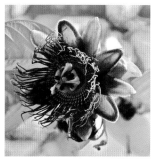

Granadilla, *Passiflora* sp.

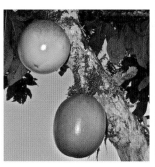

Pilchi, *Crescentia cujete*

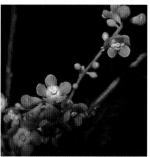

Matimuyu, *Clavija weberbaueri*

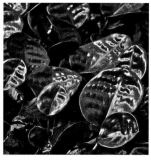

Yai sinaneñá, *Geogenanthus ciliatus*

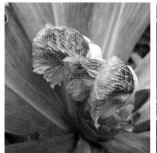

Caña agria, *Costus guianensis*

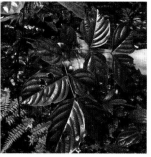

Mönse, *Cedrelinga cateniformis*

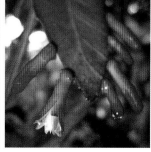

Pakipanga, *Disocactus amazonicus*

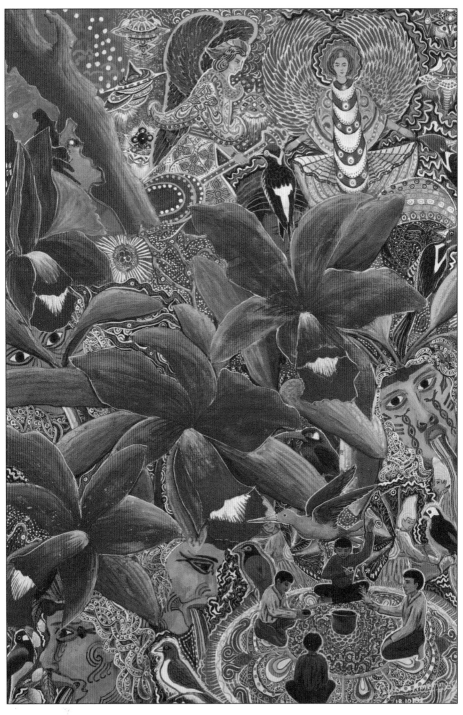

Chirapa Callu, "Rainbow Tongue," by Pablo Amaringo, gouache on Arches paper, 2001

Chapter 5

Preparing a Proper Brew

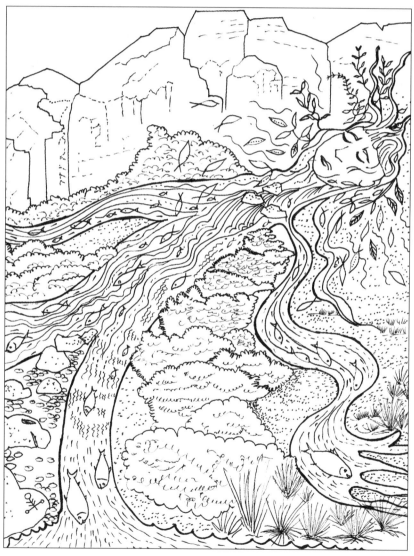

Becoming Great Nature by Merging with the Elements

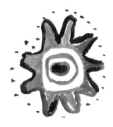

A good batch of yagé must unite the heavenly and earthly energies, and to realize this, subtle elements are necessary in the preparation. This is among the most refined essences of nature, fit to be drunk by the traditional elders. This chapter documents many of the guidelines for preparing yagé according to standards which the Secoya say come down to them from the Ñañë Siecopai, the Multicolored People of God. Note that methods as well as plant mixtures vary throughout the Amazon basin.

Sourcing and Harvesting Ayahuasca

"I have observed in using both yage and Peyote a strange, vegetable consciousness, an identification with the plant. . . . It is easy to understand how the Indians came to believe there is a spirit in these plants."
—William Burroughs, *The Yage Letters*[1]

The brew is carefully prepared from a mixture of yagé *(Banisteriopsis caapi)* and yagé ocó *(Diplopterys cabrerana)* vines. (Remember, this is the Secoya admixture of choice; people in other parts of the upper Amazon tend to use chacruna, *Psychotria viridis.*) These vines are usually cultivated in private gardens, which are reserved for this purpose and visited and cared for only by the yagé drinker. He is considered the father of the vines and stays in communion with the *yagémopai* (yagé people), the spirits of the yagé. Only with permission from their human father are the vines respectfully harvested, often after being softly sung to.

The thick central "mother vine" is usually not harvested. It is the abode of the plant spirit. The yagé vine is viewed as a house within which resides its owner, the spirit mother of the yagé. Many kinds of yagémopai or spiritual entities can live in this house, depending on the ability and grade of the yagé drinker or shaman who owns the vines and the depth of his/her wisdom. In visions, these can present themselves in multiple forms, such as a big complex insect with many eyes and many legs, or a large showy green grasshopper, or as many little people, or as a jaguar, a colorful snake, or a beautiful beaded goddess.

Usually new vines are planted regularly, and eventually, if need be, an entire vine can be harvested, including the thick central vine, but only if the shaman has not used this central vine to trap trickster spirits (something explained below). In the case of wild vines, the region where they grow will largely determine the quality of the spirits that have been attracted to live inside them.

In the Secoya and related traditions, the woody vines as well as leafy branches and offshoots of the mother vine are harvested for cooking down into a thick tea. The plants may be wild or cultivated, but it's always good (if not essential) to know something about the source of the ayahuasca as well as the admixture plants. Traditionally, students on the path find a trusted master to provide guidance and an appropriate source of sacred plants. In healing ceremonies as well as ayahuasca churches, people trust their healers, shamans, and spiritual leaders to find and provide safe and appropriately handled materials. Urban ayahuasqueros do not have a forest nearby, so they must obtain plants on field trips or from vendors of medicinal plants. They might have a small garden but it's not likely to support jungle-sized lianas.

In this regard I can offer the example of don Solon Tello, a great urban healer from Iquitos and master ayahuasquero, who owned no property in the bush and depended on friends and relatives to prepare medicine for him. On one occasion I met one of these friends, a humble elder of dignified stature. Don Solon had once healed this man's daughter, and they became friends. One afternoon while I was there visiting, he brought don Solon a bottle of medicine as a gift. Don Solon uncorked the brew and knew instantly that it was good. He held it to the light and none could shine through; the liquid was deep dark brown and syrupy thick. It was well prepared, he said. Don Solon told me if it were not for this modest man's virtuous solidarity with his healing practice, or his own son, who, at times, brought him medicine as well, he might not even be drinking. A master often relies on the inspired gifts and assistance of other people who believe in him and want him to continue his beneficial work. This was certainly true of don Solon, who did not rely on any fixed pattern or set deals to keep his practice going—only on the power of his skill and virtuous intent to attract what he needed to continue healing.

Often it will be the patient who provides the medicine. Among the Secoya as well as urban dwellers, frequently if a healer is requested to attend to a patient, those who call the healer must provide the brew. It is not always well prepared, but a worthy master can sometimes circumvent setbacks and call the spirits anyway in order to do his work.

In the case of curious Westerners seeking experiences, it's pretty much a crapshoot as to what type and quality of brew they will be served, either in a city or a jungle hut—or on another continent where bottles of already-prepared brew are brought in. There are a few reputable retreat centers in the Amazon where people come to be healed from addictions,[2] or to pursue dietas and spiritual experiences, and their stewards are known to provide quality rainforest plant medicines.

As the energy of a cook is passed to the food he or she makes, the energy and intent of the people preparing an ayahuasca brew are as important to the final product as the plant sources. (See later in this chapter, "Cooking the Plants into a Sacred Drink.") As with many things in life, one's experience often depends upon attitude (of both the maker and consumer of a commodity) and approach (mainly one's own relationship to a substance, experience, being, etc.). In all cases, regardless of tradition or lack thereof—and I mean even for the most clueless ayahuasca tourist—one must approach the plant or the drink with respect. This means not to touch it without permission of the owner, to handle it slowly and calmly when harvesting, and to avoid loud noises, disrespectful jokes, and excessive small talk, gossip, or jabber when working with the plant. As botanist and educator Kathleen Harrison notes, it's wise to model our use of ayahuasca and all plants, particularly sacred plants, "on the indigenous traditions that have a long history of using these substances to build respectful, reciprocal relationships and to achieve healing on many levels."[3]

Harrison states the importance of a plant's source in the medicine world so well that I will quote her directly here:

> [T]he source of a sacred medicine is very important. It certainly is among native people. Before using a plant, they want to know exactly who has grown it or collected it in the wild, and they want to be sure it's someone they know very well and whose intentions are pure. But it goes further than that. Let's say I'm a Mazatec shaman [of Oaxaca, Mexico] and my best friend was in the highlands and found the species he was looking for and collected some and brought them back, but along the way, a strange incident occurred. In that shaman's worldview, the fact that something strange had happened was considered a bad omen and the mushrooms would be deemed tainted; no one would take them. Indigenous masters of this type of botanical wisdom consider this kind of medicine so vibratory in nature and so absorbent of human intention and events that they take the history of a plant's origin very, very seriously. I recommend we follow their lead.
>
> In the case of ayahuasca, these are often not wild forest plants, but are grown in the shaman's garden. Who grew these plants? How pure were the intentions of that shaman as he grew, harvested, and brewed the plants? Every single brewing is a different recipe on a different day in a different pot, under a different sky. All these factors combine in an incredibly intricate mix to affect our experience. This is not something you should just get out of a bottle from somebody and not know where it came from or what happened to it along the way. It's not just a drug. It's something else.[4]

To further understand why the plant's source is so important, let me impart a few details related to sourcing and cultivating ayahuasca vines that I was enlightened about over the years. It's known that when a good master needs to accomplish an advanced spiritual healing, he might trap a harmful spirit in a place where it can do no more damage, and this might be within a yagé vine. In turn the master will lead the heavenly spirit to a new vine, one that he has cultivated in a more remote part of his garden. After this occurs, the old vine is never again used; it is left to overgrow and return to the wild, becoming the "jail" of the negative spirit. This is why the Secoya never drink from an old vine that is left in the overgrown garden of a deceased shaman. They are showing respect and also acknowledging the uncertain history of ceremonies related to each vine.

It is considered extremely dangerous to take a live cutting of an ayahuasca vine from an active shaman's garden without having been granted permission. The Secoya say that if this happens, when the person prepares the drink he will see in his vision that he is attacked and strangled. Shortly afterward, he might become very ill or die, unless the vine he has stolen from is cut down and destroyed. The same can happen if one takes a wild vine without first asking permission from its spiritual owner, as wild vines from remote wilderness areas are homes to particularity powerful spirits who need to be appeased and recognized so that they willingly give of their energy to those interested in learning.

Traditionally, when a vine is passed along from its cultivator to someone else, it is given as if in a marriage ceremony, with several witnesses present, usually two couples on each side of the benefactor and beneficiary of the vine. The recipient humbly accepts the vine, which is given over fully charged with celestial energy. In all cases the recipient would need to be a disciple or relative of the shaman, as the vines are not passed on lightly.

These are some of the reasons why in the Amazon most new students who do not have a teacher and want to drink look for a wild vine in a remote wilderness area, even though these vines cannot be touched without precaution, either. The hopeful gatherers pray to the spiritual owner of the vine and they fast. Just because the vines are growing wild does not mean they do not have an owner—wild plants always have spiritual owners or guardians. The aspirants may drink strong *yoco*[5] (*Paullinia yoco*, a caffeinated jungle vine) or a beverage called *mëto* that is prepared by mashing strong native tobacco in water and letting it settle in the sun. These drinks help one concentrate energy and facilitate the necessary contact with the spiritual owner of the wild yagé vine. One must meditate on the question of harvesting the wild yagé and actually see the spiritual owner and request and receive authorization before harvesting these vines. At this time the vine's spiritual owner appreciates soft and harmonious music, especially singing or flute music. With proper intention, it won't be long before the spiritual owner of the *airo yagé*, the wild or forest yagé vine, responds and authorizes the harvesting. The permission is received through a vision, dream, or other indication, such as colorful birds flying out of the vine, either in one's inner sight or in actuality—for example, the *jëesaipë*, *pisasá*, or *mapia*, the blue-necked tanager, paradise tanager, and scarlet tanager, respectively.[6]

A kind elder told me that once in his youth he went to a wild vine with the intention to gather some of it. He drank yoco and concentrated in order to encounter the spiritual owner of the vine. Suddenly a scarlet tanager flew down and landed on his right shoulder. It perched there for a moment, chirped some, then jumped off and flew back into the canopy of the vine. This was how the spiritual people of the yagé accepted his request and authorized him to proceed with his harvest.

SOME BOTANICAL TRAITS OF *BANISTERIOPSIS CAAPI*

Ayahuasca, *yagé*, and *ingandu (Banisteriopsis caapi)* are three of the many names for an elliptic- to lanceolate-leafed pan-Amazonian climbing woody liana whose thick intertwining stems form helixes reminiscent of DNA. A peculiar characteristic of this vine is the small extra-floral nectar-producing glands found on the underside of the base of each of its simple, entire-margined leaves. During flowering they secrete a sappy morsel that deters ants and other insects from damaging the fragile blooms. The subtly scented baby-pink flowers fade to white over the course of a few days. They attract several kinds of tiny stingless honey-bees.[7] The vine's pollination by honeybees can be interpreted as a sign of its association with spiritual life: Honey is symbolic of the nectar of the celestial realms, the essence of spiritual immortality.

The plant's flowers are said to be the "trail of the heaven people," upon which the Wiñapai descend from their celestial abodes to the Earth, in order to fill the yagé drinkers with their immortal energy. The time when the vine flowers during the summer months, when the cicadas are sing-ing, is considered to be the best time for drinking yagé.

The ephemeral five-petaled flowers are followed within two to three weeks by *samara,* winged propeller-like seeds, that upon drying turn brown and drop, spiraling gently to the forest floor. The way the seeds spiral down is considered by traditional elders to represent how the yagé toyá—the deeply symbolic energy designs or visual patternings carried by the yagé—arrive in soft, gentle, often spiraling or inchworm-like rhythmical undulations. In a similar flight of imagination, the leaves falling from the canopy when one harvests the vines are referred to as "fish swimming home" because they will transform to nourishing mulch. The image repre-sents the cycles of life and death, transformation and rebirth—the phases of the grand eternal continuum that is existence.

Another characteristic is the bark, which may come off easily or be stubborn and difficult to remove. The trait of easily removed bark is used to identify the best varieties of yagé. This is why among the Secoya wild yagé vines are not as desirable—they have thick bark that is hard to pound off—although I have heard and read in the literature that in Peru among mestizo vegetalistas who cook the brew with its bark, the wild vines are more desirable and considered stronger. The cultivated varieties such as tara yagé have soft bark that is easily removed with some moderate pounding, whereas the wild vines require much more work to prepare.

Punished by the Spirit of a Wild Ayahuasca Vine

In May of 1997, on a visit to the wilderness region of Pëquë'yá (known in Spanish as Lagarto Cocha, meaning "Black-caiman Lagoon"), I went in search of a wild yagé vine, together with one of the younger traditional elders, Agustin Payaguaje, nicknamed Tintin, and several tourists.

Near the camp, we found a large wild *Banisteriopsis caapi* vine. One fellow who had hoped to see a wild vine was deeply inspired by the stories of them being home to powerful spirits. Mesmerized by the thick vine, he began offering tobacco and praying to it to release its wisdom and power; he wanted to see the spirit owner of the vine, even if it was in a dream. As he earnestly prayed to the wild ayahuasca vine, Tintin suddenly approached and began harvesting it. Today Tintin is a much more refined master, but in those days he was still a borderline wild bush man, and he walked straight up to the vine and just started cutting down the tree that the vine was growing on, wood chips flying. The fellow who was praying stood back and his jaw dropped, aghast. With a perplexed look on his face he asked me, "But shouldn't we be praying to it first?" I too was shocked, but said that his prayers were appropriate, and then added something about the need to get going with preparation since it was a long, involved process. Cutting into the wild yagé with fury, Tintin began handing us long, heavy segments, some as thick as my leg, that we carried away to where we had set up a place outside our camp to cook it.

The following morning, after a beautiful nighttime ceremony, we packed up camp and left the area. We all began boarding the large dugout canoe taking us back to the Secoya villages on the Aguarico River upstream. As Tintin was about to get on, he felt two sharp blows to his back, one after the other, as if he had just been stabbed or shot by darts. Everyone saw it happen: he leaned backwards in agony, holding his arms to his back. No one knew what to do at the time, but we got him on the boat and left for our two-day river journey.

The entire trip I sat next to his side holding his arm, because several times he tried to jump off the boat into the swift current. I had to hold him with all my might and kept whispering in his ear, "Your mother, she is waiting for you. The old master, he will heal you soon. Hold on, my friend, hold on." I was referring to don Cesareo, to whom I planned to take Tintin ASAP.

"Yes," he would reply, nodding feebly.

None of the other Secoya seemed to even notice, acting aloof and unconcerned, as the majority of the group had little experience with such matters and most people were slightly afraid. Yet Tintin was in agony, his body twisting, and it was painful for him to sit there in one place. Arm in arm we traveled the entire trip.

Cesareo hadn't joined us on the journey this time because his niece was about to give birth. When we reached his house, we found him waiting for us, already aware that something had happened. We placed Tintin before him and Cesareo immediately started shaking a fresh leafy green bundle of leaves picked for this occasion, and softly singing over him. Cesareo sang and sang, and kept brushing him with the leaves, cleansing him, blowing and singing. Tintin gasped for air and finally relaxed. Amazingly, he was fine after that, as if nothing had happened. This was a hard-learned lesson, as well as a powerful affirmation of the existence of the spiritual owner of yagé.

Cesareo knew right away what was going on. Though Tintin was raised in a traditional setting and had participated in ceremonies while he was growing up, he simply underestimated the power of the wild yagé vines and failed to seek the customary permission-granting sign. Cesareo counseled us about how to contact the owner of the yagé, adding that now we could see why this must always be done. To mess with an old wild yagé vine is serious business.

Here is another example that I personally witnessed. I was with don Delfin, a traditional Secoya elder, friend, and maestro, on a remote rainforest hill in September 1997, again at Pëquë'yá. We were out searching for *cocawasi (Xylopia benthamii),* a special tree with a bark that splits easily into slender boards that are then used for crafting the yagé drinking crowns. Don Delfin was patiently showing me the different kinds of plants that exist in the firm-soil ridge forest we were exploring, such as the highly revered wansoka tree *(Couma macrocarpa)* with its sweet edible fruit and a chewable bubble-gum-like sap that is gathered to make the ceremonial yagé incense smudge. We admired *wirisaka (Iryanthera hostmanni)*, an understory tree with richly aromatic rust-red-colored bark worn for armband perfume during the ceremonies. And we marveled at the *watí gonzá* palms—the "spirit oil-fruit " palms that are not the ordinary gonzá *(Jessenia bataua)* palm. Their fruit racemes hang low to the ground and are thus easy to acquire, whereas ordinary gonzá palms start fruiting when the tree is quite high, and it is a major feat to climb one and get the fruits (something that indigenous people pride themselves on being able to do). Delfin noted the presence of these watí gonzá palms as an irrefutable sign that the forest is inhabited by superior spirits.

Soon we encountered a large wild yagé vine growing in a remote part of the forest, on top of a long ridge that overlooked a lake. There was not a cloud to be seen in the clear blue skies. But as we approached the vine, in that moment the sky above us began to darken. I focused my camera and took a few photos, then reached out to touch the vine. Just as I touched it, thunder grumbled from the heavens and it began to rain. Delfin said that we should leave, and this we did. As we withdrew, the clouds high above the vine and the rain shower dissipated as well, shortly revealing the clear expanse of blue sky once again. We walked a good distance before we stopped at the lake shore where we had tied up our canoe. We stood there quietly for a while thinking about what we had just witnessed. From the spurt of rainfall, mist rose from the water's surface and from the rainforest's canopy on the hills behind the lake. The reflection of the golden-white disk of the midday Amazonian sun was almost blinding. The remote Amazonian wilderness regions are profoundly mysterious places.

Praying to the Vines

When harvesting the vines and branches of yagé, one first must blow on the vine. Soft chants of gratitude can be offered for the medicine that is complete and effective, and prayers of thanks to God the Creator who governs these vines; to the earlier masters of this tradition who taught and followed the sacred ways; and to the mother of the vine and the guardian spirits of yagé, asking that they be kind in releasing their wisdom, the *deopai yagé toyá*, "good-people's yagé designs"— that it may follow the vines to the place where they will be cooked and permit the drinkers to benefit from this most sacred medicine. Here one can bring forth one's intentions. The spirits of yagé are capable of sensing one's innermost vibrations, so it is necessary to be sincere. With heartfelt prayers, the vines are spoken to, as if speaking to an old and trusted spiritual master, guide, and friend. The yagé is contented with sincere prayers, song, music, and aromatic smoke.

I am able to present three sample prayers, courtesy of the gracious elders who allowed me to record some of their rituals and stories.

In April 1993 I accompanied Taita (Father) Casimiro Mamallacta on a voyage to his purina tambu (literally, "a shelter that is walked to," but meaning much more than that—this is a wilderness region where the ancient ways are upheld, a retreat area) at Napo-Galeras. We respect-fully harvested the ingandu, the ayahuasca vine, after blowing tobacco smoke on it and leaving an offering of homegrown jungle tobacco at the vine's base. Then Casimiro kneeled before the offered materials, raised his hands in the air, looked up to the sky and prayed:

> *"Spiritual masters of this land, beings of the trees, of the stars,*
> *spiritual owner of Galeras Mountain,*
> *please look upon this moment.*
> *I am your son, and here I am with my children, your children,*
> *to prepare this sacred medicine.*
> *Please make it so that it may be strong, so that we may see clearly,*
> *so the ancient knowledge of my ancestors will continue."*

Early one morning in July 1996, I accompanied Cesareo Piaguaje to harvest yagé. He blew on the vines, first with his own breath with-out tobacco. Then up into the branches he blew the smoke of a cigar containing homegrown natural tobacco rolled in a banana leaf. He shook the vine a little and offered up some prayer through softly spoken song. I asked him the essence of the prayer and he shared it with me in Spanish:

> *"I have come to learn, great elder teacher, with a humble heart*
> *and a willing hand.*
> *Please teach me, help me to see and better know the correct way*
> *of life.*
> *Help me to be a better healer so I may be of service to the people,*
> *so that I may follow the way of service, to be part of God's*
> *highest plan,*
> *grant me strength to rise above my inertia, my lassitude,*
> *my weakness*
> *so I may be stronger with each passing day,*
> *so I may correctly follow the medicine way of life,*
> *so I may be wiser with each new day that comes,*
> *more upright, more sincere, better, more willing to serve.*
> *I come to you now, great medicine vine, I come to harvest of*
> *your branches,*
> *and ask of you, hear these words, read these thoughts, owner of*
> *these vines,*
> *may the pinta come with them, fill them with your life-giving*
> *energies,*
> *allow them to be effective so we may cook yagé."*

Don Esteban Lucitante shared this next prayer with me in August of 1997. We were sitting around one afternoon watching the river flow, and I asked him what kind of prayer he offers to the yagé when harvesting. He said his prayer goes something like this:

> *"Thank you, great medicine vine, from all my being,*
> *from the most sincere depths of my being,*
> *from my heart, from my body,*
> *from my willing feet and willing hands,*
> *from my mind and soul, from all aspects of my united being,*

from my spirit to your spirit, I thank you.
Thank you for this medicine tradition that my grandfather
taught me,
thank you for helping me to see the celestial people of my origin,
the doctor people, the medicine people of my ancestors.
Thank you."

Orphaned Vines

Another phenomenon is that of "orphaned" vines, as the elders call them. These are vines that have become part of the common world in such a way that connection has been severed with the original ancestral, ancient, and celestial spirits (something difficult to obtain and easily lost). Many vines that people purchase over the Internet, or obtain through other anonymous or questionable methods, are in this category. These orphaned vines are like empty homes. Yes, the alkaloids will have an effect when consumed, but the effects are not like those of the stewarded vines.

Once some friends from Hawaii brought our master in Ecuador a batch of ayahuasca that their friends had prepared from vines growing on an island there. When we all tried the brew, the elders pronounced it empty of pinta, although the brew was thick and apparently well-prepared, and although other Western friends who drank it reported amazing experiences. After some talking the next day, the elders concluded that it had been cooked with orphaned vines. They went on to say that the medicine is giving and wants to be utilized as a vehicle for the positive and auspicious unfolding of life. When these orphaned vines are used to make a brew that is consumed by earnest, good-hearted people who pray and sing to them often while abiding by certain guidelines,[8] and who live an upright and disciplined life, they may be noticed by heavenly spirits who eventually "see" the empty house and may allow their spiritual energy to reside within this vine. This spiritual energy can then coexist among humanity in a new and different place. These vines get progressively better and stronger, and if the drinkers are disciplined, they can meet these spirits and learn more and more, eventually becoming good healers.

On the other hand, the rightfully stewarded vines that are cultivated in remote gardens where no one but the shaman and his students visit produce completely different effects. Many things can be experienced. One sees the supreme yagé toyá, the energy patterns of the immortal beings, and one sees the immortal beings themselves that the indigenous elders and the masters see. These visions are difficult to see and are normally not even encountered in one's wildest dreams.

Cooking the Plants into a Sacred Drink

"It does not suffice to cook the vine. One must also have some spiritual contact to give one strength; and one's way of being must be appropriate because we are influenced by spiritual beings. Even though they are not seen, it is true they exist. They are the ones that have taken over these plants. They are the conservers, they take care of the plants. This is why they don't give visions to persons who don't comply with all the requirements of this so-called *ciencia vegetalista,* which in the old days was known as *alquimia palística,* plant alchemy."
—Pablo Amaringo, *Ayahuasca Visions*[9]

The methods related here are ones I learned among the Secoya, as taught by God's Multicolored People. Though these techniques were kept secret for generations, the good elders who taught me have been clear: now is the time to make these valuable secrets of nature available to those who feel the calling to learn more, because today humanity desperately needs to awaken the vision of sustainability and the new world order of true cooperation and harmony. I share this information here from a sense of moral responsibility, knowing that there are many people out there experimenting with this plant medicine and for the most part wholly unaware of the vast body of traditional context that grants a higher degree of success when traveling with yagé. I also wish to record this knowledge as history, for the elders are passing, often with no apprentices. So many secrets of nature have already been lost due to humanity's drifting—sacred knowledge and wisdom that have been handed down through countless generations is now dissipating. I hope that by documenting this esoteric knowledge of nature, it will be preserved and enhanced.

In this section I outline traditional Secoya methods of preparing two types of yagé: yagérepá, "proper yagé," and ëo yagé, "burnt yagé," the latter thickly refined until it is the consistency of honey. At the end of this section is the method for preparing a third type, a cold-water infusion, which is used much less frequently.

Outside a specific healing context, yagérepá is drunk to learn fundamental principles of the tradition, as well as to practice the sacred meditations and techniques for spiritual cultivation.[10] With this type of yagé one can experience many marvelous wonders with a lower risk of causing damage to oneself or to others.

The second type, ëo yagé, is thick and strong; it is also called *weasiko yagé,* meaning yagé that is thick like corn gruel. This can be referred to as *miel* or *payá,* meaning "honey" in Spanish and Paicoca, respectively. Today, ëo yage is principally reserved for graduation ceremonies. Only after yagérepá has been drunk many times is ëo yagé prepared and taken—usually only once or twice a year during the celestial summer when it is believed that the Wiñapai are close to the Earth and can more easily be perceived. In the old days the masters preferred to drink ëo yagé, given that it is so much stronger, the visions can be sustained, the drinkers can learn about the marvelous realities of spirit, and the healers can accomplish their work most effectively.

The Making of Yagérepá

Among the Secoya, clear guidelines regulate preparation of the medicine. They are adamant about this preparation method and insist that the guidelines be followed. I've already discussed some fundamentals of harvesting the plants. When respected, all the elements and subtle factors combine to make a potent and efficacious medicine, necessary for a positive and healing ceremony.

As mentioned, soft songs and prayers are offered to the spirit owners of the vine, asking that the pinta or yagé toyá, the energetic emanations that can take the form of visions, come out of the mother vine and follow the harvested branch vines (which are, as the elders say, "her children"). It is imperative that no one walk across or otherwise intersect the trail leading from where the vines have been harvested to where the cooking will occur. In this way, the yagé toyá sent by the mother vine can find and catch up to her children, the harvested vines. Don Cesareo would say that the harvested vines are like children calling for their mother, and the mother vine calls back to her children. The call and response continues until they find each other, and then the toyá, the pinta, arrives in the harvested vines.

If the pinta sees that the trail has been crossed by someone, it does not know which way to go, so it returns to the home vine. This manifests as a weak brew. The master will have to drink more and work harder to call the designs. Though it may be strong in terms of alkaloid content, and those who drink it will feel intoxicated, this is not the intention. The intention in preparing a proper brew is for the drinkers to be engulfed in supreme designs, heightening their consciousness and making known the reality of the Wiñapai, while diminishing the often unavoidable feelings of drunkenness and stupor.

Each elder has a distinct approach. Cesareo was adamant that if it was certain that no one would cross the path where the harvested vines have been carried, then they can be cooked that same day. If the vines are in an area where it is inevitable that someone will walk across the designs' path, then the harvested material must be placed gently on the ground, covered in banana leaves, sprinkled with water to stay fresh, and left at the cooking site for a few days. The yagé toyá will eventually find the way. (When these vines are to be cooked, the tips that have been touching the air are cut off; otherwise, say the elders, the master's throat will get dry and he cannot sing.) If the path is crossed and the yagé is drunk the same day anyway, the master drinker can call the toyá himself and the yagé can still be effective, but it means more work for him, and it reveals to him that an error has occurred in the preparation process.

Other elders shared that it is possible to hold the vines up above one's head when carrying them across an intersecting trail. Lifting them up high is thought to ensure that the pinta travels through the air behind the trail of transported vines. This simple act keeps the pinta from being dissipated and therefore this material can be cooked that same day. Domestic animals that could follow the cooks are tied up and left at home; the Secoya, unlike other indigenous and mestizo ayahuasca users, never allow their dogs to be present while cooking or at the ceremonial lodge, since they believe dogs carry Watí with them. The dogs live tranquilly with these spirits, but it is believed that these same spirits can contaminate the yagé and potentially disrupt the pinta.

As already discussed, the preferred admixture plant of the Secoya is yagé ocó, which is harvested and brought to the cooking spot following the same procedures as the yagé. Harvesting yagé ocó requires even more prayers and songs than harvesting yagé, as this plant has abundant pinta and brings a highly scintillating toyá, rich with aura and designs. Because it supplies the light of heaven or the air element (while yagé supplies the strength of the earth element), the visions of yagé ocó are more ephemeral and difficult to sustain, so deeper concentration and heightened focus on intent are necessary when harvesting the DMT-containing admixture plant. Often the prayers are made in silence. As with the yagé vines, tobacco smoke or copal incense can be offered, with the tobacco left at the base of the vine before snapping branches off, always with one's hands, never with a metal blade. The cut of the machete is said to be too "cold" for this plant, severing the fragile threads of spiritual energy that follow the vine to the cooking place after harvest. Also, the sound of its pinta awakening is said to be a snapping type of sound, similar to that made when breaking a branch with one's fingers. Regular manual pruning keeps the vine healthy and within reach, allowing the plant to regrow new shoots that will be easy to access for the next cooking. For all these reasons the branches of yagé ocó are snapped off.

Before commencing the brewing, all the pots must be clean, there must be abundant chopped firewood, and all the water must have been hauled for the cooking and for bathing afterward. One needs some candles and a flashlight in case the process leads into the night, copal incense in order to make aromatic smudge, and a small pot and/or bottle(s) to store the final product in. Other necessary items include a sieve to strain the final brew of leaf and bark pieces, some small gourds or cups, a wooden mallet to pound the vines, and long forked pieces of wood to retrieve the spent material from the pot at the end of the process. Also necessary is a pot of water with which to bathe afterward, and a set of clean clothes.

To begin, a generous wad of the *Banisteriopsis caapi* leaves is blown on and then rubbed over the entire inner surface area of the cooking pot. This is to prepare it for receiving the medicine and to soften the edge between it having been sitting around cold and now called to action, about to be heated and used.

The thickest portions of yagé vine are pounded with a wooden mallet to remove their bark, then washed in a separate smaller pot of warmed water that has been scooped out of the main pot, under which a fire has already been lit. Much of the vines' earthen brown-colored essence is released into this water, which is then poured back into the mother pot. This is done in order to capture more of the vines' essence and make a stronger brew.

After having been washed like this, the thick vines are pounded again to further awaken the spirit of the yagé, and to loosen even more its divine energy auras for release into the brew. These thick portions of vine are then placed into the cooking pot to be heavily boiled. The thinner vines are left as long as possible, and all their bark is pounded off. These long segments of pounded vine are rolled into coils or bundles that are tied together with a piece of the same vine, then placed into the pot to boil. It is believed that by leaving them long and not cutting them into small pieces, the toyá will be sustained and will not dissipate quickly. Sometimes as part of a harvest, yagé roots are pulled out of the ground, rather long and up to an inch thick; these are baked over the fire for about ten minutes before being pounded and added to the pot; the roots' bark is not discarded but rather added to the brew. Adding roots like this significantly augments the strength of the final product. One can also add some of the highest leaves and, if available, as many flowers as possible.

As I mentioned earlier in the book, not all vegetalistas pound off the ayahuasca bark. The Secoya prefer to remove all the bark because it is known to make one vomit, and therefore only the "bone," the inner part of the vine, is used in their preparation. The pounded bark is placed in a pile off to the side so it won't be stepped on. It is believed that if the cooks step on the bark during the cooking process, later during the ceremony the drinkers will vomit.

Properly prepared, much larger doses can be swallowed without running a high risk of vomiting. Understand, vomiting and otherwise purging is among ayahuasca's benefits, so it is not bad. It rids us of impurities and can be an important part of a patient's healing. However, for this specific reason, the Secoya carry out cleansings with the sunrise renewal ceremony (see "Dieta" section in Chapter 4) prior to ceremonies with yagé. For the latter, the intention becomes to stay very still and quiet, to hold in the medicine, to practice meditation, and to "see" what the master is transmitting through song, vision, and wordless teachings of the medicine. It is believed that if someone vomits at the onset of a ceremony, before the yagé toyá arrives, then the visions will not come quickly and the shaman's work is made more difficult.

The vines are boiled furiously for at least four hours, together with abundant young leaves and pounded branches of the yagé ocó admixture vine. It's imperative that the fire stay at the highest possible temperature throughout the cooking process without any reduction in intensity or heat, for which the wood must be well dried. This is why certain types of wood are preferred, such as that of the *ëné* palm *(Bactris gasipaes), guayaba (Psidium guajava),* and the *pëné* tree *(Inga edulis),* among other tight-grain woods that sustain a high temperature and burn steadily.

The cooking takes place in the ceremonial lodge, which is always removed from the village or household. It might be located behind the yagé drinker's house, or sometimes it is up to an hour's walk through the forest at a select site, like the top of a small hill or a forest glade near a bend in a stream. It is important that the cooks be upright and focused in their intentions, work rapidly, and consume no food and only a little water in the process. There should be little or no talking, nor loud noises or quick movements. The vines must not be handled roughly or thrown to the ground, in order to avoid disturbing the coalescence of the pinta. The cooks should concentrate on celestial affairs throughout the entire process. They must not leave the yagé under any circumstance until it is fully cooked, reduced, refined, allowed to cool, and stored (if it is not to be drunk immediately). Nor must the cooks take off their tunics if it gets too hot, or express complaints about the heat of cooking in the midday sun or the fasting that must be sustained through the entire day (sipping only a little water and/or eating one baked green banana at noon if need be). The cooks must all be in good health, dedicated students of the tradition, and they must have refrained from sexual activity or be celibate and dedicated to the learning of the path. If they are married, they must have refrained from intimate contact for at least five days before the cooking, and, ideally, somewhat longer.

Also it is imperative that at certain times the cooks smudge with sap- and resin-based incenses such as *kënjé* (the fragrant resin of *Dacryodes peruviana,* one of a number of trees known throughout Latin America as "copal"), *sohó* (the sap of *Hymenaea courbaril*), and *sohómanë* (an incense log made of multiple ingredients). These smudges expel negative energies and invite the presence of celestial beings. A piece of copal can also be used to start the fire, as it is highly flammable.

Smudge is applied to the freshly cut vines before they are to be pounded, and to the pot when it is taken off the fire to cool, and during the reduction process. Once the vines are cooked, they are taken out of the pot and stacked up off to one side; then they are covered with banana leaves and heavily smudged. Covering the pile of employed vine material and leaf with banana or other large leaves is what Delfin calls *cobijando,* a Spanish word meaning "blanketing." It is believed that covering the spent vines will both help the drinkers stay warm at night and concentrate the pinta for longer-lasting effect.

To improve the brew's potency, additional guidelines are observed, such as not letting the water in the yagé pot boil over and fall on the ashes. As a precaution against this, the pot is never filled too close to the top. The pot used for cooking the yagé is maintained exclusively for this purpose and stored on a base or hanging from a high rafter, not left to get "cold" by touching the ground.

Another simple factor in the cooking process, yet one of profound significance, is the respectful recognition of something that has been mentioned above, the *Wiñapai toyá ma'a,* the "always-new divine immortals designs path," or simply *toyá ma'a,* the "designs path." Cesareo told us that his grandfather acknowledged the path with two balsa logs about one and a half meters apart, with the ends farthest from the pot widening. In small holes that he made along each log, his grandfather would put erect flowers, all lined up in a row. These logs would be placed to reach outwards from the back of the fire, clearly marking the designs trail that mustn't be crossed; Cesareo requested that we do the same. This invites the divine immortals to arrive and impregnate the yagé with their supreme supernatural designs. By clearly defining where no one should walk, the most critical part of the cooking process is respected. Wood is supplied to the fire and the brew monitored only from the front of the pot. Never during the cooking do the cook or assistants walk behind the fire or cross the trail further back. Later when the brew is close to being finished, this trail is smudged with aromatic tree sap (from the sides, still not walking on it), sanctifying this strip of land in sincere hopes that the medicine will be effective. Once the brew is complete and ready to be carried to the ceremonial lodge, the same path must be respected and not crossed.

There are several other restrictions in the cooking process. Anyone who happens to walk into the cooking area must stay there through the rest of the process until the brew is finished. They cannot come and go back to the household, or the yagé will be ruined. Don Cesareo would make us throw the brew away if this occurred. Other elders say if the brew is left alone for a few days it fixes itself—the pinta gathers again and coalesces, and the yagé can then be drunk and be effective. However, I think it was good to learn from Cesareo, since he holds true to the ancient traditions, while others have drifted a little. You could say he is an orthodox old-school drinker, upholding the tradition to the T! Cesareo explained that the area where the brew is being cooked becomes like a celestial island, and if someone arrives and leaves during the process, or if one of the cooks leaves while the brew is boiling, the pinta disperses. Elements can come in but not leave until the process is completed. In my mind I could see the analogy of a hot-air balloon rising: more air can come in, but if the air exits, the balloon can no longer rise.

The reduction process requires the most surveillance, because things can go wrong if the water is allowed to boil too low. After four hours of vigorous boiling, the pot is taken off the flame and left to cool somewhat. Then with two forked sticks made of hard wood peeled of their bark, the materials are taken out of the pot and placed to one side. The leaves can be squeezed into the pot once they are cool since they hold a lot of liquid. The pot is placed back onto the fire and boiled for up to an hour, depending on how much liquid is left, then it is removed from the fire and left to cool; the liquid is strained and placed into a small pot or bottle, at which point it is ready to be served.

If the brew is being cooked to bottle for travel or to drink another night, then a separate set of clothes is brought and left at the edge of the cook site. After cooking and bottling the yagé, the cooks themselves cool down and wash with a bucket of water. They do not immerse themselves in the river or swim; they bathe on the land with the bucket so the pinta does not get washed away but rather goes into the earth and stays nearby. (The same practice is followed the day after a ceremony. It is believed that in the water there are many Watí. The elders say that when people bathe in the river shortly after drinking yagé and a piece of hair from their body floats into the water, the Watí see it as if it were an iridescent blue feather. A Watí will swoop up and grab the feather and keep it, and the drinker's energy level will drop.) When the brew is fully ready and the cooks have bathed, they put on fresh clothes and can leave the cooking area. Among the Secoya, yagé is usually drunk fresh after it is cooked, for which they put on their ceremonial tunics, necklaces, and yagé drinking crowns, paint their faces, tuck the aromatic maña herbs into their bracelets and armbands, and carry the yagé to the ceremonial lodge, where the gathered drinkers and the ceremonial guide—who have all fasted the entire day, and who are regally dressed for the event—lie meditating. Tranquil in their hammocks, they await the arrival of the cooks and their brew.

All these guidelines must be followed when cooking yagé to be served to a traditional master. Otherwise the yagé will give the master a headache and he won't see visions. It's not unusual for the brew to turn out bad, and during the ceremony the master will groan; or he'll fall asleep and snore for hours, or stay still and quiet, or he'll suffer strange body pains most of the night. If he has to accomplish a healing it will require much more work to establish and confirm the necessary spiritual connection. He will drink through the night until dawn, suffering all kinds of experiences and holding with steadfast concentration, until about 3 AM, when he will be able to effectively carry out his healing work. If there is no one to be healed and the drinking is just among students, the ceremony is cancelled, the fouled yagé is poured on the four posts of the lodge "so that the house may get drunk," and everyone goes to sleep. A new batch is cooked a few days later. Sometimes if the yagé is good and only minor flaws have occurred in the cooking method—like if a dog passed by the edge of the cooking area, or maybe someone took off his tunic during cooking—the yagé will be only partly bad; it can be left for a few days and will fix itself as the pinta gathers back into the brew. This slightly flawed preparation is hung in a high spot in the yagé lodge or placed on some pieces of wood off the ground in a corner of the house where no one walks. The energy patterns assemble again; a few days pass and it is then fit to drink.

When the yagé comes out good, it is something that brings great joy to the master, who knows immediately upon first glance that it is a good brew. The master will begin to sing soon after drinking, and sustain the songs all through the night and even well into the next day until the yagé is gone. The master is contented with the cooks and repeatedly blows gorgeous visions onto their each and every cup so they may learn and see. Like this, every three or four hours the drinkers go drinking more and more yagé,[11] learning and seeing more and more. A well-prepared batch of yagé keeps the pinta and does not get ruined easily. After the ceremony is over everyone is in high spirits, fully charged, enthusiastic, happy, and laughing! The master is already arranging for the next ceremony in a few days to continue drinking the good yagé....

But most of the time something goes wrong and it comes out so-so, as there are so many subtle variables that can interfere with making a potent and highly effective brew. This is why the elders are so adamant about staying true to the ancient guidelines in order to avoid having to suffer drunken and chaotic nights of little or no visions, only moaning and sensations of oblivion.

Preparing Ëo Yagé (Yagé Honey)

The making of ëo yagé starts the same as yagérepá, but since the intention now is to prepare extra-thick yagé, about four times more plant material is needed, possibly even an entire vine. To make this type of yagé, the following procedures are carried out. Instead of boiling the brew in only one pot, two pots filled with material are used for the four-hour boil described above. A massive amount of firewood needs to have been chopped and piled up and all the water hauled and ready for the cooking—a lot of work is involved to make this kind of yagé.

After four hours of furious boiling, the spent yagé vines and admixture leaves are piled up off to the side. The two brews are poured together. The newly produced yagé water from one pot is poured onto the yagé water of the other pot. The empty pot is then filled again with more water and more fresh, newly pounded plant material. The pot with the yagé water is also filled with newly pounded plant material including both yagé vine and yagé ocó leaves—preferably fresh young ones. These two pots are cooked at a high boil for three to four more hours, depending on the amount of water, taking caution to not boil the liquid down too low and burn the material. The pots are taken off the fire and the spent vines are removed and piled off to the side. Then the yagé waters from the two pots are added together for the process of refinement. If the liquid from the three pots is ample and there is still vine material left, more fresh pounded vine can be added in. This is brought to a furious boil for two hours, after which the pot is removed from the fire and any remaining vine and leaf material taken out. Once cool, the leaves are squeezed, but only by the cook, not the assistants, to avoid over-handling.

This liquid is then submitted to a further refining process, smudged with abundant incense and boiled steadily for one to two hours more, depending on the amount of liquid. As it is refined and reduced, becoming more and more concentrated, one has to pay close attention. Prior to the cooking process, the small pot or jug that is to be used to store the brew is filled with water and poured into the empty pot. A peeled stick is inserted and then notched at the level of the water as a marker. This is the level that the yagé will be refined down to. The notched stick is used to measure the level of the final product for an accurate reduction, and once the level of the liquid in the pot is close to the marker, the fire is lowered to hot embers.

During this final stage the cook must stand over the pot keeping a close eye on it. He must offer abundant incense smudges all around the area and on the expended vines, as well as on all the utensils and pots that have been used, and on himself. The cooks and assistant must stay quiet and serene. The reduced liquid simmers on the coals for up to an hour more, always carefully observed so it doesn't boil too low. Once it has reached the level of the notch on the marker stick, the coals and embers are pushed off to the side and the pot is left to slowly cool. The pot is never placed on the ground or the yagé honey will cool too quickly. Before it cools completely, it is strained into a small clay vessel made especially for the occasion. This is proper ëo yagé.

One small pot of yagé from the first cooking has been set aside. This is for the master and some of the assistants to drink, since the strong ëo yagé will be drunk only by the students aspiring to graduate, by two to four students at most who have gathered to undertake the graduation ceremony. The elder master and some assistants drink the yagérepá, which is quite strong and sufficient for them to sing, guide the ceremony, and care for the students. Once the brew arrives, the aspirants are summoned. The master takes the clay bowl of ëo yagé and cures it well. He sings for an hour or more, filling the strong yagé with the supreme energy patterns, celestial auras, and energy vibrations of the people of yagé.

All these traditional tactics combine to make a very powerful final batch that can be considered among the most refined substances of nature. It contains the essence of the region where it was cooked, the spiritual energy and strength of the master or adept who has prepared it, and the energetic emanations that have been blown onto it by the master.

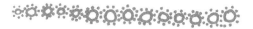

A friend asked me once if these customs or so-called guidelines were not mere superstitions. I thought about his question and responded like this: Superstitions stem from lack of knowledge; they arise with the loss and degradation of spiritual science. The yagé cooking customs can be seen as the code to a combination lock. To release the lock and open the door, to reveal the secrets concealed within, one must know the combination. The knob has to be turned to the left to just the precise point (harvest and cook the vines properly), then turned to the right to just the precise point (not crossing the designs path, staying focused on the process), and then back left (not letting it boil over onto the fire) until it opens in one's hand. Anyone can feel the difference between well-prepared medicine and the opposite. This is a subtle science that must be properly approached.

The Making of a Raw Infusion

Occasionally the Secoya prepare a cold-water infusion with the variety called *wai yagé,* which means "animal yagé." This is a variety of *Banisteriopsis caapi* that doesn't grow over a few meters in length, an ancestral strain that I have seen growing only among the Secoya. It has a thick and meaty bark and a solid stem that doesn't form the DNA-like helixes characteristic of the tara yagé varieties. It is prepared in an entirely different process. With wai yagé, only the bark is employed. The vine is warmed in water, then the bark is pounded off and pounded heavily in a large wooden mortar. To the bark is added a small amount of warmed water and abundant young leaves of yagé ocó. Only the young leaves are used in this preparation, preferably ones highest above the ground that receive full sunlight. While the preparer fasts, the wai yagé is pounded and pounded and pounded for up to four full hours. Then it is left to soak for a few more hours in the full sunlight, then strained. This yagé is almost white in color. After being cured by the master—sung over and impregnated with sacred energy and intentions—a large gourdful is drunk, usually by two people, as it is difficult to make significant quantities. My friend the Secoya elder don Rogelio Piaguaje shared with me his experience on a visit I made to his home in 2010. "The visions were pure white," he said. "This is a very strong, sacred, and ancient method of drinking yagé."

The Cofán people in Colombia also prepare a cold-water infusion. A heavy wooden pestle and a large wooden mortar hollowed from a tree trunk are needed. A lot of yagé ocó leaves are used, as many as can fit into the mortar. The yagé vine is lightly scraped, and then, together with the leaves and some water, pounded hard for a few hours. This infusion is left to sit for a few hours, at which point it is strained and is ready to drink. In a ceremonial setting just after nightfall a large gourd of this is drunk. A friend who spent time among the Cofán shared with me his experience of this. He said they prefer this method and say it is cooler for the body. They prepare it over fire and reduce it to a thick liquid only when they need to travel with the medicine—otherwise they prefer the cold-water infusion. "The raw yagé is strong as well," said my friend. "It comes on quick and passes quick. The effects last about two hours." While they are fasting and preparing the cold-water infusion, the Cofán drink a tea made of boiled pineapple husk.

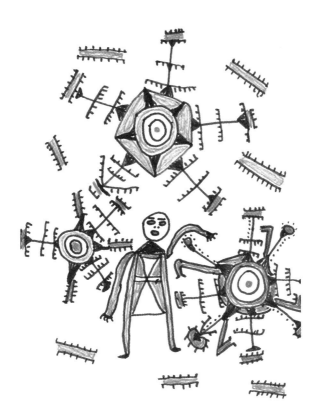

In the Trance of Yagé

Chapter 6

The Celestial Summer of the Cicadas

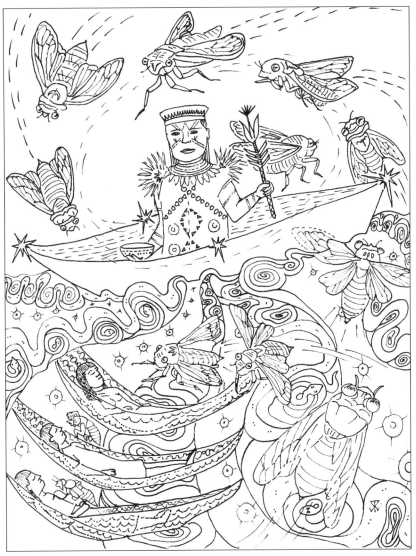

Downy Cicada Jaguar and His Canoe, the Southern Cross

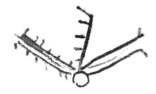

"It's normal to initiate the period of drinking with the moon before August; that's the best time for graduation. It's summertime, with its fireflies and butterflies. The spirits are above the trees, nearby; the angels move across the face of the earth. When you drink yage, you see clearly the spirits in the fireflies and the other summer insects. The drink shows them as they really are, celestial spirits, though some of them are also instructors or conductors of witchcraft. Others appear like tiny people, or like children, or like dolls."

—Fernando Payaguaje, *The Yage Drinker*[1]

After the rainy season begins to wane toward the middle of July, winds come blowing through the forest, clearing out the humidity and indicating the arrival of a period characterized by beautiful weather and spectacular sunsets. It is when auspicious insects of many kinds such as butterflies and fireflies begin to appear. During this time, different species of cicadas emerge by the thousands from within the earth where they have been sucking the sap from the roots of trees. They climb up into the forest canopy, where they molt their exoskeletons, unfurl their iridescent blue-green wings, and fill the rainforest with their shrill, high-pitched, ear-piercing emanations. Due to the appearance of the cicadas, this time is called by the Secoya *Canco'tëkahuë,* meaning "cicada season." It is a roughly forty-five-day stretch between the full moon of July and the end of August or beginning of September, at which point swarms of horseflies arrive, marking the end of the season. When the cicadas emerge is considered to be the most auspicious time for drinking yagé, being that their appearance indicates the return of the

Cancopai ("cicada people"), a particular group of Wiñapai ("always-new people" or "always-new immortals") who arrive close to the Earth every year, in order to deepen humanity's spiritual life. Elders say that at this time of the year many types of Wiñapai arrive close to the Earth, as do ancestor spirits. Many types of trickster spirits arrive as well, which, in the past, were kept away through powerful ceremonies with the aid of Cancowitoyai, "Downy Cicada Jaguar," a deity discussed below. The Wiñapai descend upon the ceremonies when subtle elements are in alignment, including deeply earnest sincerity, as well as great discipline and self-control on the part of all participants; otherwise, the Wiñapai come only to the edge of the lodge and giggle at our silly human predicament. An orchestration of multiple forces and efforts by all involved in a ceremony can lead to the confirmation of the truth of the existence of the Wiñapai as the everlasting foundation of this sacred spiritual tradition, this celestial culture, this way of life.

The interval of good weather is a much-anticipated interlude between the rainy months that occupy the majority of the year in the equatorial rainforest.[2] I call this season "the celestial summer of the cicadas," because it is during this time that the Secoya undergo their ceremonial life most fully. From the dawn of this sacred tradition, and in some cases up to the present day, the Secoya and many other Tukanoan-speaking peoples of Northwestern Amazonia have gathered to drink yagé during the time of the emergence of the cicadas. In remote wilderness places, by sacred lakes, or at the homes of shamans who had yagé lodges built for this purpose, the people congregated to drink strong yagé, exchange knowledge, celebrate life, and commune with heavenly spirits. This is the time when the students were initiated, apprentices crowned, and disciples encouraged to achieve new levels of knowledge, advancing along the great path of spiritual growth and learning. Common activities such as hunting, agriculture, and canoe building and house construction were set aside, and the people devoted themselves to the production of crafts and ceremonial attire, to sharing the many aspects of their great oral history, and to experiencing firsthand the sacred culture.

My experience participating in these gatherings was that the mood is always animated, yet calm. The assembled group is ready for its spiritual education. Yagé is boiling at one end of the ceremonial lodge; tranquility permeates the fraternity that is fasting. It is a time for cultural transmission, and the elders, when inspired, share legends, accounts of past ceremonies, and the cosmology of their ancestors. All participants have previously adhered to a dieta and undergone extensive purifications, often preparing for this season on a personal level all year long. The most common method of purifying among the Secoya is through the sunrise renewal ceremony (discussed in Chapter 4 in the "Dieta" section). Traditionally up to twenty renewals are recommended before entering the strong drinking season. These purification rituals cleanse as well as help train the student's body to receive higher doses of the yagé and no longer vomit.

Elders and students arise before dawn to consume emetic substances. The elder awakens the brew by tapping on the pot with the serving gourd. The brew has been left all night under the stars in order to gather the energy emitted by the heavenly bodies and become more potent. He blows on the brew and whispers to the medicine to arise, to waken, and to help the group arise and waken as well, to be strong, upright, and direct, like the ancestors who passed along this great tradition. The renewals are very important to undertake prior to the ceremonial season, because during the graduation ceremonies, it is considered a setback when someone vomits, especially at the onset of a ceremony. Everyone knows that the elders, or for that matter any older student, or the son or wife of the shaman, has the full right to request that a student desist from participating in further ceremonies. This happens if they see that the person has not undergone sufficient purification and/or is unwilling or unable to collaborate on the high level of everyday chores necessary to uphold ceremonial life, such as chopping firewood, hauling water, and clearing the garden sites, or simply being calm during the ceremonies. If someone is boisterous and unwilling to collaborate, the ceremony can be canceled and the drinkers go home. All participants should exhibit their highest, most virtuous behavior, and be ready to enact selfless service and to display humility in order to not interfere, and to see that the ceremony takes place as hoped for and planned.

THE WIÑAPAI, THE "ALWAYS-NEW PEOPLE"

Wiñapai translates literally as "always-new people" or "always-new immortals." The term *pai* is both singular and plural, referring to a person and/or people; it also refers to the godlike divinities and immortal beings of the universe that transcend human form. *Pai* can be understood as the immortal essence in human form. *Wiña* means "young," "tender," "new," like the pristine blossoming of flower buds. It can also refer to the burgeoning leafy growth on the tips of the branches of a plant, as well as to the downy feathers of newborn birds. The word describes anything that is flawless, pure, or uncontaminated, virtues that categorize the divine spirits of the celestial realms, who live in a constant state of renewal, and to whom each moment is like a new life.

A Wiñapai can take on any form it wishes. It can transform into an ant and walk up the side of a tree to watch you, or become the vast cloud-filled sky. *Wiñawai* (-*wai* is a plural ending) is the general term given to all legions of divine immortals, supernal, angelic, godly, or celestial beings, such as the Cancopai, the "cicada people" mentioned above; the Omepai, "summer people," who visit the Earth annually, in the month of January, as part of the universal cycles of renewal; the Jaicuntipai, "high-hill people," from inside the isolated limestone massif of Napo-Galeras; and the Jujupai, "healing people," who live within rivers.[3]

Don Cesareo once mentioned to me that in the skies where the Wiñapai live there are rivers, as there are here on Earth. The biggest one he knew of was the Sari'weco tsiaya, a word that translates as the "upper reaches of the green-parrot river of heaven." Cesareo's father-in-law, the old shaman-chief of the group, used to go to that river and fetch water; after the yagé ceremony he would have a clay pot filled with it to use for healing. This is the river where the red and white heaven boats float, the Makëhna Yowë and the Pokëhna Yowë. "Joaquina's father showed the people who lived there the way to the yagé lodge," Cesareo recalled. (Joaquina is his wife.) "They had long white hair like gringos!" These Wiñawai would come to the yagé lodge to heal the people.

Other beings of these celestial rivers include the Weco'wiñapai, the "green-parrot always-new people," who live along a tributary of the Sari'weco tsiaya. "The green-parrot people are terrifying to look at," Cesareo noted. "They look very strange. It is difficult to describe this in words." Continuing enthusiastically he said, "There is another river, the yellow river. [He did not mention its name.] Here is where the Paisuku live. They are dark black people who smoke an extremely strong tobacco—one puff and you fall over coughing. They wear crossed necklaces made of all kinds of large weapons. They never do harm, only protect; they are the most reliable form of protection that some yagé drinkers have come to know." He paused. "The place in the sky where all those rivers are is where the Secoya ancestors reside. It is their heaven. *Wati yeha aideo.*" He finished by saying, "The spirit land is very nice!"

The Wiñawai are reserved, reclusive, and self-contained; they have no dire need to make themselves known. They transcend all realms and dimensions, including time and space. To meet them and know them, to befriend them and then marry into these families, is a primary motive of Secoya yagé drinking. From listening to the elders' accounts, it seems to me that their existence is the true promise of salvation, but not as we may imagine and most likely not as we may desire. Most or all personal desires must be left behind to find the way.

Meeting the Cicada People

Among the Wiñawai of the summer ceremonial season, the Cancopai or cicada people occupy a central position in traditional Secoya yagé-drinking culture. The elders attest that these immortals dress as the Secoya traditionally dress, and vice-versa: the Secoya traditionally dress like the Cancopai. The cicadas are the terrestrial representatives of the Cancopai, whose wisdom is shimmering and vibrant. To meet and merge with the cicada people is something that can be accomplished this time of the year, when their realm is temporarily in close proximity to the Earth, hovering, as the elders say, just above the treetops.

Delfín Payaguaje, an elder adept of the tradition, related to me that the ceremonial guide among them holds the matipë, a decorated scepter tipped with the long straight tail feathers of a scarlet macaw. Along the matipë, light travels up in waves and flashes out from the top. When the Cancopai wish to drink yagé they only think about it, and piles of yagé vines suddenly appear. When the master among them holds the matipë above a pot, from the bottom of the matipë drips yagé, pulling the essence of yagé from the vines and filling the pot. Delfín added, "The Cancopai are always drinking yagé."[4]

When the Cancopai are close to Earth, the Secoya drink yagé in order to acquire the unparalleled visions produced by encounters with them. The cicada people teach in mysterious and impressive ways, confirming the existence of other realms and energy beings and granting the drinkers renewal and life-strengthening attributes. With the energy obtained from the Cancopai, one can become a healer and guide among the people. One can be healed and/or simply learn how to live a quiet and simple life of non-interference and humility. This can be accomplished after thoroughly purifying and strengthening one's body. During the summer months when the cicadas are singing, the yagé begins to flower. Celestial visions come more easily. This is why the elders initiate the youth during this season, giving them extra-thick yagé to drink for the first time. This was my experience as well, and I recall with fond and nostalgic memories the precious moments I was gifted to have among them drinking yagé during those summer months.

Downy Cicada Jaguar, Deity of the Southern Cross

Cancowitoyai's name literally means "cicada (canco) downy (wito) jaguar (yai)." Every year during this season, he travels to Earth on his canoe, which is represented by the glittering constellation of the Southern Cross, hanging low in the sky. The cicada represents transformation, down lightness, and the jaguar primal energy.

Cancowitoyai is an important figure in the yagé drinkers' cosmology. Cesareo informed me, "When Cancowitoyai arrives in his canoe, things in the room begin to transform. A bench changes into a wild boar, then a snake, then a bird, and back to a bench. Everything transforms and spins, everything changes around him when he arrives."

Tintin interjected earnestly, "Whatever you do, do not board his canoe!"

Cesareo, nodding, said, "If you board his canoe, your spirit will get caught in the multiple transformations and you can die. Then the canoe will depart and take your spirit far, far away."

The elders explained how in times of old, the masters of this tradition would carry out very strong ceremonies in which they would summon Cancowitoyai. They had enough personal energy to accomplish this and would stay steadfast when he arrived, though everything around them launched into continual spinning transformations.

Continued Cesareo, "They would talk only a little. The master of the ceremony would ask him to bring the fish and wild boar, and to leave behind the poisonous snakes and evil spirits. In this way the yagé drinkers would make abundant food available for their people while protecting the land from harm. After these ceremonies the drinkers needed to stay removed from the village and daily household for at least a few weeks. The air around their bodies was too strong and it was dangerous for them to come close to children, who could pass out and die. After the *tutu* [the strong energy] passed, they would return to village life."

Two Frogs in the Learning of the Tradition

The drinking of yagé is a reason for the elders to joyously impart many aspects of the vast cultural heritage and oral tradition. It's as if, after the hair-raising tales of meeting mythological monsters and undergoing bizarre, unpredictable experiences under the gripping influence of the yagé, the familiar stories and legends serve to bring things back to the basic educational elements of this great life-long path. Often when imparting these teachings, the elders advise the youth, especially those listening for the first time, to sit on their fists. This presses the perineum muscles and encourages the body's energy to rise up the spine. Keeping these muscles clenched is an essential part of gaining spiritual power. Sometimes students are able to overcome vomiting as a result of many renewal ceremonies, but still they can't hold in the large amounts of yagé necessary to see the celestial visions due to the fact that they keep defecating! Now the yagé wants to shoot out their rear end, for it always finds the weak points from where to escape. By strengthening these muscles at an early age, one encourages the body's ability to retain and absorb the yagé. In order to avoid defecating uncontrollably (and it's pure yagé water since the students have been fasting all day), the students are advised to wake early every day at sunrise and to clear the patio of weeds, barefoot and squatting. This also strengthens the perineum and anal sphincter muscles.

If the student keeps shitting and cannot hold in the yagé, another cure is attempted. There is a frog found in the lagoon country of Pëquë'yá called the *e'jé,* which I have not been able to identify since I haven't yet seen one, only heard about it. Elders attest that this frog has no anus and does not defecate; it survives by absorbing nutrients from the water and is never seen eating—for which reason it is believed to be effective for this cure. The frog is found the day of the fast. It is killed and then cooked over the fire and eaten at midday. Usually, one frog is enough; if not, then another is eaten sometime over the next month. Always by the second, the cure has taken hold, says don Cesareo.

The students can now hold in copious amounts of yagé without defecating, without vomiting, and without moving around too much. Like this they can see the Wiñapai. Sometimes it is inevitable after holding in very high doses that a student screams and thrashes, sometimes all through the night, to such an extent that the sitter must tie him or her into their hammock. There is always a soft, preferably cotton rope available for this purpose. Otherwise a student might run into the forest and get hurt, falling into spines or getting bitten by a snake. This is why at the strong graduation ceremonies each student that is being initiated will have a designated helper. At the beginning of these powerful ceremonies, it is very difficult for the student to handle the inebriation, which can reach a maddening intensity. This is when many students step back, after the first night or two of thick ëo yagé. For those who are determined and want to continue, another frog can help. This is the *paracoco* frog *(Bufo typhonius)*, a leafy litter toad that has one stripe directly down its back. When this frog is unexpectedly found hopping along the trail in the forest, one is instructed to pick it up gently and raise it to one's mouth, offering it some spit to drink. The frog is held before one's mouth, and after a little while it suckles the spit. Then the paracoco is placed back where it was found. Sometimes it will hop away a bit, then look back in felicity, before hopping off into the forest. Once back with its people, who are sacred spiritual beings of the rainforest, it remarks that it met a good person on the path that day, someone who gave it some delicious chicha to drink. The frog immortals then protect that person during the yagé ceremonies. They help the student to overcome any heaviness, making it possible to drink stronger doses without going off the deep end. The student sees the frog jumping on him in a vision. After this occurs, it is not that the intensity of the experience wanes, it is just that the student gets a better grip on handling it, and it is no longer terrifying. He or she learns to cope with the gripping effects of the medicine.

The yagé drinkers and everyone else are advised never to kill frogs. One can have a dream of crossing a bridge that turns into a frog leg, yanking itself in; the spirit of the dreamer falls too, and shortly after that, the person can die or get ill, but this only happens to people who harm nature, especially frogs, who are the symbols of the rainforest. People who harm nature are advised to rectify their lives as a method of purifying their imbalances. Those who do so can find themselves crossing the bridge from chaos to peace, from danger to safety, and from obscurity to light.

Only through the strengthening and integration of the body, the mind, and the spirit can the drinkers achieve the ability to hold copious amounts of yagé, which is a necessary requirement in order to see firsthand, to witness, the vast body of visions and the deeper truths of the cosmology. For this reason the youth were always made to pinch their perineum while hearing these stories, and to give some spit to the paracoco frogs on the trail. Sharing one's spit with the paracoco frog, an act seen by the Secoya as sharing one's life essence, symbolizes dissolving discriminations toward other forms of life, as well as illusory perceptions of separation.[5] By doing so, many obstacles are removed, and one finds the way along life's path, like the straight line along this frog's back.

Sacred Plant-Based Technologies of the Celestial Summer

The ceremonial season required a large amount of preparatory work in order to maintain the tradition as it was originally upheld. Besides yagé itself, the following plant technologies needed to be prepared: the aromatic pigment called *macuri;* the *jejebonsa,* a sticky, fragrant body paint; the *maña,* fragrant herbal ornaments; and the *sohómanë,* the ceremonial incense smudge log. All these are fundamental elements of a traditional Secoya yagé ceremony.

Macuri (literally "red gold") is used to paint on one's face the many elaborate types of designs the Secoya have for their ceremonies. These symbols are called *posá.* The most common include the ladder, representing the step-by-step nature of spiritual development, and the all-seeing eye of the Wiñapai, representing the wisdom that transcends time and space. Other symbols represent stars or energy vortices, or evoke particular divine beings such as the Jujupai and the Jaicuntipai.[6]

The making of macuri involves most or all of the following ingredients:

- Abundant seeds of bonsa (*Bixa orellana,* in Spanish known as *achiote* and in English as annatto), the base ingredient. From these seeds, a rich oily red pigment is obtained, which is frequently used alone as a face paint. This is also a valuable medicinal plant.[7]
- A few handfuls of *ocomaña* (*Justicia pectoralis,* known in English as carpenter's bush).[8] This small creeping herb with highly

aromatic leaves is commonly cultivated around the house sites of the traditional Secoya families.

- A few handfuls of the leaves of *gonomaña (Ocimum micranthum),* a cultivated rainforest basil.
- The bark of *mëtocua'a,* which I have not been able to collect for identification.
- The bark of *wirisaka (Iryanthera hostmanni),* a small understory tree found in hilly regions of the primary rainforest. The saplings are used to make a hand mixer called a *chuculero,* used for blending chucula, a gruel of boiled ripe plantains. At a certain level above the ground, the sapling's branches emerge perpendicularly and at regular distances along the stem, and with some cutting and trimming and bark-stripping, the stem with the stumps of the branches becomes an ideal hand mixer.

To make macuri, the leaves of ocomaña are mashed in water together with the leaves of the gonomaña, and perhaps the bark of the mëtocua'a or wirisaka as well. These aromatic ingredients are mashed by hand in a small pot with about a cup of water. Then abundant bonsa seeds are mashed into the fragrant water. After the rich oily pigment from the bonsa has been released, the liquid is strained; then it is heated in a small clay pot on a small fire consisting mainly of embers. It is brought to a simmer, using caution to avoid overheating in order to not lose any of the essential oils from the herbs and barks, and also to avoid burning as the consistency thickens. Then the macuri is removed from the embers to cool. As it cools, it hardens, forming a creamy, waxy, red aromatic paste. This is scooped onto some corn leaves, then rolled up and tied off to make a container. The macuri face paint is now ready.

Jejebonsa is a sticky aromatic paint for the arms and legs. *Jeje* means "sticky," and *bonsa* is achiote. This body paint is an amazing and ancient legacy. Today few people know how to prepare it. Jejebonsa is usually made only by the most traditional women in the village, those who support the ceremonial life of their people.

The making of jejebonsa involves most or all of the following ingredients:

- Abundant seeds of bonsa.
- A few handfuls of aromatic kënjé incense resin, also known as copal (this is the sap from the large rainforest canopy tree *Dacryodes peruviana*).[9]
- Some *antaracone* sap, aromatic and white, derived from any one of these three understory trees: *Dacryodes cupularis, Protium amazonicum,* or *Protium copal,* all belonging to the Burseraceae family.
- Sap of the *bonsáwito* tree (*Brosimum utile,* Moraceae).
- Sap of the wansoka tree (*Couma macrocarpa,* Apocynaceae).[10]

This recipe starts with bonsáwito sap, which is dyed with the bonsa seeds until it is a deep red, then put in a pot over a fire. Dried kënje resin is ground, as is the dried resin of the antaracone tree. Once the substance is boiling, the fine resin powders are slowly stirred in, and the mixture is now continuously stirred slowly and consistently. After a while it begins to thicken. Then just a few drops of the wansoka sap are added. This acts as a coagulant and the entire batch thickens even more. It is then removed from the fire and left to cool and harden. It is kept in the same pot it was cooked in, which is always made of clay and usually decorated with simple, elegant designs from the world of yagé.

The jejebonsa is warmed up a little in the sun before applying to one's body. After bathing and dressing for the ceremony, one dips the tip of a stick crafted for the occasion into the sticky sap. This is then further warmed up by rubbing it in between one's big toes. When the sap mixture is warm enough, it can be rubbed along the length of the stick. Then one uses the stick to paint lines across the backs of hands, the tops of feet, and in rings around the arms and legs. These traditional designs resemble sandals and *tefillin,* the leather straps that Jewish men wind around their arms before praying; like tefillin, the designs serve to remind the wearer of the eternal covenant between the human and the divine. Jejebonsa lasts an entire week on the body, which is the length of time during which one must take extra precaution and dietary care so as to allow the pinta or toyá that has been collected during the ceremonies to be absorbed into one's essence.

After the jejebonsa is applied, the interior of an ëné palm heart is rasped. This white material fluffs up like cotton and is then placed within a loosely woven string bag. The palm-fluff net bag is patted over the freshly applied sticky body paint, and the cottony material sticks to the design and fluffs up over the area that has been painted. Jejebonsa is highly aromatic, and the combination of sensory inputs makes for a most interesting phenomenon, as it merges the color of the red pigment, the designs, the smell of the fragrant sap, and the soft texture of the white down. Its effect in the ceremony is profound, gently nudging the mind toward a state of synesthesia, the unification and surpassing of the sensory perceptions. It is in this state that one may meet the Wiñapai.

Another use of jejebonsa was for divination. The elders speak of times when they had to revert to warfare to defend their territory. The wise master would meditate before a pot of fresh jejebonsa. Soon a large horsefly would come near, and if it flew into and got stuck in the pot, this would be a sure sign of victory in the coming battle.

A third material component of the traditional yagé ceremony is the sohómanë incense smudge log. The making of sohómanë involves most or all of the following ingredients:

- Sap from the wansoka tree, known as *wansoka witó*.
- Dried, powdered resin of the *sohó* tree (*Hymenaea courbaril*, Fabaceae). This neotropical canopy tree is a contemporary relative of ancient trees that provided all New World amber. The resin is found under the soil around the base of the tree.
- Dried, powdered resin of the kënje tree.

A few cupfuls of the white wansoka witó are boiled and stirred continuously in an old pot. An old pot is used because the sap is so sticky that the pot can never be used for anything else. The kënje and sohó resins are stirred in. The mixture is stirred constantly over a low flame until it becomes thick and black like tar. Then water is poured over it while it is still hot so it can be molded. Even if it is hot, if the mixture is underwater it can be handled without burning the skin, and it is molded before it cools into several log-shaped smudge sticks, about 5 centimeters thick by 20 centimeters long. These have a tendency to melt in direct sunlight, so they are kept in the shade or in a pot of water. During the ceremony, when these sticks are rubbed against the glowing end of a stick from the fire, the sohómanë crackles and sizzles and emits a thick, rich, deeply aromatic smoke. Since ancient times, the burning resins of these most sacred trees have been known to dispel negative spirits, and the smoke emitted from the burning sohómanë is considered to be the most effective for purifying the environment. It also used to invoke the Wiñawai. It is a great aid in accomplishing healings too, as the rising smoke helps lift off the stickiness that is the sickness of the patient. The smell grants the master the ability to merge his energies more thoroughly with that of all divine immortals, and thus accomplish a positive ceremony for the group.

All proper yagé ceremonies require abundant smudging through the night. Sometimes people are unable to move from their hammocks. The ceremonial leader groans. The yagé is strong and has the entire group immobilized in its grip. Its constricting qualities are one of the reasons the yagé is associated with diverse types of spiritual serpents—cosmic, terrestrial, and aquatic. After a while a drinker is able to slowly gather strength. He carefully obtains a stick from the fire and begins to rub the sohómanë back and forth on its embers. Sizzling, the incense emits its rich smoke. First he smudges the elders, who awaken soon after and begin to sing. Then the smudge is passed around so all the drinkers may inhale its fragrant energy-rectifying vibrations. The smoke helps to lighten and clarify the drunkenness of the yagé. Often at dawn the smudge is inhaled and blown on oneself to dismiss the pinta and enable re-integration back into the world of everyday phenomena and daily life.

Also at times, in the deep still night of yagé, one can witness the potency of the smudge. Its light, sweet, familiar smell brings the drinkers back to the countless ceremonies of the past and is thus deeply reassuring. The yagé will unclench its grip and everyone will feel better. Through the smudge, the light of the divine immortals may shine upon the lodge, recognizing it as a living altar, an occurrence that awakens all the drinkers, making their energies truly divine and sincerely effective. The smudge invites the eyes of the ever-fresh ones, the Wiñapai, to gaze upon the hearts of the drinkers and to confirm their devotion to a truthful way of life.

The spirits of the trees who gave their saps and resins may present themselves in visions. The sap of the wansoka has a rich, reassuring smell, and through it the tree transfers energies to the drinkers, who may see copious, opaque white sap oozing down onto them, flowing over their bodies, purifying and strengthening. The sohó tree may appear as shimmering diamonds of deep purple and green. The kënjé, according to Pablo Amaringo, which he called copal (not being Secoya but rather mestizo), is an empire of heavenly spirits; in a vision, he once saw a temple on a celestial island dedicated solely to the burning of its resin as a confirmation of the eternal truth that peace can reign in all realms of the multiverse.

There is still more work to undertake, and a final source of fragrance needs to be added to the ceremonial gear in order to uphold this great tradition. This is maña, an adornment consisting of herbs, painted palm fiber and/or peeled aromatic bark. The maña is bound to the arms and wrists with woven cotton bands called *ñe'ñé*. Maña is traditional among the Secoya, Siona, and Cofán people, who, not long ago, would dress every day as they would in the ceremonies, as for them there was no separation between everyday life and that of the ceremonies of yagé. Even today, the last traditional elders upholding these traditions can be seen wearing maña every single day. The aromatic herbs most commonly used for maña are gonomaña, ocomaña, and yapé *(Spigelia humboldtiana)*. These cultivated herbs are tied together in bunches. Their rinsed roots may be painted red with achiote. They are tucked under wristbands and armbands, perhaps next to longer-hanging palm fibers.

The second type of maña is made from the bark of the wirisaka. When this bark is rasped and exposed to air, it oxidizes to a deep orange brown and emits a distinctive fragrance. The third type of mañn is made of fibers from the young leaf shoot of the *ne'é* palm *(Mauritia flexuosa)* or the *a'pó* palm *(Ammandra natalia).* The leaves are peeled and the fibrous bony part discarded, leaving the long white flexible leafy strands. These are then painted with bands of red using achiote. Mañá made from palm fibers hangs down the sides of the arms, away from the torso. The Cofán wear it longer than the Secoya do, letting it hang down almost to their elbows from bands on the upper arms.

According to don Cesareo Piaguaje, the Jujupai, the doctor spirits from the realms of the water, wear mañá, as do the Macuripai (literally, red-gold people), who live in a dimension inside the gold and red streaks of sunset clouds, where there is a golden-red river.[11] Cesareo said it is possible to see these spirits' arms in one's visions, painted with jejebonsa and all fluffed up with the cottony rasped palm heart. Tied to their wrists with ñe'ñé are elaborately crafted mañá intricately wound with colorful strings, beads, and grasses. The mañá of these celestial beings are aromatic and beautiful beyond description.

The elders say they dress as they do because it is how the Wiñapai dress. Cesareo added, "The dress must be aligned with the virtues that each item represents, otherwise the objective will not be fulfilled. To dress like the Wiñapai is not sufficient: one must become like them, not just look like them."

Painted faces and aromatic herbs allow participants to recollect ceremonies of old—not necessarily the specifics of the ceremony but rather the energy that was transmitted. Rich aromas of ocomaña and wirisaka, the fragrant scents of the golden macuri and the sticky jejebonsa, all fluffed with the rasped heart of the ëne palm, contribute to triggering and then transcending the senses. These and other adornments that I cannot detail here due to limited space are intended to locate the cosmology on one's very own body. By wearing the cosmology on one's body, one becomes the cosmology. And that is another purpose of the yagé ceremony: to become the living truth, the subtle principles that are the invisible, inaudible, spiritual laws that govern creation.

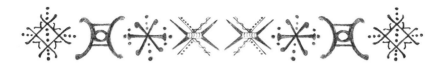

About the Secoya, People from the Multicolored River

Earlier in the book I provided a brief introduction to the Secoya people as a native Amazonian society, part of the Western Tukanoan language group. Their independent and self-sufficient way of life flourished in the jungle for hundreds of years, facilitated by the indigenous science explored in these pages. The knowledge of plants displayed by traditional Amazonian cultures is unsurpassed anywhere on Earth, in part due to the high level of biological diversity. As for their origin, the Secoya themselves will tell you that the heartland of their historic ancestral homelands extends outward from the sacred region of Jupo, where they attribute their origin and all of humanity's. It's at the headwaters of what is known today on most maps as the Río Santamaría, located in the Peruvian Amazon. From this heartland, the great expanse of the ancestral territory extended well into what we know today as eastern Ecuador and north and south to the Putumayo and Napo rivers.

The Secoya's oral history says a lot about this place. It includes a river they call Siecoyá, "Multicolored River," at the headwaters of which occurred the mytho-historic encounter with the Ñañë Siecopai, "God's Multicolored People," generations in the past. In those days, the diverse clans referred to themselves by their clan names, such as the Piojepai (or simply Pioje), the Piaguajepai ("bird clan"), and the Payaguajepai ("oily-face clan"), among many others previously mentioned in this book. The Secoya people's own authentic name for the union of all the Paicoca-speaking kinship groups, those who share a similar culture and provenance, came to be Siecopai, meaning "multicolored people." The name is derived from that of the Ñañe Siecopai, "God's Multicolored People," an encounter that deeply shaped the culture of the Siecopai.

Later, because the name of this river was Siecoyá, the missionaries came to call the people who lived there by the name "Secoya," as it was easier to pronounce. When they began to be called the Secoya they accepted it; it was close enough to their own name, and it did not seem pejorative. Not all the settlers were detrimental to the Secoya; some were helpful, ameliorating the difficulty of a life in the wilderness by bringing them utensils such as sewing needles and thread, scissors, cloth, machetes, axes, and mirrors. Before there was friendly contact, other settlers referred to them as the Encabellados, meaning "long hairs," given that traditionally the Secoya men wore their hair long, something rarely seen today.

Generations later, the lower body of the river that was called Sotoya, "White Clay River," came to be known as Wajoyá, "River of War," because of the battles there against the Portuguese invaders in the early part of the 1800s. This name was given to commemorate the valiant defeat of the Portuguese by Wajo Sará, the great cultural hero.[12] Wajo Sará lived just upriver from the confluence of the Wajoyá and the mighty Napo (the latter a major tributary of the Amazon).

Despite defenders like Wajo Sará, and despite their plant-medicine science, the Secoya have been challenged by the maladies that come with Western contact. The Secoya territory along the Aguarico River is surrounded by development. The Secoya worldview has become gravely affected. It's the same as what's happening to other indigenous cultures worldwide, as communities become alienated from their traditional lifestyles and tempted by consumer wares and ways.

Up until as recently as the 1950s, the ancestral territory of the Secoya encompassed an area of approximately 12,000 square miles of Amazonian rainforest wilderness. In Ecuador this territory included a great portion of what today are the provinces of Orellana and Sucumbios. Along the Napo, historical accounts relate that the Siecopai lived farther upriver from the modern oil-boom city of Coca,[13] where the mouth of the Payamino River flows into the Napo. Even further upriver, at a location the Secoya called Sooñá, there is a long hill with a flat ridge, where some cliffs come close to the river's edge. There lived a powerful and famous drinker of yagé who shared his medicine with all who came to learn. But the people there died like fish out of water from illnesses brought in by settlers, a tragedy thought to have occurred at the turn of the twentieth century (early 1900s), and the land lay empty of people for a hundred years or more, until others came to settle the region. This explains the Secoya people's historic and cultural recognition of Jaicunti, now known as Napo-Galeras, an isolated limestone massif located at the base of the eastern slopes of the Andes and viewed by yagé drinkers as the home of the Jaicuntipai discussed above.

To the east along the Napo River, Secoya territory extended to where the Peruvian military post of Pantoja is today.[14] The northwestern portion of Maynas Province in the Peruvian Amazon, from the mouth of the Santamaría River north to the Putumayo, was also part of the ancestral homelands of the Siecopai.

Beginning in the late 1800s, rubber tappers were the first to make major headway into the Amazon in search of its riches for export. They were followed by Portuguese conquerors and settlers. From about 1900 onward, well over ninety percent of the population of the Siecopai vanished, some from warfare but the majority from common illnesses introduced by foreigners. The contemporary jungle town of Pantoja in Peru, on the Napo River not far downriver from the Ecuadorian border, was once the location of the largest and most prosperous Secoya villages. Pantoja is said to be built over a landfill of bones. Here thousands of people died suddenly from illnesses like the common cold, smallpox, and hepatitis. With their population decline due to illness they had no immunities to, the vast homeland of the Secoya people was largely uninhabited by the 1920s. As the Ecuadorian Amazon was penetrated by oil development over recent decades, new roads opened the way for a tidal wave of colonization spilling down from the overpopulated and arid mountains and coastal regions. Simultaneously, from other regions of the Ecuadorian Amazon, individuals and families from more populous indigenous ethnic groups such as the Shuar and Kichwa escaped the overpopulated areas at the base of the Andes and followed the rivers and the oil roads to acquire new lands along the Napo and Aguarico rivers. Most of the mestizo settlers ended up near petrol frontier boomtowns like Coca, Lago Agrio, Shushufindi, and Tarapoa, which are now more like small bustling cities than towns, and growing rapidly. This resource grab and colonization of the wilderness has brought massive and unabated destruction to the rainforest.

Until the 1940s, the majority of the surviving Secoya lived in what is today Peru. Some family groups returned upriver to Ecuador to live at the Cuyabeno lagoons. When war broke out between Ecuador and Peru in 1942, the Secoya were divided by the new border. In 1972, the Ecuadorian Secoya moved from Cuyabeno to the Aguarico River, where they live today.[15] Before 1900 the population of the Secoya people is thought to have averaged roughly 30,000 individuals.[16] Today the Peruvian and Ecuadorian communities together number approximately 700 individuals, about half living in Ecuador and the other half to the east in the Peruvian Amazon.

The Secoya may once have been such a harmonious part of the natural order that they did indeed meet God's Multicolored People and strived to emulate them, but that was a long time ago. I won't say that life was perfect when the indigenous people first clashed with modern civilization. Intertribal warfare was not uncommon, but it escalated immensely with the arrival of rubber tappers, new threats, and new diseases. Between 1930 and the late 1950s, the Secoya colluded with the fur trade, participating in the wiping out of many animal communities. According to Secoya belief, though, animals don't go extinct, they just enter other realms inside the earth or the water. This is when it feels to me like people hide behind their culture rather than respect its true essence, but given the pressures they were subject to, it is impossible to judge, only to try to understand.[17]

In the same time period, the practice of avenging deaths believed to be caused by witchcraft from neighboring groups resulted in endless attacks among the native people. Yagé drinkers and tribal chiefs were always the first to be blamed for the illnesses that had been introduced by outsiders, and the whole cultural system, from all sides, fell under attack from this tremendous imbalance. Despite this, the elder drinkers of yagé that I have befriended are open and happy people who do not judge others by the color of their skin, but by the caliber of their heart. The drinking of yagé obliges each individual to heal historical and personal wounds, to surpass traumas, allowing people to live in the present moment, despite the accumulated centuries of heartache, and to awaken joy.

It does not stop here, though, because there is still no happy ending to the story. Today the Secoya, like so many native people worldwide, have largely lost their traditional identity, purpose, and ways of life, exploited as workers in multinational oil, logging, and industrial agriculture enterprises. Living in such close proximity to the colonization frontier, many of the Secoya are being absorbed into a modern way of life, into the temporary illusion that is swallowing up the majority of the globe bent on resource extraction. While the Secoya still speak their own language (Paicoca), and most also speak Spanish (Ankecoca), many speak the Siona dialect, which is similar to Paicoca, and some even speak the Cofán language due to intermarriages. Today the Secoya still grow the majority of their food crops such as yuca, plantain, and other varieties of ancestral cultigens,[18] but hunting and fishing in the region are now scarce due to deforestation for oil-palm plantations, petroleum development, logging, and overhunting. Sadly, most ways of making a living or earning money are related to the destruction of the environment and compromise the cultural identity and purity of soul of the people. Some individuals have gone so far as to participate in prostitution, which is supported by the migrant workers in the region. It is all too common to see young women who have been coerced into falling in love, only to be left with children and no husband. Despite these radical changes, many Secoya have found creative ways to get by and have taken up painting rainforest scenes, making arts and crafts, and weaving hammocks for sale. Some Secoya have found jobs in the region's social welfare ministries, such as the ministries of education and health, or as boat captains and guides for the tourism industry.

The Secoya are trapped between the devastating effects of the colonization frontier and their rich traditional past, which is proving to be as fragile a reality and as fleeting a memory as the most powerful visions of their esoteric science. But instead of detailing that sad scene, in this chapter I have attempted to portray my image of this culture as I see it in its fading colors, magic, and awe-inspiring mystery, for is there anything more awesome than experiencing the spirit world firsthand and feeling the magnificent wholeness of the multiverse? Our Western science and much of Western religion pales in comparison. But nature comes close when we attempt to fathom its complexity and beauty, so I also try to paint the rainforest with my words.

At Abya Yala cultural center in Quito there is a black-and-white video documentary of a cultural festival filmed among the Secoya in the late 1950s. Many of the elders that live there today appear in the documentary as youths. It is impressive to see how elaborate these people were in their ceremonial attire. This festival is still held every year in the month of August in the village of San Pablo de Cantesiaya.[19] Today ceremonial life is upheld by only a handful of elders and their families, who still use their traditional dress, the tunic, and the many aspects of ceremonial life, such as the maña discussed above, painted faces, and crowns. The Secoya are spiritual heirs to God's Multicolored People, possessors of a rich oral tradition, great admirers of beauty and followers of a beautiful way of life that tries to make the most of being human. Once their entire society supported and upheld this ancient ceremonial life—one that, they believe, holds a place in the world for all beings to live in happiness, peace, and freedom. A few elders still do this for all of us.

WHAT'S IN A NAME?

The history and etymology of place names frequently reveals which group of people lived there in the past. Historical names can corroborate the little-known or debated truth of a certain culture's influence over a particular geography. This is certainly true in the Ecuadorian Amazon, where many current names of places and rivers have been derived from ancestral indigenous names. Because later inhabitants found those names difficult to pronounce, they modified them to some extent or replaced them with words that sounded similar. In the case of the Secoya people, because the Paicoca words are difficult for others to pronounce, simpler names took hold that are easier for the Spanish- and Kichwa-speaking settlers who now populate the region.

Some examples of this follow. As already mentioned, the name Yasuni comes from the Secoya name of this river, Tsuniyá, the "river of the tree peanut." The river today known as Tiputini, on the south side of the Rio Napo, is known by the Secoya as Paitiñia, "river of naked people," because in the headwaters of this river lived the Waorani, whose custom was to live naked, wearing only a cotton strap around their waist in which men would tie up their penis. Tiputini seems to be derived from Paitiñia, as it is not a Kichwa, Waorani, or Spanish word.

The Coca River, where the jungle oil-boom city of Coca is located, was called Haotsiaya in Paicoca. The word *hao* is the name for the coca leaf *(Erythroxylum coca)*, a plant known globally for its medicinal qualities, native to the region. Upon meeting some of the last Secoya still living in this region, the first settlers found it easier to call the river Coca. They must have asked what Haotsiaya meant, and when shown the coca plant, they called the river Río Coca. Today where the city of Coca is found, Payaguaje and Piaguaje family clans once lived for generations. The Payamino River, also part of the Secoya ancestral lands, was once named the Payaguaje. With these examples we can see how modern-day names are often derived from older ones, which can indicate the original dwellers in these lands.

Fulfilling the Dream of a Yagé Drinker to Reclaim Ancestral Lands

In view of all this, and for the Secoya traditional way of life to survive, it became the dream of a Secoya elder and tribal leader, the late don Fernando Payaguaje (subject and voice of *The Yage Drinker,* who passed away in 1994), to gain government recognition to an important part of their ancestral homelands, the wilderness lagoon region of Pëquë'yá (Black-caiman Lagoons[20]). The Secoya are a people of the lake country, and many aspects of their culture and traditions can only be maintained in the *igapó* (blackwater lake) ecosystem type,[21] such as production of the *sënori*, the yuca strainer that is made from the bark, peeled off and woven, of the *mayë'i (Pseudobombax munguba)*. The sënori is an important utensil in the making of their staple food, a yuca flatbread called *aun* (elsewhere known as cassave). Today the Secoya live along a *varsea*, a brownwater river, where many of the plants needed to keep alive their traditions are not found, and where the difficulty of navigating the large river has made it harder for families to gather.

Fernando believed that Pëquë'yá was the last chance for the Secoya to maintain a shred of their historic and spiritual ways of life as they have done for centuries, and to experience this way of life as did the generation before him. At Pëquë'yá the Secoya families from Peru and Ecuador could unite and attempt to maintain their intimate relationship with the plant world and the lagoon regions that are abundant in fish. As noted above, the Secoya have for the most part been split in two since 1942 when the border region between the two countries was closed due to political conflicts.[22] Ancestral legends and historical memories could be shared amidst the solitude of the wilderness, like in the past, and camaraderie among the diverse family clans strengthened. For these reasons, don Fernando dreamed of helping his people return to this region, as a meeting place, a place to respect and cherish, and where the people could live as before in balance and moderation.

In 1995, an old friend of mine, Manuel Pallares, was studying biology at Quito's Universidad Catolica. While living at the university's field station located at the Cuyabeno lakes (the station is now gone, due to accidental fire), he befriended Fernando's son, Delfin Payaguaje. Delfin had lived for many years at Cuyabeno until moving with many other Secoya to live on the Aguarico River, where today the Secoya communities are located. Delfin still frequently visited Cuyabeno by dugout canoe in order to hunt and fish for his family. His father had died the year before, a natural death at an advanced age.

Inspired by Delfin's account of his father's dream, Manuel found himself attempting to help make it come true by legally recuperating the ancestral lagoon region of Pëquë'yá, which lies two days' motor canoe travel downriver from the Aguarico communities, in the direction of the Peruvian border. When I first visited the Secoya with Manuel in 1995, he was bringing cotton hammock twine for them to weave into hammocks. From the sale of those hammocks the first outboard motor was purchased to begin the voyages to Pëquë'yá.

It did not take much stirring, and soon Manuel and the joyous elders I had befriended—in particular Cesareo, with whom I shared the tightest bond—inspired me to participate in the process. This is how my five-year sojourn and adventures among the Secoya began.

I had known about the Secoya ever since I was a kid growing up in Quito. I vividly recall seeing a postcard of two smiling indigenous faces. The back of the card read "Natives of the Aguarico River"—sunflowers popping out from behind their ears, cheerful happy smiles, colorful beads draped around them. This image left an indelible impression, awakening within me the yearning to someday meet these genuine people of the rainforest. Now my time had come.

I had just completed a stint working on and off for five years in Napo Province with the Waorani on the physical demarcation of their territory, as well as on the creation of the Napo-Galeras National Park with Kichwa families outside Archidona. I was ready to explore a new region of the Ecuadorian Amazon, the province of Sucumbios, not far to the north. With Manuel's introduction and my newfound friendships among the Secoya, I began collaborating on the fulfillment of the elders' dream, organizing voyages with the Secoya elders and youth. Between 1995 and 2000 I organized half a dozen expeditions to the region. I also collaborated on hosting and facilitating the elders' and community leaders' visits to Quito. Through their dialogues there, they received recognition as ancestral stewards of the Lagarto Cocha region. Several environmental groups heard about what we were doing and criticized us heavily, saying we were bringing a people already colonized by modernity into an untouched wilderness area, and for the most part they were right. But within the greater scope of things it was important that the true ancestral stewards, which are undeniably the Secoya, be recognized, because there were other land-grabbing schemes taking place by neighboring Kichwa and Cofán communities who had settled the area only a short time before. After several visits there it was evident that these neighboring communities were not happy with the Secoya moving in. So we organized several visits to them with delegations of Secoya to facilitate dialogue. Using Marshall Rosenberg's non-violent communication method,[23] the differences were settled, and for the most part the Secoya are now recognized as having a legitimate ancestral claim over this area.

To make these voyages economically feasible, we organized tours with visitors from the United States. The first Sentient Experientials workshop retreats were epic adventures. From the modest funds raised on these tours we would purchase gasoline, food, and supplies for the voyage and accomplish some projects to benefit the village. In Sewaya we installed an HF communication radio and donated an outboard motor to the community for emergencies. Alongside a motley crew of international participants and up to thirty Secoya, we traveled downriver to rediscover and enjoy. I also worked with the community in a cultural heritage revalidation process, which produced a Secoya cosmology wall calendar and several bilingual education booklets, one on the use of medicinal plants and traditional foods with Alfredo Payaguaje, and another on the cultural migrations of the Secoya people with Celestino Piaguaje.[24]

Ultimately it was through my efforts to sustain the culture of service among the Secoya community that I was able to genuinely befriend many of the dozen or so elders who embody the ways of the traditional culture and some dedicated youth, who, over the periodic sojourns and visits I have made there since 1995, have shared with me the greater majority of the experiences and information I can provide here in these pages.

At Sewaya community I forged great friendships with Cesareo Piaguaje, whom I called *hakë* ("father"), and his wife Joaquina, whom I called *hako* ("mother"), and their son Cesar. I lived at Cesareo's house the entirety of my five-year sojourn among them. In Sewaya village, I also befriended Basilio Payaguaje, a master of the oral tradition, and his brother Marcelo, two most proper traditional elders. Upriver in San Pablo I made several friends as well, people I met on the wilderness sojourns to Pëquë'yá: Delfin Payaguaje and his wife Maria; their adult children, Alfredo, Miguel, and Lidia; Agustin "Tintin" Payaguaje; Reinaldo Lucitante and his wife Maruja; Matilde Piaguaje, an amazing and most beautiful elder; and Emilio Lucitante and his brother, the late Esteban Lucitante, a great drinker of yagé who generously shared with me countless insights into his life and experiences. I was also fortunate to meet Grandmother Lucrecia, the wife of the great drinker Fernando Payaguaje, who, undeniably, shares with him complete freedom in the realms of heaven. Another elder grandmother who left a deep impact on me was Ñeñcó Luisa, Tintin's mother, who was still drinking yagé into her great age. They say she was over a hundred years old when she passed naturally and peacefully, surrounded by her family.

After five years of efforts we succeeded in accomplishing this vision, and the Secoya now have legally sanctioned access to Pëquë'yá and are recognized by the Ecuadorian state as ancestral stewards of the region. It is located within the Cuyabeno wildlife reserve, so they have only access and not land title. Due to the difficulties of getting there, few have actually gone to live in the area. Some of the traditional elders want to move there but their children do not, and this keeps the elders from returning. Today many Secoya have strayed so far from the traditional ways that they no longer find value in a life in

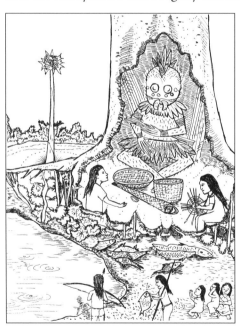

A Jurí Spirit Teaches Weaving Skills to the Secoya

the wilderness; they too want the conveniences of the modern world. The few times such people go it is only to cause damage to the local wildlife, aggravating the true purpose of the intention of returning there and jeopardizing the privilege of accessing that part of a legally protected region—one they have been allowed to enter as a traditional people to steward and care for.

Sharing the Oral Tradition from a Jaguar-Centered Worldview

As mentioned, the celestial summer is when new life is given to the recounting of the oral history. By sharing here some aspects of this tradition, I hope my readers will feel the winds of its life-giving energies, enhancing awareness of the tremendous contribution of indigenous peoples. Any sincere seeker can see how the advice and universal admonitions presented in these accounts allow those hearing the stories to become aware of many kinds of pitfalls and thus be able then to steer clear of them. Oral literature also deepens insights into the sheer magic, symbolic imagery, and beauty of the ancient sacred cultures.

In the past, before the interruptions brought on by the rubber tappers, colonists, and missionaries, the majority of the people would feel the calling to drink during these ceremonial periods, even the women and the youth from age nine and up, as it was a firm belief that through the drinking of yagé they were fulfilling the purpose of their earthly existence. While drinking, the general population would learn the ancient guidelines of their society and time-honored cosmological perspectives. Each individual came to understand his or her place, realizing there is no separation between individual and cosmos—there is only the good way of life and the deepening of one's spiritual progress. This is referred to as *ñuñerepá paiye*, "living with proper firmness," recognizing and upholding a life of dignity and integrity as the most important human function. This also acknowledges the value of upholding a devoted work ethic, and training the body to overcome lassitude. Daily life requires a continual dedication to work, and every aspect of life requires physical stamina, inner composure, and spiritual strength. When one merges with the energy of the Wiñapai, the work no longer seems like work, and one's responsibilities become life's joyous fulfillment.

Secoya oral history makes frequent reference to the iconic jaguar. According to the most traditional perspective of the Secoya yagé drinkers, the jaguar symbolizes and embodies primal energy, of which there are many types. Primal energies are pure energies of the universe, represented by the various types of jaguars. One day in August 1996, don Cesareo responded to my silly questions about the nature of things.

"Where do all these jaguars come from?" I asked. "And what do you mean when you say everything is jaguar?"

"Everything is jaguar," he reiterated, laughing. "Mouse-jaguar, grasshopper-jaguar, sky-jaguar, cloud-jaguar, star-jaguar, everything is jaguar!"

My deduction from this is that if everything is jaguar, jaguar must represent energy, and that the traditional Secoya yagé drinkers characterize the universe as energy, viewing everything—a blade of grass, each critter or object—as a kind of energy symbolized by "jaguar." It is a jaguar-centered worldview, an energy-centered worldview. In this section I share some attributes of the different kinds of jaguars (which are different kinds of primal universal energies), both rainforest cats and spirit jaguars known by the drinkers of yagé.

The Lesson of Yai Yoí (Jaguar Grunge)

The following purportedly true account, which I learned from don Delfin Payaguaje and his son Miguel, is a warning to novice yagé drinkers and illustrates some of the different types of powers. In particular, it helps distinguish clearly the powers of the earth and those of heaven. It is the story of a young Secoya man who came to be called Yai Yoí, Jaguar Grunge.

Those hearing the tale are also led to deduce that not all drinkers of yagé are upright. Some are indifferent and others merciless. This is a lesson in being careful to watch what you ask for, to not be in a rush to advance one's spiritual growth or to gain spiritual powers. The story of Yai Yoí conveys the importance of abiding by the highest way, this being the failsafe method of obtaining true progress. Lessening one's desires and strengthening one's virtues is the appropriate spiritual path but it is not necessarily the easiest way.

In or around the 1930s, don Delfin's grandfather was living in Peru in the village of Gyuiñeto. There was a fellow in the community who would never drink yagé, even though his entire family was drinking. People called him Yoí, meaning "grunge," since he was lazy and had the habit of not cleaning up after himself or following the immaculate hygiene and personal cleanliness ethics upheld by the traditional Secoya. Whenever a ceremony was being held he would go hunting and come home late, after the others had left for the ceremonial lodge. One day he came home and found that his wife had prepared some chili soup for the children, and he proceeded to serve himself some. Seeing this she said, "All you think of is food," and she tried to interest him in drinking yagé since she and others were going to drink that evening. He didn't want to and began to eat. She said to him, "What kind of man are you, only thinking of food?"

Aggravated, he left to drink yagé, even though he had eaten. He entered the yagé lodge and drank the first dose. After a while the ceremonial guide left to pee, and Yoí followed and peed too. While they were outside, when no one was listening, he asked the guide if he would blow the powers of the jaguar on his yagé for him to see.

"That's easy," said the guide. "Those powers are close by, and it doesn't take much to see. In one drink you can become a jaguar."

The novice became animated. The shaman returned to the lodge first, followed shortly by Yoí. People were in their hammocks. Soon the shaman drank another cup, and Yoí went to request more. The shaman blew onto the yagé the *yai toyácä*, the designs of the jaguar tunic.

In the morning, Yoí left and headed in the direction of his home. Not long after, the entire group that had been drinking yagé together heard a big jaguar roaring in the forest. Concerned, they went to see if

Yoí was okay, and to help if need be, but they found nothing abnormal, not even jaguar tracks. They saw Yoí's tracks where he had walked the trail, extending far past the place where it sounded like a big jaguar was screaming. Unbeknownst to the others, Yoí had entered the house of Wanteanco, the jaguar mother. The roaring they heard was him. He was roaring because the yai toyácä had been placed upon him, the designs of the jaguar tunic, and as such he had learned there how to transform himself into a jaguar. The roaring was him practicing his newly acquired power.

Some time later, Yoí was at home twining chambira palm fiber when some young people came by. They told him that a jaguar was killing people, a few here, a few there. Many people had been killed already. Yoí acted surprised and said that he had almost been killed by a jaguar too. He brought the visitors outside and showed them where he claimed to have fought off the jaguar. There was a spear stuck in the ground and claw marks around it. In fact, he had stuck the spear into the ground and made the claw marks with a toucan beak, to make it seem as if there had been a fight.

One afternoon a little girl went to pee near his house, and the jaguar attacked and killed her. The people, fed up and saddened, made a trap: a big box armed with palm stakes, a log, and a trigger, so that when the trap was sprung, the log would press the victim into the sharp palm wood stakes. They left the girl's corpse in the box, knowing that the jaguar would come back to eat it. Around midnight it came, and sure enough it fell right into the trap. When they came to see, to their utter amazement, in the trap, restrained by the stakes that were piercing its body, was not a regular jaguar but a creature with the body of a jaguar and the head of a man—and whose head was it? None other than Yoí's! Yoí's face was jaguar-like, with hefty protruding fangs. They called for his wife. She could not believe what she saw. Sure enough, he was no longer at home; he had left an hour earlier, saying he had diarrhea and was going to relieve himself. She pleaded for them to spare his life, but they insisted that if they released him he would most likely continue taking victims. He was already severely wounded, so they left him there, and shortly he died. Afterwards he came to be known as Yai Yoí, Jaguar Grunge.

The story of Yai Yoí shows that it is much easier to obtain earthly powers and tap into lower energy than to focus on and obtain the higher powers of the celestial spheres. Its lessons counsel novice yagé drinkers to reach first for those immortal energies of the supreme realms, those of the Wiñapai, which take more patience and dedication to acquire but are truly meaningful. After one has embodied these then one can learn about and handle the energies of the Earth, which can be viewed as primal or elemental energies, and use them to heal and not to harm. These energies are nearby and much easier to perceive, but as the account illustrates, without the necessary self-control or virtues of the celestial realms, one can easily be corrupted by the elemental powers. The story also illustrates another important point: Not everyone is cut out to drink yagé, and for this reason it must be a personal decision, and no one should ever coerce someone else to drink. Those who feel the call know it and go through great effort to learn.

The story raises the question of how to guide primal energies in a positive direction. The elders say that when the jaguar enters one's body, its fangs will begin pushing themselves through one's jaws. It is imperative to let only the tips of the fangs come through. Also, when its claws begin pushing themselves between the bases of one's fingers, let only the tips come through. If the fangs or claws come all the way through, the primal energy will control you, and you'll lope off into the forest and kill the first person you come across, as Yai Yoí did. This speaks to the need to control primal energy and not let the primal energy control you. Often novice drinkers can see Yai Yoí in their visions, his hands and face human, his legs and body feline. Yai Yoí does no harm anymore, he only advises novice drinkers, warning of the perils of asking for the yai toyácä before striving to see the Wiñapai. He advises drinkers not to go into the jaguar house, nor to let the jaguar into your body when still a novice. After you go to Wanteanco's house, it follows you home. You are not prepared to handle the energy and you can start doing harm, and you can kill people. If you are drinking yagé and you see Yai Yoí, it is an indication that you must be careful and should refrain from drinking for a period of time, practice virtuous behavior and good deeds, and be cautious.

It is believed that if you start seeing visions of aggressive or rambunctious jaguars, then it can be much more difficult to see the visions of the heavenly realms of the Wiñapai. Once you have established a firm relationship with the heavenly immortals, you can learn all about the primal energies of the Earth, the different types of spirit jaguars, and how to use these energies to heal and to help humanity.

Spirit Jaguar Allies

This is not to say that all spirit jaguars are dangerous. They are representatives of vastly diverse types of primal energies. There is a friendly jaguar that acts as a trustworthy guide to the novice drinker—the Paiyai ("people jaguar") or Toyáyai ("designs jaguar").[25] When novices see this spirit jaguar, it is an indication that they are approaching the celestial visions. This modest jaguar demonstrates no offensive behavior. He is elusive and shy and slightly playful; he can be all white, or painted in colorful designs. He shows how to traverse the difficult, narrow path to the houses of the Wiñapai. He leads sincere students to the water world, where they can meet the Jujupai and learn how to heal. This jaguar can enter your body and then bring you to his house, where you see him as a human being. This jaguar is calm and good-natured and is not to be feared. He teaches how to heal and gives only good advice; he is pure medicine. Nevertheless, it is always advised to not want to see this jaguar either, to concentrate only on the celestial realms. The Paiyai never tricks anyone, but if you want to see him too much, you can trick yourself. A master drinker of yagé can blow the *Paiyai toyá* onto your cup when he deems you ready. To earnest students studying independently with no master, the Paiyai arrives on its own accord, not needing to be called; once the students are ready it appears as a true friend and shows them the way. The student only cultivates virtue, concentrating on and invoking only the Wiñapai. When the student's sincerity is firm enough, then it is the Wiñapai themselves who send the Paiyai to allow the student to progress.

There are other jaguars that can visit heaven as well. These can be seen in visions and at times found in the forest in physical form. They are the Airoyai, the spotted forest jaguar, and the Neayai, the black forest jaguar. Most earthly jaguars are actually gentle beings that live out their lives aloof in the wilderness, never harming people. Only when they are possessed by a sorcerer do they attack and do harm. Some forest cats have never traveled to the heavenly realms; instead, they meet the dangerous jaguar spirits and can then harm humans. Once they start doing damage to people they are soon hunted and killed. From the Secoya perspective, the "physical" jaguars found in the rainforest are themselves spirits, and like humans, have relationships with other spirits that will ultimately manifest in their behavior.

Types of Jaguars to be Avoided

The elders relate that among the spirit jaguars, several are extremely dangerous and must be avoided at all costs. Their existence is a phenomenon of the world of yagé, one we know little about. They can present themselves to people who use yagé for superficial and transient matters, for self-aggrandizement, overindulgence, and excessive personal gain, or, for that matter, any convoluted digression from the original sacred and celestial use of the medicine as taught by the Ñañë Siecopai. The most dangerous is the Sëamëyai (enthrallment jaguar). This one is the most aggressive, and it dedicates itself solely to killing and eating people. *Sëamë* means to be enthralled, enchanted, hypnotized, or completely obsessed with something, to think only of that thing and nothing else. The Ma'tsimayai is the "red-poison jaguar," also known to kill without anyone's orders. It is extremely dangerous. It always moves very rapidly and it is reddish in color. There is also the Neatañë yai, the "black-shadow jaguar." This one flies through the air. It kills people and was used in the past by shamans to attack enemies. These dangerous spirits appear near the Earth during times of war. The graduated yagé drinkers of old knew how to help move them away, back into remote spiritual regions, so that the people wouldn't harm each other. This was known as the science of creating peace among humanity, a spiritual art for the most part now lost, as few if any yagé drinkers know how to slow down and defer the movements of these dangerous spiritual powers. When people choose peace, these jaguars eventually leave, as they don't like it close to the Earth and prefer to stay far away. Only when there is war do they come close.

Various Spirits of the Medicine Path:
The Designs Boa, Hoofless Deer, and Healer's Bumblebee

Among the many deities and supernatural powers that the yagé drinker must meet is the Toyá Uncucui, the "yagé drinkers' designs-boa." The Toyá Uncucui can present itself in various ways, descending from the sky or rising from the water or the earth. Once a Secoya youth shared with me what he had witnessed in the morning after a particularly powerful ceremony. I could see the utter amazement on his face as, still animated from the yagé, he explained in great detail what he had seen.

"I was looking up into the sky," he said. "It was blue, with fluffy white clouds. Suddenly it came writhing down in graceful motions—a tremendous, richly saturated blue-sky boa. Along the length of its body ran painted designs, dotted stripes of yellow, white, and green. It came down from the heavens to just above where I was standing and then pulled itself slowly back into the sky."

Cesareo had been listening, and he commented, "The Toyá Uncucui is one of the master teachers of the world of yagé." He went on to explain that when one is first learning, this is one of the many ways it can present itself. It appears, showing itself in its immaculate glory, and then returns whence it came.

Tintin interjected, "When one advances on the path, the Toyá Uncucui beautifully opens up the world of visions, so one may become a healer."

Cesareo continued, "The Toyá Uncucui is the ally of the healer. It never does harm." He went on to explain how people who do harm can never see the Toyá Uncucui, not for all the money in the world. This mythic and supernatural spirit only reveals itself to the earnest, good-hearted, and disciplined. The Toyá Uncucui is covered in designs of intense color; these designs are pure medicine, pure healing energy. It is a manifestation of the uncontaminated elemental energies of the water, the earth, and the atmosphere.

Miguel Payaguaje spoke up. "The Toyá Uncucui initiates the student onto the path of healing and opens the way to experience the visionary realms. It has three main ways of doing this. The first way is that it approaches slowly and places its tongue in your mouth. In awe you open your mouth, and then it swallows you whole. After an agonizing digestion experience, where you must remain very calm and quiet, it shits you out. Then your spirit goes flying like a bullet off into the vastness of space, passing through sky and clouds, popping into heaven, revealing to you the tremendous visionary realms. Sometimes people start screaming while being digested. They scatter their energy and don't witness getting shat out. This slows down the process of learning, so it's best to stay calm and quiet. The second way usually occurs to people already well advanced on the path. The Toyá Uncucui appears and peels itself open. Out of its body comes a shower of saturated light that engulfs the drinker, displaying the magnificence of the visionary realities. The third way is when it opens its mouth and spills onto you an aura of colors that permeates you entirely. Some elders have said that three design-boas appeared to them, one each from the sky, earth, and water, and from the mouth of each came this light, forming a triangle of saturated light, protecting the drinkers while simultaneously opening the visionary realms for them to learn, experience and see."

Another ally of the healer is the Ñamase, a spirit that in all regards resembles a deer but without hooves. It has soft furry stubs where the hooves would be on a regular deer. It walks over the ground as if walking in the air. At times the yagé drinker calls this spirit in order to heal certain types of illness. This spirit has a long tongue that it uses to consume the illness. Unperceived by the patient, it unrolls its long tongue into their mouth. The tongue goes deep inside the person, gathers the illness, and extracts it from the patient. Then the spirit swallows the illness. Within its body, the Ñamase transforms the illness into a harmless substance. After a while it regurgitates this substance, and with its long tongue it rubs it all over its own body, beautifying its hair. This is why this spirit has a very beautiful pelt. The student graduating as a healer needs to learn to call this spirit in order to help him heal. It's necessary to take precautions when summoning the Ñamase, though. There is another spirit, the Ñamase Watí, that lives in the forest, closer to the human sphere, and it can harm people.[26]

Another ally to the healer is a bumblebee spirit. It is only seen in visions of yagé and is called Wiñapai Ñamero, the always-new people's designs bumblebee. In a vision, it comes buzzing toward the student. As it flies overhead, it sprinkles a shower of misty water to purify the student's aura in preparation for meeting the Wiñapai. It comes as a precursor to greater visions. It can also carry the spirit of the student into the celestial realms. Later one can call the Wiñapai Ñamero and ask it to sprinkle its water over the patient so they can be healed. It looks like a bumblebee but is actually an Ujápai, a spirit doctor.

When the Jaguar Mother Comes Sniffing: Graduation Ceremonies with Ëo Yagé

The following occurred after Cesareo was obliged to kill many forest jaguars when he was a young man. He had no choice since they were continually attacking him. In one day he killed three. These jaguar-killing stories would always make my stomach churn. My passion for nature and love for life run deep, so it hurts me to hear about these kinds of things occurring, but in the Amazon life and death are intimately interconnected, and to learn, one needs to be open to attempting to understand truly what is happening.

Cesareo left Ecuador for a while and went to drink yagé with a great-uncle who lived in Peru. There he underwent several important graduation ceremonies with extra-strong ëo yage. He needed to strengthen his spirit, because back home in Ecuador his jealous brother-in-law wanted him dead and kept abusing his spiritual powers to possess innocent jaguars and make them attack Cesareo. Literally every time he'd go hunting he would be attacked by aggravated jaguars.

With ëo yagé, the inebriation came on suddenly, just like his great-uncle had told him to expect. Then Cesareo was suddenly in the home of the Jaguar Mother. She approached to look at him, sniffing him out, and she offered him sugar cane. He politely refused. She offered him a gorgeous young wife. He kept his head down low, without even looking. Politely, he refused, with the most modest movement of his head, almost as if he were frozen still. Soon the Jaguar Mother's mood changed. He had passed these temptations, these spiritual tests. Now she began dressing him, and she brought out a tunic and placed it over his arms. It was too small. She was laughing now. She placed another tunic on him. He held his arms stretched upward. Again it was too small. She swiftly lifted this tunic off and replaced it with another. After admiring it, they agreed that this was the perfect fit. It went down a tad long, just over his ankles. Then they were playing and laughing, rolling through her jaguar-spotted banana patch. And he awoke from the visions. His great-uncle chanted until the dawn, and Cesareo observed the older man's wisdom.

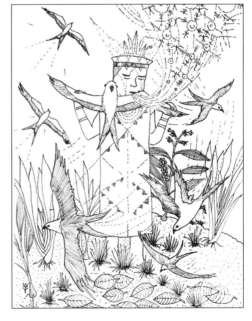

Blowing Songs through the Wing of a Swallow-tailed Kite

After a few weeks his great-uncle said, "Nephew, in order to confirm this energy, we are going to try again. Are you ready?"

"Yes," Cesareo nodded earnestly, "I am ready."

Again they gathered the materials—yagé and firewood—and began to prepare a second round of ëo yagé. Again his great-uncle gave him the same advice, and they proceeded to drink the brew. Cesareo thrashed most of the night, to such an extent that he cut up the areas between his toes from grinding them in the strands of his hammock, but he witnessed a second time everything his great-uncle wanted him to see. Just as described above, the phenomena recurred. A few weeks later Cesareo asked his great-uncle if he could go hunting. When one drinks strong yagé, the custom is to not eat any meat and not go into the forest for at least a few weeks. This time had passed and his great-uncle agreed. He lent him his muzzle-loader and the young man left for the forest to hunt an agouti.

Later down the trail the following events occurred. Cesareo spotted an agouti and was just about to shoot it when he saw the ears of a large jaguar popping up from behind some leaves. Just then he heard a branch breaking behind him. He swung quickly around and to his relief he saw his great-uncle, indicating with his chin that Cesareo should look forward. When he turned around again, the large jaguar was coming toward him. The jaguar came and jumped over him, and there he was for a third time, in the home of the Jaguar Mother, Wanteanco. Again she offered him sugar cane and he declined. Then she again suggested to him the notion of taking a young wife, and he modestly declined this as well. Then she placed on him and removed several times a tunic until the proper fit was found. Then they went rolling, laughing, through her banana patch. Soon afterwards he awoke to find himself there with his uncle in the forest near the house. His uncle said, "Now you can return to Ecuador. You have passed the test and you have acquired the energy. When you return to Ecuador and your brother-in-law hears that you have returned, he will again send jaguars to attack you, but they will be like dogs. You won't feel afraid of them, and they won't come close, either."

It happened just as his great-uncle had predicted. Upon returning to Ecuador, Cesareo soon began encountering jaguars in the forest because his brother-in-law heard that he had returned. Now, though, they wouldn't attack him. It was as if they recognized him. They would snarl, but they wouldn't attack. Not long after, the brother-in-law was murdered by a colonist. Since that time, Cesareo has rarely encountered a jaguar in the forest, and when he does, they are tame. They look at him serenely and continue on their way.

A Yagé Drinker Moves His Family into a Lake

Halfway down the Aguarico River between where the Secoya live today and their ancestral lands of Pëquë'yá is a lake known among the Secoya as Socorá, meaning "sunken lake." Presently this part of the Secoya people's ancestral lands has been settled by Kichwa speakers who call the lake Zancudo Cocha (Mosquito Lake). Here is the story of why it carries the name "Sunken Lake," related to me by Secoya elder Basilio Piaguaje.

A drinker of yagé and his family lived upriver from the lake along a small creek. One of his relatives, a young woman, had been hit by sorcery from other people down river and she was getting skinnier and skinnier, sicker and sicker. The shaman didn't know how to heal this type of problem. Though he tried and tried, she was not getting any better. The young woman went into a state of despair. She was near death and she wanted so badly to continue living that out of desperation she started saying bad things and uttering foul language. Others heard this and laughed at her. The shaman asked them to refrain. "How can you laugh at someone on the verge of death?" he asked, adding, "All this is very bad." He asked for help from the cousins of the young woman, and they went to a ridge some distance inland from the edge of a lake where there is an ancestral Secoya burial site. Near this spot they built a small thatched hut. In a hammock tied to a pole they carried her there, and in this spot the master could attempt to heal her again, this time away from the village.

Once they were there it was evident that the young woman was not getting any better. The next day when dawn arrived she proclaimed that she did not want to live any longer. She asked, "How can I live like this with people mocking me?" She had lost her will to live. Sorcery and sorcery accusations were racing through the villages, spurred by the arrival of the rubber tappers and the illness they brought. Many people were dying, and the yagé drinkers were being blamed. The shaman was highly disappointed with what was happening. He said, "I, too, have had enough. We're going into the lake."

The yagé drinker had a special affinity with Rutayo, the goddess of the water world.[27] It is she who governs the water, as well as the atmosphere, particularly the wind. The shaman concentrated his powers and, in his meditation, summoned Rutayo. Soon she came, and with her, strong winds began to blow and heavy rains to fall. At that moment the entire family and community of the master drinker of yagé began to sink into the lake. Everything around them including the earth there at that location where they lived sank into the ground. Water filled the region, and the yagé and food gardens were all washed away by the floodwaters. Right as they were going into the lake, the shaman and the young woman's cousins turned to look at her. She said, "I can't live any longer."

They asked her to come with them: "We are going to a new land without sin where we can live like before." There was no energy left within her, and when she attempted to lift herself up to go, she fell back into their arms and died. At that moment her cousins began mourning her death, and everything began sinking. Not just the area where the shaman was, the entire area began sinking into the water as well as the entire village. Many people were drowned, including the sorcerer who had attacked the girl and all his family.

At that moment many other things were occurring. Some of the people who were sinking in the water saved themselves by transforming into birds. They burst up into the air, flying out from under the water as birds. Some flew out transformed into the bird called *umu,* the olive oropendola *(Psarocolius bifasciatus),* while others flew out transformed into the *sëo*, a type of cacique *(Cacicus cela)*, a bird that is closely related to the oropendola. Both these birds are very intelligent and mimic many other birds' calls. A woman drinker of yagé flew out of the water transformed into a *wecó*, the mealy Amazonian parrot *(Amazona farinosa)*. Some people transformed into different types of fish, such as the large round *pai'puñu*, a relative of the piranha (*Colossoma macropomum*, known in Spanish as *gamitana*), and the *tupuwani* (*Vieja* sp., known in Spanish as *vieja*).

Where the shaman and his family lived, the house items and utensils all transformed into different animals. The *tokawa*, a large wooden pestle shaped like a half-circle with two grips at the flat edge, used for mashing yuca tubers, also became a pai'puñu, whose form it had resembled. The *toowë*, a long wooden trough used as a mortar together with the tokawa, became an añapëquë, a massive mythical fish with magnetic powers over water. The sënorí, a large woven strainer mentioned above, transformed into a *pë'e*, a black caiman *(Melanosuchus niger)*. The *jije'pë*, a square strainer used to sift yuca flour, transformed into the *hehan*, a kind of ray. The *meme'ñá*, a round basket used to hang the aun (the yuca flatbread, a.k.a. cassave) transformed into the *ñanami*, the freshwater stingray (*Potamotrygonidae* sp.). And like this all the Secoya utensils were transformed into animals of the water realm.

When the shaman and his family gathered in the dimension under the water, they were in human form. He organized them to go on a special mission to collect the other people who had transformed into fish, and turn them back into humans. The plan was to go fishing in a canoe. As soon as a fish bit, they were to yank it up and throw it into the canoe without looking at it. Like this they went catching and throwing the fish behind them, one after the other, the fish piling up in the canoe. When they turned around after the last one was pulled out, the fish were all people again. The fishermen asked, "How's your mouth?" Some of the former fish wiggled their jaws and replied that they hurt a little, but otherwise they were fine.

To me, while it might stretch the imagination to consider this real instead of fanciful, this story illustrates the depth of the human spirit and potential achievement of this indigenous science: to be able to transform oneself and one's family into beings that can live within a lake to escape colonialism and evil sorcery. This is none other than a fabulous feat, and it is something the Secoya believe occurred. Regardless, it's vital to stretch the limits of our imagination, to think beyond our limited perceptions and expand our perspectives, to not be afraid to dream and even less afraid to enact our dreams, one step at a time, bringing us all closer to what we can imagine as Heaven on Earth!

Chapter 7

The Deep-Forest Perspective of the Waorani

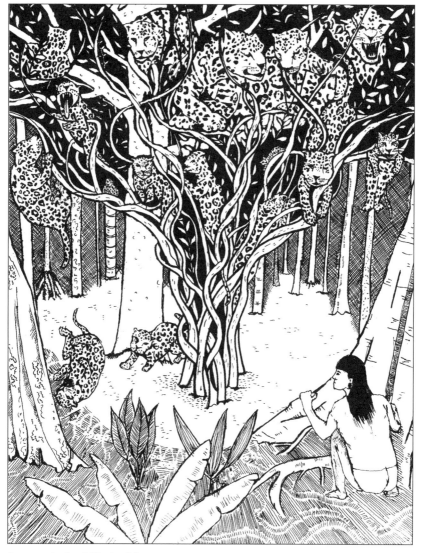

Jaguars in the Miiyabu Vine

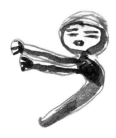

"Men, women, and children spend a great part of their lives slowly exploring the forest."
　　—Laura M. Rival, *Trekking Through History: The Huaorani of Amazonian Ecuador*[1]

To attempt to understand the Waorani is to begin to understand pristine human nature. Their animistic worldview sees that all living beings are sentient; this is reflected in the Waorani people's essentially egalitarian way of being. I hope these glimpses into the life of an independent people, who have protected the rainforest for generations, will inspire respect on their behalf.

The Waorani have maintained themselves in a state of isolation, even from other indigenous groups, not participating in trade or intercultural exchange, for a period spanning possibly hundreds of generations. Their unique language, called Wao Terero, meaning the "people's idiom," is unrelated to any of the region's neighboring indigenous languages, and it is distinct in grammar, phonology, and vocabulary.

I make no claim to being able to communicate any kind of ultimate truth about the Waorani. I'm just sharing honestly what I have seen, heard about, and experienced from living among them. I was fortunate to have spent four years with the Waorani between 1990 and 1994, when I collaborated as a volunteer on a project that accomplished the physical demarcation of their legally granted homelands. The anthropologist Dr. Laura Rival had introduced the team I worked with to Moi Enomenga, a conscientious youth from Queweiriono village who made possible the work we undertook. Dr. Rival's books and studies are mirror-like reflections of their way of life. Her insights offer an important perspective on original human nature.[2]

Meñeiriwempo: Protector Deity of the Waorani People

The date I will never forget, as it was the day that marks a leap year: February 29, 1992. The location was the bank of a small wilderness creek, a tributary of the Shiripuno River called Gueyemonpare. I was with a handful of elders and some Waorani youth, as well as my North American friend Mashuri. We had organized a camping trip into the bush to study medicinal plants. The elders happily agreed to show us their realm, and Mashuri and I were in full collecting mode. We had brought all the necessary supplies for pressing herbarium specimens, which later would be dried and mounted at the National Herbarium in Quito, in preparation for a proper identification of each plant. We had also brought a copy of *Neotropical Rainforest Mammals: A Field Guide,* by Louise Emmons, and on our first morning in camp we paged through it with the Waorani, writing down their names for the animals. Elders and youth alike enjoyed flashing through the pages, laughing and rattling off names and adventures spent with particular forest animals, acting out in great detail aspects of their experience. As soon as we turned the page to where the forest cats were illustrated, Mengatue pointed to the jaguar image and exclaimed, "There he is, there he is! This is my son!"

That evening, Meñeiriwempo, the Jaguar Guardian, came. Mengatue starts clawing and puffing and rolling on his back. His chanting is powerful. The others are all asking questions in an urgent tone of voice: "Meñeiriwempo! Tell us what you think happened!" And Meñeiriwempo responds in a long, relaxed tone, slowly releasing his words, which are his treasures, through which many types of knowledge are made known; he says it like it is: *"What-happened-is-this,"* all in one stretched-out word. Talking almost like singing—an emotionally-loaded soliloquy that use words simply as a means to allow the energy of creation to flow, to come forth, to be made known. The jaguar shaman continues enunciating, invoking this particular tone and mood almost as a joke, a serious joke. It's simple and utterly primal—it is the wizardly way of poetic vocalization particular to the *iroinga,* who among the group is closest to the spiritual world. The Waorani believe that an iroinga embodies eons of experience, including unbroken contact between the tribe and its protector spirit; this is someone who has sovereignty over nature and a communion with the realms of the spirit, and consequently is able to divine and heal with ease. Only under the jaguar trance will an iroinga heal, only when he is possessed by the protector deity of the people, Meñeiriwempo; this is when he is the spirit's true representative. Otherwise, in everyday life, an iroinga is much like any other traditional Waorani.[3]

Meñeiriwempo, speaking now through the iroinga, was delegated by the creator to help the Waorani maintain and defend their territory, a land that was ordained and delineated by a goddess (see Chapter 8). The current territory of the Waorani is about one-third its historical size, which previously encompassed approximately 8,000 square miles between the Ëwengono (Curaray) River in the south, and the Doroboro (Napo) River in the north, with visitation rights further north to Unki-yabe (Napo-Galeras) Mountain. The Waorani were able to manage a huge ancestral territory thanks to Meñeiriwempo. Many of the iroinga have passed on now, but the jaguar is cunning; it wishes to find new human representatives to make its love for its people known. The sole purpose of its existence is to see that the Waorani are protected, which is its covenant with the creator.

Meñeiriwempo grumbles and the iroinga sways back and forth. His chant is rhythmic yet sullen, lumpy with power. He starts up a high-pitched oooing and smooths it out, long, long, long, then suddenly, sullenly and drunkenly, he is talking to the people. He will begin to thrash around in his hammock, or maybe he will be lying on his back on the ground, growling and blowing, scratching at the air. Many kinds of sensational wonders are evoked during those trances, and as a listener one is humbled in silent awe. Many times Meñeiriwempo has seen where the settlers and oil workers are intruding and sent warriors to defend the territory. Expectant mothers come and he touches their bellies; if it's close to the time of birth and a baby's head is not pointing down, he growls on it some and it turns around, ready to be born easily.

Here is a summary of a translation of a section of the recording of Meñeiriwempo speaking through Mengatue from that night in 1992:

> I see the top of a mountain—there's a mountain, there are lights coming, so I'm going there. I can see over that mountain there's a different kind of tree that grows on those slopes, but down in the valley there's a city of lights and I can see there. I can see that there's a salt lick—all the animals in the forest, different kinds of animals, come to the salt lick in the early morning. The animals have come on all the different trails, and when the sun hits the trails, the mud dries up. Here's what's happening to the young Waorani: they're leaving our village, they're going to that place, they're taking in the salts from the lick—but they're taking too much and they're getting bloated, their stomachs are filling up. They fall over, as if dead. They're not dead but they don't remember that they're Waorani. They don't know how to get home anymore, and they live lost in that city of lights.
>
> There's a cure: Another Waorani who knows the way home can find them. He can say, 'Look! You're a Waorani! You're lost! Do you want to find your way home?' If he answers 'Yes,' quickly scrape his tooth. Put the tooth rasping in water mashed with one leaf of miiyabu [ayahuasca] and give him a sip of that to drink and he'll then know. He'll remember the way home. He'll remember that he's a Waorani. He'll remember the ways of his ancestors and he'll find his way home.

This is a worthwhile message for us modern people too, where "home" can be defined as a life in balance and reciprocity, in consciousness and love. We must all find our way home.

Songs of Hidden People

At another moment in the same jaguar trance recording, Meñeiriwempo said he was hearing songs. The singers were from a remote group, the Wiñetare. This group's name means "*Blue Tanager Clan*."[4] They live in isolation from everyone, are thought to be matriarchal, and reject any contact with outsiders or other Waorani.

Meñeiriwempo sings a Wiñetare song:

> We are Wiñetare, we are like the blue tanager.
> Like this bird we are, hopping from branch to branch.
> We never stop, not for one moment,
> always in motion, always singing,
> never in one place for too long,
> like the blue tanager.

> When we're alive,
> We're like the shimmer on the surface of the river.
> When you look at the river and see the glistening light on its
>   surface—
> That's us. That's how we are when we're alive.

Meñeiriwempo reports that he transformed into an ant and got up close to a Wiñetare warrior who was sharpening his spear and chanting to ward off outsiders. Meñeiriwempo sings the song the warrior sang:

> Who can come to the house of the jaguar?
> Halfway they think, "My family! They will see me never again."
> They change their minds and they return.

Two Waorani Set the Clouds on Fire

The Waorani say they come from Namokapoweiri, a triangular constellation that can be found near Orion's Belt. The name means "star cluster." In ancient times, the stars were much closer to the Earth, just above the treetops. A simple ladder joined the Earth with Namokapoweiri. On this ladder the Waorani would ascend and descend at will.

On Earth some Waorani were curious to see what would happen if the clouds were set on fire. They tied cotton wads to the end of poles and set them aflame. The flames rose up into the clouds, and to the people's dismay and amazement, the fire ran higher and higher into the heavens. Soon the whole sky was ablaze. Fire and blazing rocks fell everywhere, killing nearly all the people and burning up the forests.

Only two families survived, one that hid in the buttress roots at the base of the *bubeka* or kapok tree *(Ceiba pentandra)*, and the other that ran into a garden of *cagiwenca,* sweet potato *(Ipomoea batatas)*. The ladder burned up and the stars rose higher and higher to the place where they are seen today, shimmering at a great distance in the night sky. The Waorani lost the ability to return at will to the stellar origin, and from this day forth they became bound to the laws of nature, to a life on Earth and all that entails.

The legend could not be a more clear warning. Curiosity, but more specifically, over-stimulation of the intellect, separates one from the reality of totality. Why is this so? Because one must transcend all dualistic thoughts in order to experience the absolute realms of existence. From this perspective we can see that according to Waorani thought, the only sin is duality. In the days "when the heavens shimmered just above the treetops," people were one of the immortal treasures of the universe. This is why the Waorani could move effortlessly between the Earth and their stellar abode, because heaven, Earth, and humanity were one and the same.

Then comes the thought of "What would happen if we set the clouds on fire?" Setting the clouds on fire represents what is happening today, the overdevelopment of the intellect. At the very least, it was the act of separation from the whole. They wanted the cause and effect of things to be known, to see if the laws of universal retribution hold true, so they stepped out of bounds to see what would happen. The results were catastrophic, and the world was purified almost instantly after these doings (see illustration, "Setting the Clouds on Fire," p. 218).

The way I see it, the bubeka tree in this myth represents the tree of life. These people were saved for they adored the tree of life, not the tree of knowledge, which can be confused with the tree of life. To adore the tree of life means to deliver oneself to the seen and unseen forces of nature and to know they are deeply interconnected and, ultimately, unseparated.

Followers of the tree of life integrate their internal energies. They avoid the overdevelopment of any one specific area, striving to achieve a complete and balanced integration of their spiritual-intellectual, physical-energetic, and sexual energies, as the tree is an integration and unity of its roots, trunk, branches, flowers, and fruits. By doing so they integrate their entire selves thoroughly with great nature, with heaven, Earth, and humanity. This is the true meaning of chastity— the avoidance of desire for what one does not have—for if one is and has everything, then there is nothing to desire. This is why the early missionaries sometimes said the indigenous people were the true followers of Christ.

That the other family was saved in the sweet potato patch is symbolic of being in tune with the substance of the Earth. The sweet potato is a plant whose tubers give life the option to continue. It represents a society that has tapped into the abundance of the Earth by cultivating it, by adoring it. The tubers, which must be planted, grow within the earth, so their sustenance comes from within. In other words, they are guided by spirit through the depths of their selves.

This way can be seen exemplified among the old Waorani, who refuse help of any kind from any human. They believe that to accept help is to compromise their autonomy. Waorani are able to survive alone in the forest from an early age, as early as eleven years old, and are capable of amazing physical feats. For example, they have extraordinary tree-climbing skills and can scurry up giant canopy trees and run across their branches as easily as they strut along the forest floor. I have seen this on several occasions. Mengatue

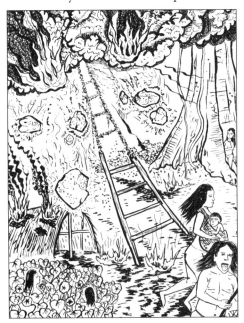

Setting the Clouds on Fire

himself was perhaps the best of the tree climbers I saw. Kue, a brother of Babe the war shaman, would swiftly climb to the top of large canopy trees when gathering fruits, hunting monkeys, or taking a look out over the forest in order to find his way back home following a classic all-out run after game in the bush.

Insights into the First Contact

Until the late 1900s, Waorani contact with the outside world was minimal. And since the early the 1900s it has not been friendly. Initial encounters with the modern West occurred during the rubber boom at the turn of the twentieth century. Later Waorani warriors fought a battle against Peruvian soldiers encroaching into their territory in the early 1940s. During this time they experienced internal war as well. According to an article on Waorani violence, "Although the oldest members of the community at the time contacted [circa 1980] could remember periods of peace interspersed with periods of violence in their youth, the Waorani had been convulsed with a nearly continuous period of raids and vengeful counter-raids for at least four decades prior. According to Wao oral history, the alternation of periods of violence and periods of peace stretch back as far as they can remember. Tracing back through the genealogies, over 60 percent of the deaths were violent ones."[5]

In the 1950s there were problems between oil prospectors and Waorani—then known to outsiders as *Aucas*, a Kichwa word meaning "savages." The novelist William S. Burroughs, an intrepid early traveler to the Amazon, wrote to his friend the poet Allen Ginsberg in 1953: "On the boat I talked to a man who knows the Ecuador jungle like his own prick. It seems jungle traders periodically raid the Auca (a tribe of hostile Indians. Shell lost about 20 employees to the Auca in two years) and carry off women they keep penned up for the purpose of sex. . . ."[6]

Such skirmishes and crimes passed largely unnoticed outside the forest. But, as anthropologist Norman Whitten puts it, in his book review of Laura Rival's *Trekking Through History: The Huaorani of*

Amazonian Ecuador, "In 1956 the Huaorani . . . speared themselves into international history by killing five Summer Institute of Linguistics (SIL) personnel who attempted to 'contact' them by landing on a beach of the Curaray River."[7] The event is famous and led to an evangelical mission among the Waorani and ultimately, in 2005, a film (*End of the Spear,* directed by Jim Hanon).

On the demarcation session there came an elder named Yowe, who had been present at the spearing of the missionaries. He told me that at first the Waorani wanted to be friends. It was only that suddenly one of them started defecating blood. This thrust him and his companions into a state of panic. In the book *Through the Gates of Splendor* (Elisabeth Elliot, 1957) there are photos taken not long before the spearing occurred. Nenkihui, whom the missionaries idealistically nicknamed "George," is photographed squatting, eating a hamburger. The foolishness of their approach is clear when one contemplates the implications of offering an aging hamburger to a wilderness tribesman. Not surprisingly, he got an instant case of diarrhea, which he and his companions saw as an act of sorcery. Yowe said that one of the Waorani, Nampa, was shot and killed, something the missionaries make no mention of in their version of the occurrence.

Then came the head-on collision with modernity when oil production in the jungle really started to boom in the 1970s, and some of these images started reaching people around the world: roads plowed deep into the heart of a recently contacted indigenous people's homeland, thousands of trees toppled, the way opened for colonization and pillage, where hidden people, never before seen, live in voluntary isolation. Noise pollution from the pipeline construction and then operation of the drilling rigs and other machinery echo in the pristine rainforest. Adding insult to injury, well sites scattered along the oil road into the Yasuni wilderness are given the most sacred names of the Waorani people, such as Iro (shaman or spirit master, irrefutable authority), Daimi (rainbow—the Waorani consider it a sin to point at the rainbow with one's finger, and instead they wiggle their nose), Nenki (the sun), and Apaika (the moon). The wanton biological and cultural erosion occurring due to human impact is indeed the great predicament of our times.

Waorani speared their way into world news again in 1987 when the Tagaeiri, a splinter group within the tribe, killed Alejandro Labaca, a Capuchin bishop, and Inés Arango, a Capuchin nun. The reason for this was made known many years later, when, in 1995, a member of the Babeiri clan, living at the very end of the oil road, kidnapped a Tagaeiri woman. When asked about the spearing, she said that the women pleaded with the men not to do it, but that only days before the missionaries had arrived, a tree had fallen, killing a child. Padre Labaca and Hermana Arango were speared to avenge the death of the child. It can be said that they arrived there at the wrong time. Their deaths were influential in the granting of maximum protection status to the Tagaeiri area, meaning that it is a part of Waorani territory off limits to the oil companies.

A Waorani woman sings:

> "In wartime the clouds hang low and we're all sad. We'll never see our families again. When there's peace the sun shines and we're happy. We love peace and it is what we most desire."
> —Conta Baihua, Queweiriono village, 1993

The Right of Non-Contact

> "Non-contacted groups are not a threat to anyone, except to intruders; they only want to be left alone. As I argued some years ago, we need to invent a new human right for all the groups still hiding in the Amazon forest: the right of non-contact."
> —Laura Rival[8]

In April 2013 while I was writing this book, news broke of more killings. Some Taromenane—members of a hidden group that no one knows whether to categorize as Waorani or not—had speared to death two traditional Waorani elders, Ompore and Buganey, the previous month, leading to a brutal retribution. This event took place outside the area called the "intangible zone," which is 3,000 square miles in size, in the heart of the Waorani ancestral homelands, completely off limits to everyone—to oil companies, to loggers, to colonists, and even to Waorani who have accepted the outside world. This place is for the hidden people, who have the right to non-contact. The fact that they still feel the need to carry out spearing raids shows that the area is too small. In May 2013, the United Nations requested that Ecuador ensure that the intertribal killings stop. Ecuadorian President Rafael Correa made an earnest plea to the UN requesting advice on what to do, saying the oil operations have nothing to do with it. The occurrence is so complex that I thought it better to add as an endnote a significant portion of an April 14, 2013, interview in *El Comercio* newspaper with Miguel Angel Cabodevilla, a Capuchin priest, activist, and friend of Alejandro Labaca.[9] According to news releases and videos taken by Waorani on cell phones, an elder Waorani woman witnessed the attack. The woman told authorities what the Taromenane were saying. They cannot handle the sound emanating from the oil rigs, an evil, demonic noise reverberating deep into the jungle, scaring the wildlife, making food scarce. They can't bear to see the trees being cut and strange crops planted in their lands. Also, behind them are the Wiñetare, who are their traditional enemies; they can move back no further. Essentially the Taromenane are being pushed between the impact of the extractivist assault on the rainforest on one side, and an enemy hidden tribe on the other side.

It remains a mystery (at least to outsiders) why exactly the Taromenane speared Ompore and Buganey.

It is evident that more than any other indigenous culture of the Ecuadorian Amazon, the contemporary Waorani are facing cataclysmic changes. Not only this, they are a people known primarily through the stories told by their enemies, convoluted distortions of the truth fabricated by those seeking to subvert them. Personally, I was given the opportunity to see them as a fantastic people from whom we have plenty to learn, and who want to live in peace like anyone else.[10]

The Origin of Those Who Ate Their Father

Mengatue related to me the following legend, pertaining to the creation of the human races. Long ago, a Waorani man desired his brother's wife. He couldn't resist the temptation and followed her to the garden. He watched her and was just about to attempt a sexual encounter with her when he saw her go to the river's edge. She pounded on a root that came out of the water and a boa came up, slithered between her legs, and began copulating with her. He went away and told his brother what he had seen, and suggested that he secretly follow her to the garden himself. The next day, the brother did this. Sure enough, the boa came out of the water and slithered around her legs and her whole body. The husband jumped out, killed the boa, and pulled it away.

Several weeks later, while the woman was back in the garden, she went to look at the rotting body of the snake. She saw maggots in the decomposing spine. Her eyes watered and itched a little bit, and she rubbed them. When she opened them again, she saw that the maggots in the dead boa had turned into little boys and girls of different races. They were all saying, "Mama, Mama!"

"These must be my kids," she thought. And she brought them home. She and her husband started raising them among the Waorani. There's a large game bird called a *bare* (Salvin's curassow, *Mitu salvini*), which sings mysteriously. The children heard its call and divined a new insight from it—that their Waorani father was not their true father, but in fact had actually killed their true father. They decided to take revenge. One day they waited for him when he was coming back from hunting, and leapt on him all together and killed him. Then they cut him up, smoked his meat, and ate him. From the teeth of their boa father, which they found in the garden where it was slain, they were able to craft all kinds of technology, including boots, guns, and metal tools that they used to make canoes—things the Waorani had never seen. They stole the Waoranis' plants, put them in the canoes, and moved downriver. That's how the *couode* came to be, the people who are not Waorani, the people who destroy everything. They're the people who ate their stepfather, the people who cut everything up, the maggots, those who follow no moral order.

When my group of peers and I got to the Waorani territory they called us *wabeka* Waorani, "people from a different place." Essentially they recognize three types of people: the Waorani, the wabeka Waorani, and the couode, murderers engaged in destroying the world. It is important to note that these designations are not racially bound, but depend on one's way of being. Which kind of person are you?

The Good Way of the Ancestors

The Waorani I met were always carrying on about *"Waaponi durani bai!"* Waponi means "good," and *durani bai* means "the Way of the Ancestors." I later came to understand this term to be as encompassing as the Taoist use of "the Way" (Tao) to describe the path of life that is the ultimate reality.

Wepe, a great traditional elder who adopted me as a son, sat sharpening his spear one day. I asked him to tell me about durani bai. "Durani bai," he said, "is like the tip of my spear, which passes through everything."

The term refers also to the era when the heavenly realms were not separate from the Earth. I was able to see that the Waorani live in a very immediate state of the now. Their word for future time, *baane,* also means "tomorrow," and anything that happened even three minutes ago is *duube,* meaning "long ago."

The Waorani are exceptional human beings, master ecologists and paragons of behavior in terms of relating to material existence. They have a penetrating quality of observation and keen sense of perception. I'll never forget the depth and intensity of how the Waorani, especially the elders, peer at things, looking, trying to understand through a penetrating, stealthy gaze.

The Waorani barely sleep at all, they have so much energy. Our camp cook Pirawa always slept like the true old-time Waorani, in a squatting position under two broad palm leaves that he had tied to a small tree above him to keep the rain off. In the middle of the night he'd wake up slowly, joyfully, start cooking, directing his long slender fingers in a graceful way. Often the Waorani would stay up all hours in the camp laughing. Never would the fires go out in the night.

Today many Waorani have deviated from the durani bai. That's why they're being wiped out, or so a lot of elders I met believed. When Waorani deviate from the durani bai, they compromise their autonomy and their history. Part of their traditional way is to adapt to their environment, but now there are all these new things in their environment, like oil companies, and all kinds of other confusing negative influences.

Working on the Demarcation of Waorani Territory

The Waorani language is relatively simple and it stuck to me naturally when I volunteered to help with the project to officially demarcate Waorani territory. I was able to take part in this effort when one of my professors recommended me to people at Australia's Rainforest Information Centre, which was contracted to undertake the demarcation. This trail-blazing project was masterminded by Australian Douglas Ferguson, who acquired support from different aid organizations to accomplish the work.

The demarcation of Waorani territory involved a core group of a half-dozen foreigners like myself, periodic other volunteers, and many members of the Waorani tribe. Over four years, in ten demarcation sessions, we created 130 kilometers of boundary lines around critical areas of the Waorani territory most vulnerable to colonization. During the entire process I collaborated as a volunteer, and I looked forward to each demarcation session with an ardent fervor. To spend time with the Waorani elders in the wilderness, though not easy, was a powerful experience for me.

It's hard to forget the run-in I had with wasps on one of these demarcation sessions. (Snakes I barely got to see.) Ducking through the vines, my backpack got caught on a branch. When I yanked it, a wasp hive came falling onto me, swarming with black *minkaye* wasps that sting like hell. For four nights I couldn't lie down, I was so swollen. On another occasion more than fifty of them stung me simultaneously on my solar plexus, leaving it swollen to half the size of a volleyball. The Waorani would laugh, saying, "These are injections so you won't get sick!"[11]

Often the jungle grew so dense and dark that it was necessary for the *macheteros* to chop tunnels into the vegetation with their machetes, and then let the axemen in, who would cut first halfway into all the smaller trees before the largest was felled in such a way that all the trees would fall together in one thunderous crash, and everyone would leap back as the entire canopy rained insects. Then, the macheteros in the rear would slash through the fallen canopy, and the axemen would move forward again, entering a new tunnel, as the macheteros in the front burrowed on, and the cycle began anew. The government topographer followed along, making the respective measurements.

Preferring the quiet of the forest, I was fortunate to cover the necessary post of helping plant rows of native palms in the wake of the clearing to create a living boundary marker. I was always with one of the elders, Koba, who would arise early and speak to the trees. He said things like, "the trees are our friends; they listen when we speak, they help us stay new." His advice to me: "Rely on the trees."

Over the four years we must have planted at least fifty thousand palm trees. Koba and I spent the days together collecting palms, and our camaraderie grew daily. We would scour the nearby forest in search of useful palms, then uproot carefully the babies to fill our baskets, returning to the line to continue planting, planting, planting. Several times we'd find wild fruit tree sprouts and plant them as well. We carried the palms in Waorani-style palm-leaf baskets and planted them every few meters along the boundary, with the goal of creating a straight line of long-lived canopy palms, all of which are useful, some with fruits, and a trail that functioned as a clearly visible, low-maintenance demarcation.

At one point during this volunteer effort, I got involved with overseeing the relocation and indemnification of thirty Shuar families who had colonized Waorani lands. This was another baptism by fire. I wasn't sure what exactly I was getting myself into until after it occurred. We went to where there were Shuar settlers living inside the territory. They spoke no Waorani and the Waorani no Shuar, and I was the only one who spoke Spanish in our group, and the Shuar spoke some Spanish, so I laid it out swift and direct to the community leaders. I said, "I'm here on a government program to demarcate the Waorani territory and you all are inside their adjudicated lands. In ten minutes you'll never see me again, and you'll have only those aucas." I indicated the Waorani behind me, who were shouting while they knocked over the Shuars' banana plants. "My suggestion is," I went on, "accept the deal." It was impressive to see how fast they accepted. They packed up their belongings in that moment and moved out before our very eyes. Then the Waorani set their homes ablaze. Prior to our arrival, these Shuar had been contacted by the Shuar Federation (at the urging of Douglas Ferguson), which supported the demarcation project, telling the families that if they did not leave they would be disowned by the Federation; and they knew if they stayed it would mean war. Given that the work we were doing was under contract with the state, the displaced Shuars were given a tract of community land inside the colonization corridor along both sides of the Via Auca oil road. After the Shuars moved out, we came through, clearing the boundary line. Here Koba and I planted only the spiniest thorn bushes.

I did a supply run to the town of Coca with Koba on one occasion. Thirty years earlier he had speared people where we were walking on newly-created streets that not long before had been verdant green rainforest. People stopped in their tracks to stare at us passing by, a gringo and an auca. The Waorani were notorious for their spearing raids. Few Ecuadorians had seen a Waorani so close, and the sight of a traditional elder like Koba immediately generated respect. Short and stocky, he wore his black hair long, cut straight across his forehead to well over and behind his ears. The emblematic feature of the Waorani people are the large stretched ear lobes, where during festivities they wear white-painted balsa earplugs.

In the years I worked with the Waorani I was able to make several trips to visit them at their homes, where I made audio recordings of their myths and teachings. I had these tapes in an apartment I was renting in Baños. Every time I came out of the jungle and went back to the house, a young Waorani named Niwa, who was probably about eleven at the time, would show up, somehow knowing that I would be there. He'd hitch a ride on any plane happening to land in his village's airstrip and hop a ride to the town of Shell. Then he'd hop a bus to Baños and without any coordinating arrive just when I would get there as well. As a result of his work on translating my tapes, I am able to share the Waorani mythology presented in this book.

Village Life

The best advice I received before my first visit to Waorani territory was given to me by don Casimiro, my friend the Kichwa elder, who told me to bring lots of candy, enough to give two pieces to each Waorani. I thought about this and tried to find the meaning. Finally it made sense. Because they are an egalitarian society, it was imperative that everyone get the same gift. Instead of candy I brought several rolls of nylon fishing line and plenty of fish hooks, cheap but useful. I was able to give a strand of nylon and two fish hooks to every Waorani, men, women, and children alike. I'd put a stick through the hole in the nylon spool so it would spin, and hand the end to whoever's turn it was. The faster they could run, the longer a piece of nylon they'd get. When they got far enough away I'd cut the cord and everyone would burst out laughing.

When visiting their villages, I always had the group of kids hurrying to stay right alongside me. At Queweiriono village, Mengatue, this entourage of Waorani kids, and I would set out for all kinds of adventures, going from house to house to drink *peneme* (chucula, sweet banana gruel) in the morning and *tepae* (yuca chicha) in the afternoon. The people are always active, always weaving, always making crafts, always in motion. I saw no laziness.

At night the kids would all sleep with me. I could feel my blanket moving over me, back and forth, all night. There were many of them, and not all fit under the blanket. The kid at one end would be left without a piece of the blanket and would pull it over himself. This left the kid on the other end uncovered, who would soon wake up and in turn pull the blanket back. A friend of mine who joined me on one of my visits to Queweiriono village brought a sleeping bag with him. One of the kids tried squeezing himself into the sleeping bag! My friend was not as generous as I and kicked him out of the bag, where he returned to huddle up among the mob sleeping with me.

It was always special to spend time with Mengatue and the flock of kids. It was his duty, when they were playing, to protect them. He was always poking around where the kids were playing, at times plucking poisonous snakes out of the bushes. I saw him once pluck a snake right out of the rafters of a house with his hands, yanking it down, breaking its neck between his clenched fingers and throwing it down on the floor dead. It was a highly poisonous bushmaster. This was at dusk, in the shade of a hut. Making his mastery known was natural for Mengatue.

Becoming an Iroinga

Mengatue told me how he became an iroinga. Gomo was his childhood name, and when he was young he became ill. An uncle of his was an iroinga named Pengunka. (Pengunka was named after the ibogaine-containing *Tabernaemontana sananho,* a tree the Waorani value as a medicine.) Pengunka put Gomo in the casing of a palm flower that when it falls to the ground has a form like a small canoe. The uncle soaked his nephew in water and healed him, saying, "You'll be a healer like me when you're older."

Much later, Gomo was married with children of his own. One day, he got a sharp pain in his neck, then fell and rolled down the hill behind his hut. (The Waorani traditionally lived on top of hills high above the rivers, though nowadays they live on the river like most Amazon residents, and have come to depend on fishing.) When he got to the bottom of the hill, a big jaguar that was there roared. Suddenly he was in the den of Meñeiriwempo, the Jaguar Guardian. She gave Gomo cooked wild boar from her own fire. She then cut off all his hair with her teeth.

A black jaguar was continually prowling about the outskirts of their fire, and Meñeiriwempo kept chasing it off. After that the Jaguar Guardian roared and Gomo was back near his family hut at the base of the hill. To him it seemed like he'd been gone only a short time, but for his family, he'd been gone an entire week.

That afternoon, Gomo was lying in his hammock. He began to feel the same pain in his neck again. Suddenly the Jaguar Guardian came into his heart. She made him chant, "I'm now coming to you through Mengatue." From that day on Gomo became known as Mengatue, and for decades he was a fearless defender of the territory as well as an effective healer, a preternaturally skilled guide, and a true friend.

Meñeiriwempo, the Jaguar Guardian, continued to come to Mengatue, in trance states in which she possessed him; afterward he would have no idea what had happened. Meñeiriwempo comes to other iroinga as well, to keep the people close to their ancestral energy, though many youth refuse to listen. Her counsel is too severe at times, because she wants to protect the Waorani people and keep their territory intact. And to try to accomplish this now in the face of colonization and oil development would mean reverting to old tactics that can't work in a new world. Despite the problems that surround them, many youth are lifting up their culture again, to live with joy. But others have gone to work for the oil companies and illegal loggers, warring against their forest and their people, acting out the crazed forces at play today in their territory.

Meñeiriwempo says she wants the Waorani to be as one, like long ago, before the fights broke out. The group once lived in peace, and then, a long time ago, some Waorani learned to make magic love potions with which they stole others' wives, and war broke out, and the situation has not calmed down yet. Back in the time of peace, there had been no end to the wilderness, and the people thought the world was flat.

POWER ANIMALS OF THE WAORANI PEOPLE

The *keñgiwe,* the harpy eagle *(Harpia harpyja),* is one of the world's largest eagles. The Waorani like to keep it as a pet, near the longhouse. The Waorani say it is like them, because it can break free of captivity and still make it in the wild, even if it was stolen from the nest as an egg or hatchling and raised by Waorani. It has no predators but man. In 1994 on the Cononaco River, I was fortunate to see one in the wild. All the birds were singing as usual, when suddenly this white-chested, black-collared eagle flew up out of the jungle. It came up over the river and perched on a tree. It sat there. The entire forest went silent, and it whistled—three faint tones.

The *meñe (Panthera onca),* in English known as jaguar, is another power animal of the Waorani, who consider themselves people of the jaguar. Some iroinga after exuviation of their human bodies roam the deep rainforest as a white jaguar. And then there is obe, the green anaconda *(Eunectes murinus).* A giant spirit obe is believed to challenge Waoranis when they die. If they are fearless, they may continue along the forest path, but if they are afraid, they fall back into the world in some reincarnated form.

The *deye,* the white-fronted spider monkey *(Ateles belzebuth),* is honored for its extraordinary abilities to climb. Birds such as the bare, today an endangered species, are still hunted as food but also sought for their fluffy white crissum feathers. The *wiñe,* the masked tanager *(Tangara nigrocincta),* is honored because it is frisky and active, and it is sought for its azure-blue feathers. The *yawe,* the white-throated toucan *(Ramphastos tucanus),* is admired for the pure red color of its crissum feathers. The *ëwe* (scarlet macaw, *Ara macao*) and the *tobe* (the mealy Amazon parrot, *Amazona farinosa*) fly high, have beautiful colors, and are seen always in pairs. These birds arrive in groups to the fruiting trees, and while they eat they knock down food for the *amo,* the collared peccary *(Pecari tajacu).* In a song sung at festivals, the birds represent Waorani women and the peccaries represent Waorani men in a traditional dance. Everyone sings: *"We are the Waorani, the people of the rainforest."*

Origin Myth of the First Miiyabu[12]

Long ago when the sky was still close to the Earth and the stars glistened just above the treetops, the first miiyabu vine was born. In those days there was a huge *degihue* tree (yellow pau d'arco, *Tabebuia serratifolia*) that rose high in the sky, its trunk glistening golden in the afternoon sun. Up in the branches of this towering tree hung many nests of the *menka* bird, the olive oropendola *(Psarocolius bifasciatus)*.

A group of Waorani walking through the forest came upon the tree, and since it was the season when the menka raise their young, they said, "Let's climb into the tree and take home the young birds to raise." The menka has long been a favorite Waorani house pet, in part because of its ability to mimic human language.

The tree's trunk was so wide and tall that the men climbed a neighboring palm and laid a pole from its crown to the lowest branch of the degihue tree, making a bridge. Once the Waorani were up in the crown of the big tree, though, it became clear that most of the menka nests were too far out on the branches and impossible to reach. Not everyone who had climbed up got a bird to raise.

As the Waorani climbed down, the second-to-last became jealous that he didn't get a bird. He crossed the bridge, then kicked the pole off the branch, making it impossible for the last Waorani up in the tree to climb down. The brother-in-law of the man stuck up in the tree sent the group back to the village, then stayed behind with the stated intention of making a new bridge at the top of the palm.

This man was a powerful iroinga named Inuito. He told his brother-in-law, "Don't be afraid. There's going to be a flash of light that will fill the sky. A large serpent is going to appear. Its head will be anchored in the clouds and its tail will touch the earth. Its skin will look like a rainbow. You hug this boa tight and come sliding down to the ground."

The man in the tree nodded and said, "Okay, okay."

Inuito slid down the palm trunk, back to the forest floor. After a moment, he raised his hands. He stood in silence, looking deeply into the sky, and then he winked. A tremendous flash of light, brilliant beyond description, illuminated the forest and the heavens for an instant. There was no thunder, only a silent flash. As soon as it was gone, the giant rainbow serpent was visible, its head in the clouds and its tail hanging all the way to the ground. It hovered there, uniting Heaven and Earth.

The man in the tree was terrified but Inuito encouraged him to hold on tight and slide down quickly. The man did as told and slid down so rapidly that all

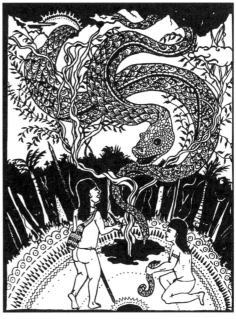

Origin of Miiyabu

his hair blew off. As soon as he got to the ground, Inuito handed him a *caanda,* a palm-wood machete, and told him, "Quick, quick! Cut off the tip of the tail!" (see illustration, "Origin of Miiyabu").

The man did this, and in the blink of an eye the boa slithered upward and vanished into the clouds. On the ground was a small pool of blood. The two Waorani men stood looking at it for a while, then met each other's eyes. Inuito spoke with his finger to his mouth: "Nothing is to be said of this. You do not know my name." With this phrase Inuito was repeating, in symbolic language, his demand that his brother-in-law not reveal what he saw. The iroinga went on, "Within two full moons, return to this spot. A plant will be growing where this blood spilled on the earth. This plant will be called *miiyabu.* Take a branch and plant it somewhere else. Once this plant grows up into the trees, then you can tell the people what happened to you today. You can tell them what you have seen, and you can tell them my name."

His brother-in-law was awed but nodded in agreement. Then they went back to the village.

Two full moons passed, and Inuito's brother-in-law went into the forest to the place where the blood of the rainbow boa had spilled on the earth. To his amazement, there was a vine growing, just as Inuito had said. As instructed, he broke off a branch and took it to another place, where he planted it at the base of an *aunghue* tree (inga, *Inga* sp.).

Soon the branch took root and began to sprout leaves. On a return visit the man found it doing well, with clusters of fresh lime-green leaf growth, and next to it, to his amazement, was a tiny jaguar, the size of a mouse, which ran quickly into the forest. After a few days, when the bewildered man came back, the vine had grown significantly. To his even greater amazement, two small jaguars, a male and a female, crouched at its base, one on each side of the vine. They were the size of house cats, and they too darted into the woods instantly (see illustration, "Jaguars in the Miiyabu Vine," page 211).

The vine continued to grow well and wrap itself around the tree. The man returned one day to find two more jaguars nonchalantly resting at the base of the miiyabu vine. These were the size of large dogs. They had a cub with them. These jaguars looked at him and walked away slowly at first, then ran, stopping some twenty meters away to look back. They growled a bit, then walked into the forest.

The man was bewildered. "Where are these jaguars coming from?" he wondered. "Is the miiyabu attracting the jaguars, or are they coming out of the plant itself?"

On his next visit he encountered a female jaguar the size of a deer with two beautiful cubs. She growled as the man approached and he froze before beginning to step backward, looking in her eyes. When they were out of each other's sight he turned and ran away as fast as he could.

He approached the place slowly a few days later, wondering what to do next. There by the vine were two large, full-grown jaguars, male and female. The vine was thicker at its base and bigger now, reaching high up in the canopy of the tree. The man did not dare get too close. He watched from a distance then left.

Returning with extreme caution some days later, he peeked into the

clearing. He saw that the vine was loaded with bright flowers. Unbeliev-
ably, many jaguars were there on the forest floor and playing among
the branches. Up in the tree, rolling around, inebriated, were a male
and female jaguar, fully grown and tremendous. All the jaguars were
rejoicing, delighted by the smell emitted from the leaves of the first
miiyabu. The sight made the Waorani dizzy, and he wondered, "How
am I ever going to look at this plant up close?"

Then he thought, "I'll catch some game and leave it nearby. When
the jaguars smell the meat, they'll go to eat. Then I'll run up and grab
some leaves." He carried out this plan and was able to rush in and
grab a branch full of leaves. When he was a sufficient distance from
the jaguars, the man stopped and began to observe the leaves of this
peculiar vine.

He rubbed the leaves together, then inhaled their smell. The fragrance of the miiyabu penetrated his entire body. Curious what its
effects might be, the man began walking through the forest, noticing
nothing in particular. He decided he might as well get some game for
his family. Suddenly a big troupe of monkeys appeared. It was as if they
didn't see him. The man caught several with his *omena*, his blowpipe
with poison darts. A little further into the forest, he easily shot several
game birds from a group that flew right up before him. He returned to
his house with more meat than he had ever bagged in a day.

"This plant is an attractor plant—this is what must be going on,"
the man speculated. "That's why the jaguars were attracted." His next
thought was: "Well, if this is the case, why wouldn't it attract the opposite sex to me as well?"

It just so happened that there was a festival coming up, and soon he
would have a chance to experiment with his new "attractor plant." At
the festival, he lay in his hammock. The miiyabu leaves were wrapped
in a little bundle. He opened it and mashed the leaves a bit. The smell
filled the area, and soon a young lady caught wind of it. She ran over
to the man in his hammock, jumped on him, and started fondling
his sexual parts. Meanwhile, other women were getting whiffs of the
miiyabu and running over to the hammock, piling on and trying to

have sex with him. Even an old woman cried out, "I want some, too!" and crawled over to the crowd.

The man managed to close up the bundle. He tried to push off the ladies but couldn't. It was agony. But soon the smell of the miiyabu dissipated, and as suddenly as they had jumped on, they jumped off him. Realizing what happened, they scolded the man in embarrassment as he ran off into the forest, back to his house. From the excessive sex his penis was damaged, and he left in agony.

Some insights and commentary to the myth: The blood dripped from the supernatural boa fertilized the earth and enabled the vine to grow. If we look at blood as the medium through which life-giving oxygen reaches all extremities of the body, then we make the connection that miiyabu has the ability to bring forth new life or make life more abundant. Like this it brings life closer to the supernatural realms, where things are infinite and inextinguishable.

The jaguar is the animal that most frequently represents primal energy in the Amazonian cosmologies. This peculiar plant is like a guardian at the gate of an enormous power emanating from the center of the cosmos.

In the realms that transcend time and space, good and bad are relative concepts, and only energy exists—refined, supremely sublime yet infinitely powerful, self-containing, self-renewing, self-sustaining. In the relative three-dimensional world, this energy can have both positive and negative effects, depending on how its release is channeled. For this reason, the instructions for handling miiyabu from the elder Waorani are clear: Watch your thoughts before touching miiyabu. Many people are not strong or wise enough to use it beneficially, and they carelessly ruin their lives and the lives of others. Whenever you touch this plant you must be aware of what you are thinking, because that is what you will attract into your life. This is why the Waorani seldom touch this plant.

"When you touch this plant," Mengatue clearly stated, "spirits come to your side as if they were your children. If you get angry at someone they can go and kill that person. It is very dangerous. If you are touching this plant you must not get angry. This way no one will be harmed and your life will not be ruined."

The Subtle Use of Miiyabu

The Waorani use of miiyabu (*Banisteriopsis muricata,* a variety slightly different from the *Banisteriopsis caapi* used by others) is peculiar and unique. They do not use consciousness-altering plants, though they have names for the ones that grow in their territory and knowledge of their powers. Up until recently, no Waorani smoked tobacco or drank fermented beverages.

But to increase a youth's hunting skills, an elder places, only once, some miiyabu leaf tea in his own mouth and passes it through a tube made from a toucan esophagus to his student's mouth, who takes a few sips. After this, the youth begins a dieta consisting only of young yuca tubers and the petohue *(Jessenia bataua)* palm pulp from the stomach of toucans and spider monkeys that he and the elder hunt. During the entire duration of his diet, which can last several months, the student whittles blowpipe darts and spends his days hunting in the forest. Also during this period, the food he captures he gives away. When he can begin eating new foods, the elder first passes some of the new food from his mouth to the student's mouth. After this he can eat those foods. Over some time the student develops extraordinary hunting skills, including being able to call the animals and to endure long days with little food. This practice can be seen as a unique cultural trait specific to the Waorani.

There's another unique and most subtle Waorani use of the miiyabu. When a child is born, the umbilical cord is cut with a sharp piece of bamboo. With a leaf infusion, an elder washes the navel of the newborn. Most families just use *wigagen,* the garlic vine *(Mansoa standleyi),* but families with iroinga in them use some leaves of the miiyabu as well. The iroinga say that this will allow Meñeiriwempo to find the individual when he or she is older and prepared to handle the energy.

With a topic like this there really is no beginning or end. Once, near Cacataro in the headwaters of the Shiripuno River, a Waorani returned to camp, animated and charged with life. Inspired, he related how he had encountered a white jaguar. I was told that several Waorani had seen this white jaguar close to where we were. Elusive, it had shown itself only a little, then slipped into the forest. We were near a large hill where in ancient times a powerful iroinga had lived, my companions said. The white jaguar was his spirit, moving through the forest, watching.

Postscript to Chapter 7

I sent this chapter to Dr. Laura Rival for her comments, admittedly at a late date in the publication schedule. She graciously replied with relevant comments, but I was unable to incorporate one of them due to the complexity of the changes and our stage of design. So I want to add an important clarification here.

The chapter discusses the concept of an iroinga, a Waorani shaman or individual with special access to spiritual guidance. Dr. Rival helped me understand that it became evident to her during her fieldwork that there are two basic forms of Waorani shamanism, *iroinga* and *meñera,* and that very little has been documented in this regard. Dr. Rival said that because Mengatue embodied the Jaguar Guardian, he was a meñera, not an iroinga. Iroinga are another branch of individuals with even higher levels of achievement such as dominion over nature and many other kinds of supernatural powers. In the legend of the creation of miiyabu presented above, Inuito is an iroinga. Among the Waorani this distinction is not made clear unless one really digs deep into the culture, and for the most part the two words, as I heard them, can be used somewhat interchangeably. In actuality, though, as Dr. Rival indicates, meñera and iroinga are distinct branches of Waorani shamanism.

Chapter 8

The Eyebrows of the Andes

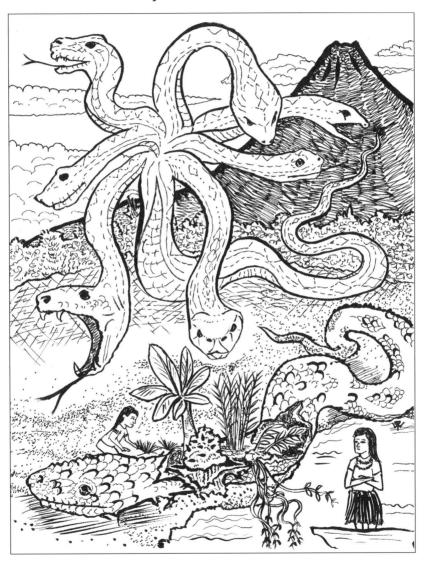

Atacapie Slays Shiu-amarun

"The Amazon River rises in those jungle-covered sharp ridges and deep canyons almost always enshrouded in mist. *Cejas de la montaña* (eyebrows of the mountains) they call that country, and well named too. . . ."
  —Manuel Córdova-Rios, *Rio Tigre and Beyond*[1]

When speaking of the mighty Andes and the so-called "eyebrows" country at the range's eastern base—the Tropical Wet Forest region—I am first obliged to give homage to the Apu, the Mountain Lords, the ice-capped everlasting sovereigns of these great lands, on whose forested slopes manifests the most marvelous biological diversity. These towering authoritative mountains, which rule without ruling, which provide for all equally without hoarding, where multitudes of plant and animal species exist, are why this book is here! Reaching high above the thick-hanging clouds, into the azure firmament, the Mountains *know!* And the mountains, by virtue of their constancy, grapple with the union of strength and gentleness, form and formlessness. And it is due to their steady, unchanging essential nature that the Apu are held as sacred, sometimes fierce sometimes calm, in a land where everything is changing, including the people's reverence for the mountains as the ways of old are replaced by throwaway consumer culture. Yet despite it all, the mountains hold together with unequaled might, making evident the truth of time as a continuum of past, present, and future, in the felt presence of the moment, as one unified reality.

The Perspectives of the Condor and King Vulture

"The most dangerous worldview is the worldview of those who have not viewed the world."
    —Alexander von Humboldt (1769–1859), German naturalist
        and explorer

Let's imagine a condor flying over these mountain tops, as the spiritual masters of not long ago did in their visions, quests, and dreams. We can see some peaks in northeastern Ecuador. First there is Cayambe, which in the Quitus language means "Origin of Youthfulness" or "Origin of Life," on whose summit rests the only glacier on the equator. Then comes Antisana ("Most Sacred Heights" or "Beacon"). It last erupted in 1801, sending a lava flow that formed Papallacta Lake, today's principal water supply for the city of Quito. Crowded nearly to its snowline with tropical vegetation and diverse birdlife, the expansive wilderness region surrounding Mount Antisana is home to the largest remaining population of Andean condors. Along this eastern range of the Andes, clouds and slow-rising mist clothe the mountains and shroud the expanse of forest, especially at the hours of dawn and dusk when the landscape is held in a close embrace by a soft lambent light and blanket of quiescent stillness. . . .

The condor travels east. The landforms drop in altitude, revealing a different perspective. A rugged landscape marked by lakes snuggled within escarpments and ridgelines gives way to humid valleys robed in clouds and forests thick with vegetation. The rivers cut deep gorges. Here the condor meets the king vulture, and both ascend in spirals, floating atop gusts of rising warm winds. Far below live the endangered mountain tapir, the rare spectacled bear (the only South American bear), the pampas cat, the Andean fox, the Andean porcupine, the puma. These are all iconic species of this great land. Bird species that have found their niche in these cloud-covered high-altitude forests include the bearded guan, crimson-mantled woodpecker, long-tailed sylph, and the grass-green tanager, among so many others.

Eastward, toward the Amazon, younger volcanoes are still active, on whose steep verdant hillsides and unruly ridgelines myriad species make their home, comprising the mega-biological diversity that marks this region. This mountain is Sumaco, "the beautiful." The word *sumak* in the Kichwa language signifies the most beautiful anything could ever be, as beautiful as heaven itself. It can be heard in Ecuador's national adage, Sumak Kausai, meaning "Beautiful Life!"[2] Like Cayambe, this mountain is located at zero degrees latitude, farther to the east yet still directly on the equator. Sumaco last erupted near the end of the nineteenth century. And it was there on the slopes of Sumaco, a Kichwa legend relates, that long ago the battle occurred between Atacapie, the seven-headed boa, and Shiu-amarun, the glistening fertility boa. This confrontation brought forth many sacred plants used today among the Amazonian Kichwa people. (Read the complete legend in Chapter 3, "Origins of Ayahuasca.") It is believed that here in the wilderness of Sumaco Volcano, Atacapie still lives, hiding in a lake.

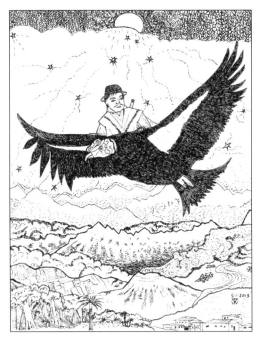

From the Condor's Perspective

These majestic giants east of the Andean divide have stretched the meeting place between rainforest and mountains, forming vastly diverse and complex geographical and climatic opportunities along the equator, all of which intensify the region's biodiversity. Here, as the Earth flows, as all living beings undergo transformation, the North Andes Plate is being squeezed between the faster-moving South American and Nazca plates, and the region is marked by frequent volcanic and seismic activity. In these uppermost regions of the Amazon, along the green and lush *cordillera real oriental* (the royal eastern ridge) of the great Andes, the creases in the mountains' foothills have acquired the curved shape of a human brow. In this particular area one finds the highest concentration of plant species per square meter and the richest diversity of terrestrial ecosystem types known anywhere. No other region in the world surpasses northwest South America in its biological diversity, and it peaks here in the "eyebrows" of the Andes. Proof of this claim is found when one compares the species counts of the Neotropics—the tropical regions in the Americas—to other tropical regions of the globe. As a result of commendable efforts by certain factions of the Ecuadorian government, large areas have been set aside as national parks, including (to name only a few), Cayambe Coca National Park, 1,556 square miles; Sumaco Napo-Galeras, 798 square miles; Yasuni, 3,793 square miles; Llanganates, 848 square miles; and Sangay, 1,999 square miles (newly bisected by a road joining the Andes to the Amazon). Here in a relatively small geographic area are 8,994 square miles of protected wilderness. Nevertheless, stronger protection for this patrimony is clearly necessary. These protected areas face many threats, such as colonization, logging, mining, oil drilling, and intertribal warfare. For example, in Yasuni National Park, hidden peoples and tribes contacted only in the past fifty years live atop massive natural gas and oil deposits. As they continue to defend their way of life, they come into the crosshairs of the twenty-first century.

Tremendous wilderness areas on indigenous land holdings are sadly slated for sacrifice. The people have been given back their rightful lands, the government insists, but as Moi Enomenga, a Waorani leader, put it, "They have given us our lands, but they have kept our blood."[3] The government retains drilling rights, and the great majority of the Ecuadorian Amazon has already been doled out in oil and mining concessions. In the face of this, many indigenous communities have threatened to engage in outright civil war, and there has been much unrest.

Famed ecologist E.O. Wilson has written, "The 6th great extinction spasm of geological time is upon us, grace of mankind. Earth has at last acquired a force that can break the crucible of biodiversity."[4]

Studies performed by a group of scientists from Duke University in 2012 demonstrate that eighty percent of the most vulnerable regions in the Tropical Andes are currently unprotected.[5] This is even more disturbing when one considers the high rates of endemism (meaning globally rare species found only in a limited region), especially in the areas between 1,500 and 3,000 meters' elevation. Duke researchers concluded that if enhanced conservation measures are not implanted by local government, we run the risk of losing many species to extinction in less than a decade.

The Tropical Wet Forest: A Conservation Priority

Throughout tropical regions of the Earth, the Tropical Wet Forest is a threatened ecosystem type. In Ecuador it is found only within a narrow band, 30 to 70 kilometers wide, running north-south along both the eastern and western slopes of the Andes, between the altitudinal gradient of 400 and 650 meters (approximately 1,300–2,130 feet).[6] Endemic to the narrow band of Tropical Wet Forest are 27 species of trees such as *Theobroma cacao*—yes, that's right, wild cacao, the source of chocolate—and *Ocotea quixos,* known locally as *ishpingu,* the finest Amazonian cinnamon; also *kamotoa,* a giant emergent canopy tree *(Gyranthera amphibiolepis)* that was assigned its botanical species name as recently as 2012 and is today vanishing due to unregulated and illegal logging.[7] This band of opulently flourishing forest is like the glistening gemstone necklace of the Pachamama, the Goddess of the Earth.

The warm clouds blown westward over the Amazon basin from the Atlantic begin to condense at the base of the Andes, resulting in a significant surge of annual rainfall levels. With approximately 4 to 8 meters per year (that's 13 to 26 feet), this is one of the wettest areas on Earth. The U.S. botanist Alwyn Gentry discovered that where rainfall increases, endemism and biodiversity do too, and with this in mind, we can understand a little more why there is so much of both in the Tropical Wet Forest. Any lone ridge top with a spike in annual rainfall levels can harbor rare, locally endemic, and in some cases site-specific plants. Gentry summarized the task of protecting unique forest types: "From a conservation perspective, to avoid massive extinction it is not only important to conserve patches of the major forest types, but also to conserve individual or semi-isolated habitat islands."[8]

Within Ecuador's system of legally protected areas,[9] the Tropical Wet Forest is an under-represented ecosystem type. Given its outstanding attributes, it has not received the recognition or legal protection that it rightfully deserves. Most likely this is because the region where the Tropical Wet Forest is found lies squarely in the path of the major development that is occurring; the lack of protection is also the result of a lack of information and understanding. Areas that actually are "protected" have been pillaged by illegal logging. Also, many government and conservation planners and biologists have lumped the Tropical Wet Forest type with the Tropical Moist Forest type found at lower elevations. In the upper Amazon, the Tropical Wet Forest is being sacrificed to the roads and the booming growth of small cities such as Jambeli, Tena, Puyo, and Macas, among others, and the activities that occur near them, such as unregulated logging, continual failed attempts at cattle ranching, and production of high-investment cash crops such as coffee for export, cacao for the global chocolate industry, and *naranjilla* (*Solanum quitoense*) for fruit juice. These crops deplete the forest and the soil fertility and fall to blights in a relatively short time. All require heavy pesticides and deforestation. The complex, little known, biologically dazzling and rare ecosystem that is the Tropical Wet Forest is unrecognized, undervalued, and in the way.

A short distance to the east and below 300 meters' elevation, one enters a different ecosystem type, the Tropical Moist Forest, where annual rainfall is less than half what it is in the Tropical Wet Forest. These lowland Amazonian rainforests stretch to the Atlantic. They too are magnificent, but there are more species per hectare and greater endemism closer to the base of the Andes and in the piedmont region such as Yasuni National Park due to increased annual rainfall levels.

Napo-Galeras: The End of the World Jaguar Mountain

Before my first visit to Waorani territory, I was introduced to don Casimiro Mamallacta, a traditional Kichwa healer and family man living in the outskirts of the jungle town of Archidona, by his daughter Mercedes, whom I met at the Jatun Sacha biological station.[10] During the years that I was collaborating on the demarcation effort and in between the work sessions, I lived with don Casimiro's family rather than go back to Quito. In addition to sharing with me many insights into the traditional ways of the Napo Runa, the Kichwa people from this part of Ecuador, he introduced me to a place he had known since childhood, the native forests of the Napo-Galeras region, a most mysterious area nestled in the midst of the "eyebrows of the Andes," and, as I was to discover, it is a place held sacred to three regional tribes. The isolated limestone massif rises up out of the Amazon lowlands just before the incline toward the eastern Andes. Don Casimiro's family members are the mountain's ancestral stewards on its western slopes. As my friendship with him grew, he recruited me as an ally of the mountain, and we worked together to gain protection for this sacred place that today is one of Ecuador's most recently declared national parks.

April 1993: One night at the Mamallactas' homestead after a few hours of sleeping soundly in my hammock, I was awakened abruptly by Casimiro. "Let's go!" he kept saying. *"Let's go!"* I groggily came to and in a partially conscious state started to comprehend the scene. It was about 11 PM, and Casimiro had just managed to pull himself away from the village. As always, the men there had insisted that he be invited for a few shots of sugarcane moonshine, known locally as *jatun manila warmi,* "big rope woman," or *guanchaca.* These days, many of the village ties are maintained through the men's drinking sessions, and a family leader like Casimiro gets poured full of the unbearably strong juice whenever he comes within range. After making all the toasts he excused himself and stumbled up the dark jungle path home. That's when he crashed drunkenly into my hammock and started enthusiastically encouraging me to get my stuff—"Let's go!"

I had no idea where we would be going at that hour, but Casimiro knew the path so well that he could walk it in full darkness and after his obligatory moonshine-drinking. We quickly covered a lot of ground, walking eastward.

I pieced together that we were walking the first leg of a three-day foot-journey to Casimiro's purina tambu, his wilderness retreat or ceremonial "place that is walked to," which is the literal translation. The month of January typically has more clear days than any other in the upper Amazon, and Casimiro takes advantage of the opportunity to get to his beloved stomping grounds as much as possible, setting out without thinking twice. Most of the year, because of the high elevation of the place, there's a tendency to experience thick fogs or persistent storms, making the journey much more difficult. Casimiro spent several years living in the Mamallacta family's purina tambu as a boy, where he was given a traditional upbringing by his grandmother—including strong doses of tobacco juice through the nose and potent bark extracts. He has made regular trips there over the course of his life.

We didn't pack any food, but the next day we came across some palm hearts along the trail. After the second day we reached the banks of the beautiful Pusuno River, the "River of Bubbles," and there we ate a couple of small armored catfish that Casimiro obtained by reaching his arm deep into an underwater crack in the limestone bank. Hiking nonstop on muddy jungle footpaths requires a huge amount of energy, and everything we found to eat seemed increasingly delicious. On the third day Casimiro surprised me by digging up some six-month-old mashed chonta palm fruit powder that he had conveniently stashed for a future visit. This is a marvelous food prepared especially for long foot-journeys. Stored in the anaerobic environment of a clay embankment, the palm fruit powder cannot ferment, and it stays lush and incredibly nutritious. This material was so fine that when I picked it up it sifted through the cracks between my fingers, leaving a golden cloud and a hypnotic aroma. Just looking at the golden dust was giddying. Mixed with water, the powder turned a deep orange color with a rich, oily consistency. It was enchanting even for a passionate chicha drinker like myself. The Mamallactas knew I loved chicha, so they dubbed me

Asacutu, "chicha howler-monkey," a nickname that made everyone laugh. The hunger we were feeling took the drink to a new level. The nourishment from the chonta fruits gave me strength and energy to finish the walk. We were heading to the summit of the mighty mountain of Napo-Galeras itself.

Napo-Galeras is a special place that very few visit. "Here we come for spiritual reasons," Casimiro explained, "for making prayers when people are ill, or for making spiritual quests to cultivate strength and spiritual power in order to help people in need." In the past people visited Galeras only as respectful pilgrims.

Traditional Napo Runa culture bears a rich heritage of oral literature. Life is informed by a thorough understanding of humanity's place, both ecological and spiritual, in a more-than-human world. An important locus of their spiritual geography is Napo-Galeras Mountain or, as it is called in Kichwa, Izu Mangallpa Urcu. The name may be glossed as End-of-the-World Giant-Earthen-Jaguar Mountain. *Urcu* is "mountain." *Izu* means the end of a cycle, a time of transformation, an apocalypse. *Allpa* is the name for "earth," while *mangallpa* has several meanings, including clay pot and big jaguar—which signifies primal energy, the raw power of pre-human stages of development.

In the creation epic of the Napo Runa—the Kichwa people (*runa* means "people") who live around the Napo River—there are extensive tales about Kuilluru and Duceru, the hero twins who brought humanity from the period of a more ancient, inhospitable world into the current timeframe in which humanity flourishes. Before their heroism, the villages were constantly plagued and people were killed in great numbers by the Mundupuma, the "world puma." The twins came up with a plan to save the people from the Mundupuma's constant menace. They found a cave in Galeras and prepared a rock inside with a thick coat of sticky beeswax. Then they took stringed instruments and started playing beautiful music, luring the giant Mundupuma into the cave with them. "Come and play music with us!" they called out joyfully. The Mundupuma came in and sat down on the rock they had smeared with beeswax, and they handed him a drum. As the story goes, they quickly jumped out of the cave and threw a huge boulder in front of the opening. The jaguar, stuck in the beeswax, could not respond quickly enough to jump after them. The jaguar roared and thrashed, furiously trying to get out and banging on the cave walls. The boulder was too heavy to budge and he remained sealed in the cavern. The people were finally freed from his constant menace.

Far from being fossilized, oral history and its symbolism are a living part of contemporary Kichwa insight. These mythic understandings, widely known among natives of the area, continue to grow and respond to current events. In the 1950s came a key moment in Napo Runa history—the construction of the first roads into the area by international oil companies. They say that in those times, you could still hear the Mundupuma inside Galeras Mountain, a deep booming like thunder that set the earth trembling for miles. This phenomenon was common while the roads were being made, and it stopped shortly afterward and has not been heard since.

Some people suggest that the Mundupuma has left its confinement in the cave, and that we are seeing a prophecy being fulfilled. This interpretation explains the arrival of cultural and ecological decimation in the area, but leaves some aspects of the story out, for at the time of judgment the emergence of the Mundupuma is believed to lead to the destruction of offending humanity *only*. Those living upright lives will be spared, to live freely with the land that will again become a place without sin. Surely the oil companies brought an unprecedented force of destruction to the upper Amazon, yet the impacts of these activities have affected good and kind people as well as wicked people in their onslaught of the indigenous peoples' homelands, and for this reason there are doubts that the prophesized judgment day has yet to come. To some it seems that the order of the cosmos taught in the legends must have been disrupted or changed for this to happen, and I heard others say that the Mundupuma must have died, asphyxiated in the small cavern, before it could come out and fulfill the prophecy.

Don Casimiro, whose family has a particularly intact tradition of oral literature, tells another aspect of the original legend—that in the period before the Mundupuma emerges, it will go to sleep inside the cave. When it awakens it will fulfill its purpose, emerging to devour the offensive people within humanity. Despite the varying interpretations of how the current crisis fits into the story, to Kichwa speakers living around Napo-Galeras the Mundupuma is real, a latent force inside the sacred mountain, waiting to emerge and play its role at a crucial turning point in world history.

Lessons of the Mountain: Powerful Spirits and Places

Casimiro says that at Galeras one should walk in quietude, avoid joking altogether, and be serene and respectful at all times. Like many of the lessons associated with this mountain, this requirement teaches the integrity that must be summoned to act responsibly on the psychological frontiers of human life. Remembered as reliable history as well as symbolic advice, stories set in Galeras are anecdotes from the powerful no-man's land between the exclusively human and the totally wild, where everyday life touches a realm independent of human consciousness and influence, a realm governed instead by the wild, ever-present physics of mythic nature. Because it's home to powerful spirits such as the Juri-juri and Ingaru Supai (both ardent protectors of the wilderness), the Chullachaqui (the one-legged spirit who teaches plant medicine), the Amazanga Supai (the luminous force of nature that can appear as a ball of light like a moon), and the Kayu Runa, the "Lightning Man" that lives in the waterfalls, Galeras generates respect. In essence the entire mountain of Galeras is seen as a place where the mythic realms are unlikely to succumb to human relegation to the "beyond," and pilgrims have to be psychologically prepared to deal with that experience. Not only in legends but also in personal stories and modern experiences, visitors are forced to face the delicate psychological space that occurs when conscious and subconscious are forced together. Respect is a precondition that precedes and overshadows intellectual understanding—expect to respect first, and then possibly to understand later.

One vivid story relates how a mute man who was brought along to Galeras on an expedition with boisterous and disrespectful hunters witnessed them all having their eyes sucked out by the Juri-juri Supai. The mute was instructed by the hunters to make a fire. Without embers, the man had to revert to using the ancient method of banging two quartzite rocks together over a small pile of dry tinder. But everything was wet and he wasn't having any luck with it. After hours of frustrating work with nothing to show, the man noticed a wisp of smoke rising from a ridge on the far side of the valley as the mist cleared. So he headed there to ask for some embers, and upon arriving, to his amazement he realized that it was not another person but a Juri-juri Supai, appearing as a venerable grandmother. How did he know? Her firewood was human bones.

She offered him some chicha and he drank. "You're a good person," she said. "This I see." She gave him some embers to start his fire. "Just after sundown," she added, "you must climb a large tree near the camp and tie yourself up on a branch. Do not come down for anything. Tonight my children and I will come. These people who are hunting are mocking the dead animals, disrespecting the fact that killing animals is a solemn act, necessary only for one's survival. For this reason my children and I will be coming tonight to suck some fruits."

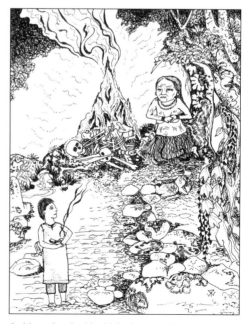

Asking the Juri-juri Mother for Embers

The Juri-juri Supai Mama (mother of all the Juri-juri spirits) could see the hunters' actions and knew the nature of their thoughts. They did not have the proper respect needed to be entering and especially to be hunting in Galeras. The mute man received the embers and returned bewildered to his camp.

The hunters came back with the spoils of their hunt to find a fire burning nicely. While cleaning and roasting the meat, they began to joke and make fun of the animals. "Look at that charbroiled monkey—looks like you, ha ha!" They continued to mock the lifeless animals. The mute tried to get them to stop, urgently mumbling, "Hmmm, hmm!" but he had no way of explaining what he had seen and heard. All he could do was wait until dark and then climb a tree as instructed.

Just before dawn, as he slept fitfully in the branches, the gentle rhythms of the insects were abruptly interrupted by a sudden tremendous blast of wind. He heard violent screams from the camp below. Wide-eyed, he stayed firmly tied to the tree as his campmates were attacked. After the sun rose he climbed down and found the hunters panicking, screaming, and crying as they groped around the camp. Their eyes had been sucked from their very sockets. "Can anyone see?" they called out. For a while he didn't know if he should make a noise, but finally the mute answered with a *"Mmmp."* They pled with him to take them back if he could see the way. He tied them in single file to a vine and set out for Archidona, several days' journey away, with the sightless hunters stumbling along behind him. Not only had their eyes been devoured, but also their cooking pots and the metal blades of the machetes had been consumed, leaving only the handles. Even the footsteps they left as they walked around the camp had been consumed by the furious spirits.

After a day of hiking down the mountain, the group came to the Pusuno River, to a spot where the yacu yutzu trees grew along both banks, their flat crowns of branches reaching across the water and forming a shaded canopy. To the mute man's surprise (for only he could see), hanging from the trees like ripe fruit over the river were dozens of finely decorated clay pots. He stood awestruck a moment, gazing at the strange scene, and then continued on toward Archidona.

Back in the village, the mute Kichwa was left in a state of shock, unable to shake the psychological trauma of the experience, and unable to communicate the horrible scene that had played out below his perch in the tree. He went to see his friend the yachac, who offered to prepare ayahuasca to help bring the mute man back to balance and to cleanse his mind of the horrifying images. During the ceremony, the healer saw in visions everything that had occurred.

The healer asked the mute if it was true that where the travelers had crossed the Pusuno, mysterious clay pots were hanging from yutzu trees. His friend nodded. The yachac told him he had a plan. The mute man with a stick in the sand drew for him the designs on one of the pots and with his hands he showed the width and height of the pot. After the pot was fired, the yachac drew the designs onto the pot, just as the friend had indicated to him. Once the pot was finished, the mute man nodded enthusiastically, indicating that it was very good. After purifying themselves adequately, they left with the pot, and after a few days' walking they arrived at the location. All the clay pots were still there, hanging over the river. Very carefully, the shaman crawled out on the limb over the river and gently replaced a pot hanging there with the one he had made. Then the two men left, taking the spirit vessel with them. (See the book's opening illustration.)

Once they got back, the shaman and his wife marveled at the pot and thought they would make some chicha in it to see how it turned out. Soon it was ready to drink, and it was delicious, the best they had ever tasted. What was most impressive is that as they drank, the level of the liquid in the pot did not go down, but always stayed full. The yachac and his wife were generous and they shared the chicha with many people.

Sadly, though, some thugs in the village felt threatened by what they could not understand and decided to take it upon themselves to look a bit more into the matter. They went to the yachac's house while he was out in his garden. One brute reached his hand into the pot. His hand became stuck there and he started screaming. He pulled and pulled and couldn't yank out his arm, so he grabbed a pole and smashed the pot. The chicha spilled out everywhere on the earthen floor. The yachac

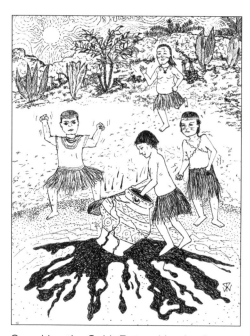

Smashing the Spirit Pot and Losing Its Magic

ran from the garden, shouting, "I shared generously with everyone, showing the good way, and now none of us will have this great drink again!"

Later the elder drank ayahuasca and saw in his visions that the pots over the river were gone. He returned to the spot to see, and sure enough, there were just the yutzu trees. The only thing hanging over the gently flowing river were the long branches.

There are so many stories relating to mysterious occurrences and powerful places at Galeras, such as the lake where the Kayu Runa, the Lightning Man, was petrified. The remains of one giant rib and one testicle can be seen. It is said that without fasting, though, the place can't even be reached—thick fog and clouds enshroud the mountain, pelting the traveller with rain and driving him back with wind. When one fasts, though, the way is clear, and pilgrims would come to meditate on the banks of this sacred lake where a special pair of ducks swim. Gazing at the powerful presence of the remains of the mythical being's rib and testicle turned to stone, meditators can achieve a deep connection with the forces they embody to achieve spiritual growth.

Here is another most amazing tale. Many generations back a sage out in the jungles of Galeras was fasting, and a man appeared whose face was painted with the blue/black temporary dye called *witú* obtained from a tree by the same name *(Genipa americana)*. He said to the sage: "If you bring me a boa I will make a fire here on this beach and I will show you something." It was too odd a request to deny, so the sage went and hunted a fairly large boa.

When he got back to the spot, he met the man again. It turned out that the form he had seen was a manifestation of Kayu Runa, "Lightning Man," the spirit of lightning who lives in the waterfalls. Kayu Runa had laid out a long pile of rocks along the edge of the river. "This is my firewood," he said. "Lay the boa there on top." The sage laid the boa out on top of the rocks.

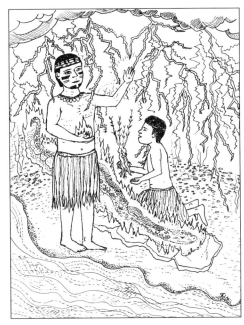

Kayu Runa, "Lightning Man," Gives the Snakebite-curing Tuber

Kayu Runa raised his hands and blinked and lightning crashed down onto the rocks, which exploded in flames then turned red hot and glowed like giant embers. The whole boa was charred almost instantly. This occurred on the new moon. Kayu Runa said, "Come back when the moon is half grown and look here where the heart of the boa has burned. In response to your deep love for the people, and your devotion, you have received this gift to help the people."

In two weeks the sage came back and found growing in the heart of the boa an unusual plant, today used to heal snakebite. This rare plant is cultivated only by some elders among the more traditional families. It is called *machakui wishuk*, meaning "snake tuber," and I have not yet been able to identify its genus or species. The plant resembles a stunted, pygmy ayahuasca vine, growing in small patches to a height of no more than 30 centimeters. After three or four years it produces a ginseng-like root tuber, shaped like a little person or sometimes two, curled together in loving embrace.

Unkiyabe: Galeras Mountain in Waorani Tradition

The Waorani call the sacred Galeras massif Unkiyabe, "Long-house Mountain," because its shape is similar to the traditional Waorani *unku*, a leaf hut or long house. They also refer to it as *Eygaweyaboga*, "the mountain where eygaweyabe grows," referring to an extremely rare Galeras endemic species that they describe as belonging to the mythological realms.

Tribal traditions of the Waorani, Kichwa, and Secoya have coexisted for hundreds of years, sharing the sacred spot. Casimiro always stuck to his purina tambu on the western side of the mountain, respecting the eastern side as traditionally pertaining to the pilgrimages of the fierce Waorani people, whom the Kichwa know as the Aucas—savage, uncivilized, deep-forest dwellers. Even on the western slope, Casimiro and his grandfather were chased off the path by spear-wielding Waorani several times in his childhood, and Waorani presence there has a long history, though that history is now largely forgotten.

As the only mountain coming out of the true geologic floor of the Amazon basin, the isolated limestone massif stands as an impressive monument, overlooking the entire lowland expanse of the Amazon. From its eastern crown, the view encompasses the greatest expanse of rainforest that can be seen at one time without an aircraft, a verdant stretch with the Napo River snaking through it. Situated on the western edge of the low-altitude jungle basin, the top of Galeras receives the first light of the sun each day in the upper Amazon. It is from this point that the Amazonian dawn begins as a faint glow and slips down into the mist-covered forest.

Since traditional societies align their cosmologies with nature, it is not surprising that this unusual elevation that brings the jungle closer to the long-awaited illumination of the celestial realms has a profound place in all cultures that have been historically aware of it. Waorani legends teach that in ancient times a sacred woman appeared from the forest to the Waorani and showed them the boundaries of their homeland. To the south they walked to the Curaray River—the

Ëwengono, "River of Scarlet Macaws."[11] There she and the people left a food offering. "This is the southern border of the place where you can live," she told them. Then they walked to the north, until reaching the Napo River, the Doroboro. "This is the northern border of the place where you can live." Then they crossed the Napo, over to Galeras Mountain, to Unkiyabe. "In times of crisis," she explained, "when things become bad, you may leave your territory and come to Unkiyabe. Here is where you shall come to pray." She cautioned them that when making a journey to Unkiyabe, nothing should be taken back from the mountain.

All around the Waorani, as they stood on the slopes of Unkiyabe, were big tame jaguars lolling peacefully on the branches of the trees. The Waorani prayed there for the benefit of their people, that they might be able to live a life in peace. There was one mischievous Wao among them, though. The fragrant leaves of a particular plant caught his attention. This was the eygaweyabe that gives the mountain one of its names. "I wonder what would happen if I took this back to the community," he thought, disregarding the warning of the holy woman. He broke off a branch and took it back and planted it in the village. The plant took root and grew. When it got about three feet high, out of the plant leaped a giant jaguar, which killed half the people. The survivors chopped the plant down, and the bloodthirsty jaguar loped back to the mountain. Another legend attests that a Waorani family escaped the ravaging torrents of a great flood by fleeing to Unkiyabe.

Jaicunti: Galeras Mountain in Secoya Tradition

At the turn of the twentieth century the Secoya inhabited regions along the Napo River close enough to easily see Napo-Galeras rising from the lowland rainforest, receiving the first light of day.

Amazing stories are one of the legacies of a philosophical system that teaches the need and techniques for a particular form of gnosis that opens the door to life's mythological dimensions. The indigenous people's awareness of and involvement in this obscure dimension of physics constitute an impressive, if not astounding, contribution to human culture.

The Secoya call Galeras *Jaicunti,* "High Hill." Between heaven and earth, Jaicunti is home to the Jaicuntipai, the spiritual immortals who live inside the mountain in an alternate dimension.

My teacher and friend Cesareo Piaguaje related the following. Years ago, when he was training, he was seriously injured by the malice of a jealous sorcerer. He was given bad yagé to drink, which "broke his crown"—not the physical one he wore during ceremonies, but worse, the spiritual one. He lost his ability to see visions and thus to heal.

Cesareo's teacher was an albino Secoya drinker named Juan Gringo. He is fondly remembered in a number of stories that are still told among contemporary Secoya elders. He was the descendant of a unique Secoya bloodline—the grandson of a man who had married a Tsia-yapai, a mythological water person, and people say that Juan Gringo inherited a spiritual ability to enter into the world of the water. When his student had his crown broken, Juan Gringo gave him strong yagé, well cured and blown on, and introduced him through the visions of yagé to the Jaicuntipai, the immortals of the high hill of Napo-Galeras.

After ceremonies and a rigorous dieta, one morning at 9 AM a hole in a tree opened like a cave's mouth. Juan walked in first and then invited young Cesareo to enter. Ducking their heads to clear a vine that was dangling across the opening, they found themselves in a different world upon entering. Guava trees grew slanted to one side, and a small winding path led through them and up and over a hill. From the top of the hill they could see the village of the Jaicuntipai. They looked down on eight houses—according to the Secoya yagé drinkers' spiritual perspective, there are eight original lodges that the Creator himself made for the Jaicuntipai to dwell in. The ancient buildings shone like new; the roofs, though made of thatched palm leaves, glimmered like metal. When the Jaicuntipai saw the two men coming, they called out, *"Look! Look!"* Preparations were made and several inhabitants hurried out to meet them. They wore traditional tunics and immaculate beaded crowns, perfect circles with no signs of a beginning or end.

"Who is this that you're bringing?" they asked Juan Gringo. He introduced Cesareo as his nephew. With no delay, they gave him a new designs crown, because stashed in the rafters of their homes they have dozens of these. Then they performed a marriage between Cesareo and a young woman of the Jaicuntipai. This woman became his spiritual wife, a social category recognized by Secoya society.

Upon returning home, in addition to having recovered his ability to see visions, Cesareo entered a new period in his life. From that point on, he says, his spiritual wife has come and occupied his body during the ceremony of yagé, enabling an incredible range of healing that was impossible before. The Jaicuntipai, like the Jujupai of the water dimensions, are doctor people. They are associated with extensive healing powers and they teach many forms of healing.

Modern-Day Adventures in Caretaking a Sacred Mountain

August 1991: One day while I was living with the Mamallactas we received a troubling piece of news: a long ribbon of land had been clearcut into Galeras. Casimiro immediately started out walking, taking me along.

After a day's hike we came to the Pusuno River, where we ran into the cleared area—a familiar sight recognized as the first step of a new road's construction. Casimiro wept when he saw that the road was planned to cross the headwaters of the River of Bubbles. Flowing through the Mamallacta purina tambu, the Pusuno is an idyllic river that flows crystal clear over a grooved limestone bottom; it's home to a large population of river otters that can often be seen playing. The gash of the road was beyond out of place—it was obscene. We followed the ribbon of cleared land for another day and camped on the lower slopes of Galeras.

During the evening we heard a distant *"Woooo!"*—the call Runas commonly make to each other in the forest. Up the trail came a cousin of Casimiro's who had heard about our departure and hiked quickly for two days to catch up with us. We stayed up late around the fire that night, listening to his stories about special places he had discovered in his wanderings in the jungle foothills of the Andes. His strong and wiry body showed his dedication to the dieting, and he told us of a place of spiritual power where an unusual rock glowed with various colors. This boulder, he said, could only be reached by following a river's course and climbing past several waterfalls. To a passer-by it would appear as any old rock, but to a pilgrim who had come fasting it could be seen to pulse inside with flashing lights of red, orange, and green. He would go there often to fast, and he had learned incredible songs as well as techniques for healing a variety of ailments. His fascinating information made a strong impression. This was my introduction to a science through which the Runa understand the power that can be found in certain stones called *curirumi,* "golden stones," or *piedras vivas,* "living stones."

That night we had a rare concert when we heard several jaguars screaming from the top of the hill opposite us, like fierce bulls bellowing. Our small camp was a tiny oasis of humanity in a massive, independently willed jungle where jaguars roared in the dark. They stayed on the ridge across the Pusuno and after a while fell silent. We began talking about the jaguar. Casimiro's cousin noted that jaguars have a well-developed position in Napo Runa thinking. As ferocious predators capable of easily taking a human life, effortlessly overwhelming any physical resistance that even the most prepared could muster, they inspire the people to use all their ingenuity to survive. Past generations of advanced spiritual masters, he told me, developed sciences that drew on their subtle knowledge of the mythological workings of the ecosystem and addressed this problem specifically. Casimiro said that when he was a boy there were still some elders who could give a selected person a non-physical *uchu corona,* meaning "chili pepper crown," during an ayahuasca ceremony; after some dieting, its power would stay with the person. The coronation would affect the personal energy of the subject in such a way that jaguars in the forest would consistently avoid him. Casimiro received this in his youth, and to this day, though he has lived his whole life in the remote wilderness of his motherland at Galeras where there is a relatively dense jaguar population, he has never been molested by these forest cats. This is the legacy that enlivens Kichwa culture—a science which, however lofty it may seem at times, pragmatically informs and empowers right relationships to the natural world.

Part of what makes Galeras so special to the tribes of the Ecuadorian Amazon is that although it is a gateway to the spirit world, it is set firmly and undeniably in this physical one. Like any contemporary natural treasure, it stands silently vulnerable to the subjectification of nature for human interests. This road cut was made because the Ecuadorian army found the landmark to be an ideal spot for a small radar-monitoring station. Its interesting position overlooking the Amazon basin makes it a good point from which to scan for low-flying planes, including those involved in the illegal drug trade from Colombia.

In this case, though, Casimiro was able to stop the project. We contacted the military and organized a meeting with the officials in charge. Ecuador's army, fortunately for us and for Galeras, maintains a surprising respect for the indigenous population and is loyal to its needs when possible. Most of the army is comprised of indigenous peoples, and it has relied heavily on the service of tribal units trained in their cultures' warrior tradition. Although a small radar camp was established, the army agreed to access it only by helicopter, and forbade the few cadets stationed there to hunt or disturb the wildlife. Soon after, we learned that Galeras had acquired a small degree of protection in gaining the official designation of *"bosque protector"* or "protectorate forest." A contractual agreement was made, through the Park Service, that the Mamallacta family be recognized as caretakers of the mountain's western slopes within the limits of their traditional purina tambu. These conditions set the foundation for the newest period in the seven generations of stewarding Galeras—the proper integration of the End of the World Jaguar Mountain in the spheres of modern national and international policy.[12]

Establishing and Protecting Napo-Galeras National Park: A National Patrimony and International Treasure

To secure greater official protection for Galeras, a devoted team of activists and indigenous residents decided to seek national park status for the whole mountain. With the western area largely protected by the Mamallacta family, whose land is part of the Pueblo Kichwa Ruku-llacta, we shifted our efforts and worked to gain designation for the eastern side of the mountain as well as a rich lowland area known as Wairachina Sacha. However, colonists were already established in parts of the mountain's eastern base. Casimiro, conscious of his boundaries as caretaker of the western side, gave us his blessing but declined to participate actively due to the social conflicts likely to ensue. Idealisti-cally, I committed myself to the project, and although I had secured some support from the Rainforest Information Centre, I proceeded to get a baptism-by-fire in the world of grassroots rainforest conserva-tion. As anyone involved in this work knows, there are many competing interests and perspectives when it comes to Earth's natural resources and riches.

My education started with a wake-up call to the realities of the Kichwa cultural crisis in Napo Province. Although many families, the Mamallacta among them, have preserved an inspiring heritage through their adherence to traditional values, contemporary Kichwa society as a whole has been deeply impacted by centuries of oppression. Before the arrival of the missions in the 1500s, it is believed that dozens of distinct cultures and language groups, now lost, flourished at the eastern base of the Andes. Then came generations of forced acculturation in which the use of Kichwa—a highland Incan language that had previously been used by the Amazonian tribes only as a common trade language—was promoted by the new authorities. The lives of many became dictated by their oppressors rather than informed by their ancestors. Today, though many Kichwa retain a rural jungle lifestyle, they often live in ways that directly oppose the cosmology of their elders. As time goes on and transmission of the complex tradition becomes increasingly inhibited by the pressures of assimilation, more empty cultural space appears in the younger generations—a vacuum that consumes the traditional culture from the inside out. When a particular aspect of the culture is lost, television marketing and unsustainable land-use practices are pushed into the gap. I learned to value even more highly the contributions that traditional Kichwa families like the Mamallacta (and the Santi and the Pilco in the highlands[13]) have made in their struggle to maintain their way of being.

I first thought that the indigenous groups would be our greatest ally in protecting Galeras, yet many insisted that the recently homesteaded land was their ancestral right. This attitude has become common among modern Kichwa throughout the Amazon, helping them justify the colonization of other tribes' territories somewhat as if it were a continuation of the expansion of the former imperialistic Incan empire.

A federation of settler communities, in order to gain political votes, already had its own plan for Galeras and, like us, had petitioned the government. They wanted to subdivide the mountain in long strips and award land titles to each of the communities at the base. When those of us wanting to preserve the entire mountain as a national park first crossed to the eastern side of the mountain to investigate demarcation of a national park boundary, we were met by a violent party from the communities that sent us running back down the trail to safety.

From our perspective, we had all relevant interests in mind—protecting the sacred mountain for everybody and everything, keeping it from getting overhunted and colonized. The sad reality was that in the current competitive and impoverished environment, our efforts were generally misinterpreted.

At one point we even managed to relocate nine colonist families from a wilderness area to the outskirts of an existing village, contained within the first line of colonization. Ultimately a rare win-win situation that had to be handled with delicacy, this was a perfect solution—less colonization in primary forest, and the colonists returned to the village infrastructure, which they preferred anyway.

Then in 1994 with opposing petitions for the protection and subdivision of Galeras, the Ecuadorian government had the final say—specifically the Institute of Agrarian Reform and Colonization. It was a critical time, when thousands of hectares of land titles were being given out to different indigenous communes. Fortunately, the ruling came down on the side of protection, thanks in large part to continued recognition of a deal with USAID in 1984 that built the bridges for the Hollín–Loreto road, after an earthquake damaged the main road to the northeastern oil fields. These bridges were paid for in exchange for the Ecuadorian government securing basic protection on Sumaco Volcano and Napo-Galeras massif. In the agency's words, a nationally designated area "cannot be cut up like a piece of cheese." A German aid organization that had donated significantly to the country was also influential in urging the Ecuadorian government to enact park status, and in 1994, these two mountains became the Sumaco/Napo-Galeras National Park.

Our work wasn't done yet, though (it never is), because Ecuador's infamous bureaucratic bumbling and lack of continuity led to new maps being drawn that did not reflect reality on the ground in Galeras, including locations of existing communities and even appropriate natural boundary lines such as the Pucuno River to the north. Now with the help of Rita and Ramon Mamallacta, two of Casimiro's eldest offspring, we worked to convince the government of the accuracy of our maps and to bring their information in line with ours. We set out for each village to get their input and support, and to continue collaborations for future land use, stewardship of the national park, and boundary acknowledgment.

We continued to try to revive the memory that Galeras is sacred to the Kichwas and to other jungle tribes as well. Although Casimiro had stayed home, Cesar Mamallacta, an eloquent elder in his late seventies, came along and championed the cause. He would make us cry with his speeches, standing before various communities confused about conservation: "Look, we come in the name of the forest, of the plants, of the animals, of the trees that are being wiped to extinction.

We are the indigenous people—we are the protectors of the land, not its destroyers!"

I'll never forget our last night at Galeras after a month of boundary-ascertaining, collaboration-seeking meetings and a journey along the eastern slopes of Napo-Galeras including the lowland sector of Wairachina Sacha. Our last camp was pitched at a most beautiful spot that overlooked a river and offered an impressive vantage point. Throughout the last weeks of the walk, we had often noticed a white hawk majestically circling overhead. Shortly after we settled into that last camp, we realized we were sitting directly under the white hawk's nest. We spent the afternoon watching it come and go from its home. This, too, was a delight and an auspicious sign to us, and the camp was full of happiness for the way things had been going.

Rita Mamallacta returned to camp with a massive log of ayahuasca vine, two feet long and ten inches thick, that she had been gifted by an elder in the community, with instructions that we should cook it there in camp and drink. Having helped Casimiro brew ayahuasca plenty of times, I volunteered to prepare it for the motley crew of Kichwa Indian friends and some foreign volunteers that comprised our team. There was no elder shaman among us, but Rita insisted that it was okay to drink. She said that it would be auspicious for us to drink it given that we are protecting this sacred place, so undeniably we would be gifted spiritual learning in exchange.

That day while hiking I had found a wild variety of *Psychotria viridis,* and I went out to harvest it for the preparation. The trail led me past a startling specimen of *pungara* tree *(Gutiferea iridea)* loaded with yellow fruits. An important food for monkeys and birds, the tree had burst into full fruit undetected—none had yet fallen to the ground—and the branches were heavy with the delicious fruits. It was an impressive and strange sight to find in the forest, where food can be scarce. Fasting in light of the preparation of the brew, I savored the aroma and restrained myself from climbing the tree and feasting on the fortuitous bounty.

It was May 15, 1994, the conclusion of a powerful and productive experience walking the eastern edge of Galeras. The process seemed to really catalyze the relationship of the neighboring communities, who were warming up to the idea of the mountain as a sacred place that ought to be preserved intact.

I can recall vividly the experience I had that night.

The brew came on very strong. I found myself looking at a large waterfall, then looking, close up, at a bird flying in the wind. Soon I found myself seated in a circle of people, a large group like a meeting. There were representatives of many different indigenous cultures from around the world, some that I recognized and others that were totally new to me. A Waorani, from his place in the circle, got up and started to sing "Kayahue," a traditional song that succinctly embodies the essence of the Waorani worldview. When he sat, another stood up, a man from a culture I'd never come across before. He sang a beautiful song that seemed to come from the heart of his culture, expressing through the music and not words the significance and identity of his people, their relationship to the physical and mythological worlds. I sat there silently, grateful to be present at such a gathering. When that singer sat down, another young man stood up. I was struck by the elegance of the beautiful, intricate designs painted on his face. He began quietly to sing his song, so incredibly slowly yet simultaneously filled with great strength, letting the presence of the song fill the place with a powerful feeling. Listening, I was made somehow to understand that the essence and effect of this song was the perpetuation of forms, the Holding-Everything-in-Place as we know and see things to be. The song was sustaining and perpetuating the entire web of life and the structure of experience, entire galaxies centered on the gravity of the slowly unfolding melody. . . . I was awestruck, and in my emotional response, positive as it was, I started to objectify the song, longing to learn it myself. As soon as that desire showed up, the vision and the song were scattered and the pieces slipped away. I woke up and found myself sitting in the cool stillness of the night amongst the trees.

Early the next day, we were ready to break our fast. When two of us went to find the pungara tree that I had encountered the day before loaded with fruit, it was nowhere to be seen! It wasn't far from our camp, right on the trail, but we looked and looked for at least an hour and could not find it. I surrendered to the notion that it must have something to do with the mysterious master I was given the gift of being able to set eyes upon briefly, and it was impressed upon me again that the rainforest is indeed a place of mystery.

Wairachina Sacha, Rainforest of the Purifying Winds

Part of the Galeras National Park campaign (1990-1994), a finished report and proposal to protect 3,700 hectares (approximately 8,880 acres) of Galeras' precious piedmont Tropical Wet Forest, was apparently lost in the bureaucratic shuffling from the Ministry of Agriculture to the Parks Service. This left an important area of biodiversity and wilderness with a less-protected status than the newly designated national park. To say the least, I was disappointed to see the negligence of indifferent bureaucrats bungle such hard-won grassroots achievements, especially after surmounting such challenges as accusations of carting off the world puma in a helicopter to a zoo in Quito, threats of murder during the process of relocating the settler families (afterwards they were very happy with me), and near-riots, as when we were ousted from Santa Rosa de Arapino village on our first attempt to enter the area. After all this we had finally achieved a ground-level demarcation of the area and acceptance among the local population for its protection.

In 2010 I was inspired to return to the area. I concentrated my efforts and submitted an even better and more well-researched report and petition requesting the inclusion of this lowland Tropical Wet Forest in the adjacent national park. This is a critical opportunity to preserve a unique and priceless forest type that is underrepresented in conservation acreages, while also making the park a pole for sustainable local development.[14]

Thanks in part to this more recent report, the area is currently designated on official government maps as Patrimonio Forestal. Located on the eastern slopes of the Napo-Galeras cordillera (as well as the equator), Wairachina Sacha is one of the last representatives and probably the most significant stand of Tropical Wet Forest life zone remaining in the Ecuadorian Amazon. Its conservation could save the intact gradient of ecosystems from lowland tropical rainforest to the summit of Napo-Galeras massif at 1,770 meters above sea level.

Sacha is the Kichwa word for "forest." A *wairachina* is a leafy broom rattle that healers use in ayahuasca ceremonies to cleanse their patients, to move energies, and to provide rhythmic accompaniment for songs (generally made from a shrub called in Kichwa *surupanga;* Latin name, *Pariana radiciflora). Waira* means wind, and in this context with *china,* meaning "to teach or transmit a power or an energy," the term can be interpreted as wind teacher or transmitter of cleansing energy, invoking the power of wind in the translated name "Forest of the Purifying Winds." In the reserve, which we are proposing be designated a higher protection status, is a river called Wairachina Yaku—River of the Healer's Leafy Broom Rattle—from which the forest takes its name.[15]

Inventories here in the Tropical Wet Forest show over 300 different species of tree per hectare, as compared with 180–220 species in the already-megadiverse moist rainforest nearby to the east, at a slightly lower elevation. In 1991 I collected some plant specimens near the summit of Galeras and had the chance to share them with master botanists from the Missouri Botanical Garden who were studying in the area. They affirmed that several of these were new species undescribed by science. One of them was an impressive tree, its trunk about three feet in diameter, and it flowered in beautiful waxy purple blooms. It was a previously unknown species of the genus *Blakea.* In 2010 I returned to the area to revisit the past work, and while there I collected another few hundred specimens. This time they were analyzed by Dr. Carlos Cerón, a distinguished Ecuadorian botanist who is curator of the Central University Herbarium. Seeing that several of the specimens I had brought to him were new to science, including a never-before-described species of palm (in the genus *Aiphanes*), he wanted me to take him to Galeras. We arranged an expedition when he had a window of opportunity for a field trip, and a few days later we were there, this time exploring an area lower on the slopes, in the heart of the Tropical Wet Forest. Here is where Dr. Cerón made a most impressive observation. Seeing so many species in the cacao family (Sterculeaceae), more than he has ever seen elsewhere, he convincingly announced to us that this region should be considered the origin site of *Theobroma cacao*, the chocolate tree!

Wairachina Sacha hosts the giant armadillo *(Priodontes maximus),* the giant anteater *(Myrmecophaga tridactyla),* its smaller relative the northern tamandua *(Tamandua mexicana),* and the even smaller silky or pygmy anteater *(Cyclopes didactylus),* known locally as *flor de balsa,* balsa flower. Six types of cats make this rainforest their home, including the largest in the hemisphere, the spotted jaguar *(Panthera onca);* the lesser-known, elusive margay *(Leopardus wiedii);* the oncilla *(L. tigrinus);* the ocelot or dwarf leopard *(L. pardalis);* and the jaguarundi or eyra cat *(Puma yagouaroundi).* Large boas are still found in this region, and many kinds of monkeys such as the saddleback tamarin *(Saguinus fuscicollis),* a species exclusive to the Tropical Wet Forest. Also found here is the kikanjou *(Potos flavus);* the bushy-tailed olingo *(Bassaricyon gabbii);* the elusive cacomistle *(Bassariscus sumichrasti);* tapir, peccaries, endangered Salvin's curassows, and three types of deer.

On this 2010 visit we saw that a new road was being built. It was painful to see. The road would have already cut across the entire area, in an attempt to push all the way through to the Napo River below, if it were not for the tractor having gotten stuck in the mud while attempting to pass a steep creek. In my report I was able to highlight the virtues of the forest and include the opinions of both scientific and cultural specialists, such as Dr. Cerón and the Mamallacta family. Amazingly, the government responded to this report and local objections and halted this road attempt with a four-year court injunction.

For this Wairachina Sacha region to gain the necessary maximum protection, and for this initiative to truly work, the surrounding communities must be involved and supported as well. This would be a model of the integration of national and local government working for megadiversity and sustainable regional development (much as we see happening in Costa Rica surrounding Corcovado National Park). To align with the rainforest communities and work toward creating

sustainable economic alternatives such as improving cacao production, producing native guayusa tea and other medicinal products, and
ramping up ecotourism is a valuable investment of time and energy.
This will be a vital step forward in the shift toward cultural heritage
revalidation, sustainability, and rainforest conservation.[16]

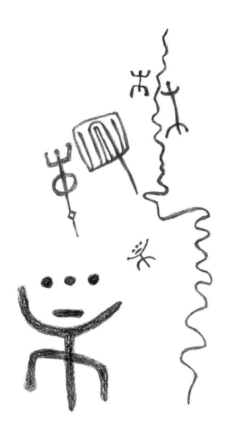

Petroglyphs made by the hero twins who
became the planet Venus

Chapter 9

Lineage Holders of the Traditions, Deep Forest and Urban

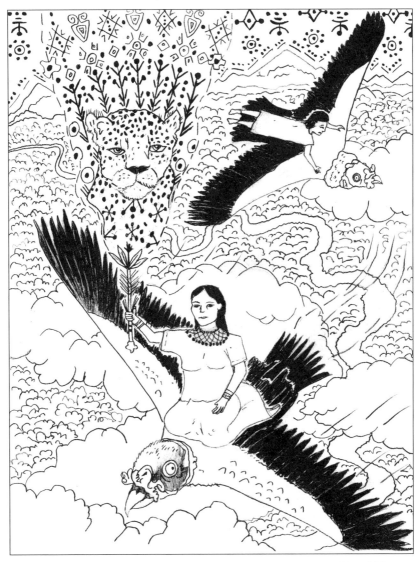

From a Secoya Legend: Returning Home on the Backs of the King Vultures

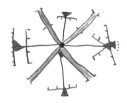

"People of self-delivery, if inspired, try to discover the profound secret of being absolute, which is where true freedom lies. An absolute being can light up the meaning of all worded and wordless teachings of all the ancient great minds in one instant."
—Hua-Ching Ni, *Workbook for the Spiritual Development of All People*[1]

In this chapter I recall some inspirational elders and their families, stewards of a few spiritual and cultural traditions of the upper Amazon. Some of the most remarkable experiences of my life have been with them. I hope these brief glimpses will help round out my presentation of the region's indigenous science by portraying a few cameos of the people who embody its purpose, potential, and power. There is a universal essence common to all of them that transcends languages and cultures.

During the years I worked on the demarcation of the Waorani territory between 1990 and 1995, in between my usual month-long stays with them I spent quality time with several Kichwa families, including the Mamallacta family on the outskirts of Archidona in Napo Province at the base of the Andes, and the Santi family near the jungle town of Puyo, in Pastaza Province to the south. Later, between 1995 and 2000, I spent time among the Secoya and made periodic journeys in Peru. Because I wrote so much about the Secoya lineage holders earlier in this book, I won't add more here—this space is for the mestizos, the Kichwa, and the Waorani.

Urban Ayahuasqueros of Peru

In 1997, sacred-plant experimenter and writer Terence McKenna asked me to find out for him what a foreigner had to do in order to operate a floating Amazonian research station in Peru. As a result of this quest (which was ultimately fruitless), I found myself in Iquitos, meeting Kenneth Symington, Terence's friend, who had translated a book on ayahuasca and Amazonian thought called *The Three Halves of Ino Moxo*. We met by accident (if accidents exist) at the Pascana Hotel, and this led to some epic adventures. Kenneth introduced me to don Solon Tello, at whose home I met and befriended his disciple Rafael Tuesta Rios, another most proper, good-hearted, and humble urban ayahuasquero. To search for ayahuasca was not my intention when I traveled to Peru, but it must have been meant to be, since I inevitably met these good elders who generously shared with me their knowledge of *la purga* (ayahusaca) and facilitated many of my experiences with these different aspects of traditional Amazonian medicine. It was in Peru where my friendship with the visionary artist Pablo Amaringo began, and where I met the urban ayahuasquero don Laurencio Paredes, who is the father of Dimas Paredes, one of don Pablo's students.

Don Pablo Amaringo

To have met and been don Pablo Amaringo's friend was a great joy and blessing, one I will be forever thankful to have had. The legacy of his visionary art coupled with his tremendous insights made known through his two books, along with his magnanimous personality, have enriched my life and the lives of so many others. Long after he quit drinking ayahuasca, he exemplified the urban ayahuasquero tradition of using the plant medicines to heal people effectively and with the true spirit of dedicated service in the ever-changing conditions of modern urbanization. The following is just a small glimpse into his spiritual attainments and his unfailing generosity.

When Pablo was still a teenager he ran into some trouble with the law after having used his artistic abilities to counterfeit money. His character was unformed and he was still weak, he told me. To evade incarceration he fled into the jungle. This was the beginning of the path that led to his six years alone in the wilderness.

Don Pablo's father had sent him to visit an elder maestro, an aya-huasquero who lived alone in a remote part of the forest. To Pablo's utter amazement, the maestro lived with two jaguars. Pablo did not notice them until later, when he walked into the forest at the edge of the patio to urinate. They were lying under the house. He stopped dead in his tracks. The ayahuasquero laughed and said not to fear, they would do him no harm. He had found them as cubs in the forest and raised them. Their mother must have been killed by hunters.

After some time living with the maestro, Pablo left for a dieta deeper in the forest, one that would occupy about six years of his life. During this time when he was alone in the wilderness he never once built a fire, nor did he see any people. He ate only roots, raw fruits and nuts from wild trees, vines, and leaves from bushes. He followed groups of animals, eating only what they ate. He followed peccaries, eating the fruits and nuts they ate and the roots they would dig up and eat. He followed flocks of parrots, feeding off what they would send to the ground from the canopy above. He slept mainly in the canopy of trees, always in different trees, as he was constantly on the move. Some nights he would sleep on the ground, and sometimes, so as not to get cold, he would sleep squatting (like Pirawa, the Waorani camp cook).

"The years passed in this way," don Pablo told me. "Eventually I learned to live in nature." A long pause led me to understand that this was a great feat, one arduously attained. "I became like a fish swimming through the currents," don Pablo went on solemnly. "The fish does not recognize the difference between itself and the currents. It is one with nature."

As a healer and person of spiritual merit, don Pablo was truly detached from the petty problems of life. Once he received a call from the local authorities. An impoverished woman who had many children and no husband had squatted on his property. (It was a jungle property that he hadn't been to in a while.) She found out from neighbors who the owner was, and placed a legal demand on him, saying that he was taking her property. In fact, it was she who was squatting on his property. He told me he was fond of the property; he had once lived there and grown food there. He had done some fasting there as well, and he even had a land title for the place, as it was relatively close to town. But seeing that she had so many children and was in need, he simply signed the land title over to her and walked away untroubled.

Laurencio Paredes and the Phoenix Encanto

A student named Dimas Paredes at Pablo's Usko Ayar School of Amazonian Painting was the son of a healer who lived a few blocks down the street in Pucallpa. Dimas invited my friend Matt and me to participate in his father's ceremonies. His father and a disciple drank the medicine three times a week. Since we were staying at don Pablo's home, it was important to receive his consent, I told Dimas. When I asked don Pablo if we could participate, we were encouraged to go. Don Pablo said that don Laurencio was one of the great local healers and that we would get a powerful firsthand view of urban ayahuasca shamanism.

The very next night we were at the shaman's home, ready to receive the medicine. We both marveled at how this opportunity had opened up for us. Neither Matt nor I went to Pucallpa looking to drink ayahuasca; we were planning to spend three weeks with don Pablo at his art school, learning and practicing painting.

Dimas introduced us to his father, who said little and sat there sternly. Dimas interrupted the silence, enthusiastically asking his father to show us his *encanto,* a word that means "enchantment." Don Laurencio, shrugging slightly, laughed some and leaned over to open a drawer, saying, "Ahh, yes." He retrieved an item and brought it closer for us to see. He held it in his hand; he would not place it in mine.

Dimas explained, "You don't know how lucky you are to even be seeing this."

In don Laurencio's open palm was a beautiful phoenix made of metal. Its long graceful tail feathers were extended backward, its face turned back to regard the tips of these regal plumes.

"Father," Dimas said, "bless them with your encanto. They are here to drink with you in the ceremony tonight. I have invited them. They are living with don Pablo."

"Open your arms," the master said, "and hold them outstretched to the side." He passed the charm over my back from head to foot, while blowing. I felt shivers going down my spine. Then he blessed Matt as well.

In don Laurencio's ceremony, the purge was strong. It shook me violently, peeling open in all directions with flying layers of light in piercing golden colors. Amidst the explosion of energy, I saw ruffled feathers, white, crisp, and very close to me. In an instant I had become a large guayacan tree *(Tabebuia serratifolia),* standing firmly. My arms outstretched were its branches, and on the branches sat eight squabbling scarlet macaws. As I realized that I was no longer me but a tree, in an explosion of screeching the macaws jumped off me, flying away with outstretched tail feathers. I returned to my senses and came out of the vision.

The ceremony concluded, and at nearly two in the morning the lights were turned on. The master's disciple whose name I never learned looked at me and said, "You saw." A smile was gleaming on his earnest face. I nodded. No words were needed. He knew what I had seen.

Many years later I received a letter from Dimas. He said his father had "left this physical plane." He was in his early nineties. Dimas wrote that for six months after his death, don Laurencio returned every night to teach his spiritual wisdom to his children and students. After that period of time, he let them know he was finished with his instruction, and he did not return.

Mr. Sun

"Mr. Sun" was my nickname for don Solon Tello. *Sol* means "sun" in Spanish (the urban language of Peru), and the syllable *-on* at the end of a word means "big," so his name can be interpreted to mean "great sun." The wordplay is apt: his was a generous, radiant way of being. Don Solon passed into the higher spheres in 2010 at an advanced age.

In Iquitos, Mr. Sun lived calmly. His urban setting on an inner-city street offered the sounds of motocars and a radio blasting from the neighbor next door. Many children were rushing about preparing for school and running out the door one morning when I arrived at his home. He was sitting on the porch in a rickety rebar rocking chair wound in plastic twine, smoking a fat *mapacho* cigarette made of strong native tobacco. We had met once before, when Kenneth brought me to his home one night for a ceremony.

As I sat there by his side I felt I was in the company of an old friend. The day went by quickly talking with don Solon, and we fasted on the days of a ceremony, only smoking some mapacho, which greatly helps one endure the all-day fast, but the tobacco must be black and properly cured. Western-style corporate cigarettes or even natural tobacco of another kind is not the same as the authentic mapacho (or masu, tobacco logs, as they are known in Ecuador). Sitting on his porch, we watched people walk by on the street, and our conversation oscillated between everyday occurrences and supernatural realities as we discussed world events in one moment and different kinds of spirits in the next. Don Rafael, his disciple, sat calmly by his side, nodding.

He told me about a goddess whose cloak is made of butterfly wings; then about the Llypian Yachai, a polka-dotted green octopus that wears a golden-yellow crown and has eyes of glass that can see everything; then about the Aceroruna ("steel people"), giant robot-like beings of celestial metal that hover in the air just above the tree canopy and are able to control the weather. These ayahuasca phenomena he saw and learned about from his teachers, great sages of the Lamista people, with whom he dieted for years as a student in the wilderness.

Mr. Sun shared with me, too, how his skilled master had many ways to help people. On one occasion during his initiation a notorious brujo was causing havoc and harming many people. Don Solon's master used the power of the volcano to cover up the visions of the sorcerer, rendering him harmless. Don Solon went on to explain that in the science of ayahuasca, when you can't see, you can neither harm nor heal. It requires many dietas and a rigorous training and initiation to learn to really see.

Afternoon came around and Mr. Sun's children and grandchildren returned from work or school, laughing and content. People cooked dinner and ate their meals; they all showered, one after the other, in the tiny stall just off the kitchen. The crowded but functional home consisted of several little bedrooms along one side, plus the kitchen, dining area, and front room. There must have been twenty people living there, yet the space was all well-kept and clean. There was hardly anything in the front room except for a table, and to my amazement a reproduction of one of don Pablo Amaringo's ayahuasca vision paintings on the wall. Don Solon commented, "He is our very own. I marvel at what my country has produced." He was proud to be Peruvian. Despite the poverty and hardships, he loved his country that he called the "motherland." He added, "This is a land of creative people."

Sometimes don Solon would travel. His friendships were diverse, and his good reputation was widespread.

Don Solon had eleven children, none of whom had learned the science of ayahuasca. In many ways, he said, he preferred that they not learn, as the path is simply too fraught with problems. He wanted his children to live simple and ordinary lives. Each has studied diligently, and now they have their own professions.

"To drink," don Solon noted, "is a beautiful thing. The challenge is to deal with the sorcerers who want to topple you. For this, you need to sleep with one eye open. In my heart, I have never had enemies. But others are jealous of your abilities, and they test you. This is the major problem. This is why I taught my children to study and to work. To become a healer and ayahuasquero is an innate calling: if you are meant for this path, you will follow it, no matter what others say, no matter the challenges you are obliged to undergo. That's how it was for me."

A charming and friendly woman well into her sixties attended to us marvelously and gave us a great breakfast after the fast and ceremony.

I took her for don Solon's wife, but she was actually his ex-wife, as she told me after I'd been living there for a few days. It hadn't worked out between them, she said, but she loved him like an uncle. His apprentice Rafael (who also lived in don Solon's house) was her brother. She invited me to meet her current husband. "He's over here," she said. Lo and behold, behind a curtain in the back of the kitchen was a whole separate section of the apartment. This section opened out to another street; in the middle, the two sections shared a kitchen. The man and I shook hands and smiled.

Back in don Solon's half of the house, several generations of people drifted around—husbands who had married don Solon's daughters, wives who had married his sons, each with their own little room where they slept with their children and babies. In the weeks that I lived in his house, I saw only joy and happiness and a willingness on everyone's part to be helpful, and to generally keep to their own space. Even though there were so many people there, it felt like there was always enough room! This was an amazing thing to witness, something that gave me some faith in humanity again.

The first time I met don Solon, I arrived late to his house. I had been invited by Kenneth to participate in his ceremony. Welcomed into his home just after dark, we shook hands and entered the kitchen, where we sat. Don Solon sat before his picture of Maestro Jesus, his sacred rocks, his bottle of Agua Florida perfumed water, and his bottle of ayahuasca, which he referred to as *purga*. Soon a small cup of brew was passed my way, and a soft voice began to rise up through the room, a whispering that strained our ears to hear; through this concentration I suddenly became utterly present. Don Solon's prayers were spoken with so much earnestness that I felt profoundly humbled to be in the presence of his ceremony and prayers. All the other participants seemed to feel the same.

Don Solon never failed to invoke Christ of Bagazán of the city of Iquitos, and el Señor de los Milagros, the name of Jesus associated with a miraculous painting venerated in Peru. At every session he had his bottle of camphor water and his mapacho cigarettes. After his prayers were made to *Dios todopoderoso* (God almighty), to the saints, and to the ancient masters, he would pray and bow to the four cardinal directions, then serve the purga. He would sing beautifully from the onset to the end of his ceremony, accompanied by rhythmic movements of the *shacapa* leaf fan (his was made of the aromatic plant ruta, *Ruta graveolens*). When someone needed to puke, they'd let it out on the shower floor that was off to the side of the kitchen. A large parrot perched on a stick in the kitchen was the continual witness of his ceremonies while the majority of his family slept in rooms nearby.

My friend and I left just after midnight, so I didn't imagine the social dynamics of his home at the time. Once don Solon invited me to live there with him, I began to see his family life. Watching him conduct his ceremonies in this setting sent questions racing through my mind. How could he hold ceremonies in such a crowded space in a city? How could he live with his ex-wife, and even more so with her new husband and their new kids? None of the complexity around Mr. Sun seemed to perturb the calmness of his mind—not the loud music from the apartment on the left, nor the loud and obnoxious motocars cruising by, nor the TV and radio blasting from the apartment on the right into late hours of the night, nor his wife's new husband or all the kids swarming around. At night when everything settled down, he would sprinkle holy water on the kitchen floor and lay out a woven palm mat. Out would come his portrait of Christ, his healing stones, his bottle of Agua Florida, and his revered bottle of purga, and like that the ceremony would begin.

He never rejected a patient and would heal at any hour of the day or night when needed. He worked for many years in the Takiwasi drug-addiction treatment center in Tarapoto, not far from Iquitos, helping to heal people. He was much loved there and become well known as a great healer for the effectiveness of his cures. He never prioritized his economic needs over his mission as a healer.

Rafael Tuesta Ríos Sees the Origin of Ayahuasca

At one point while we were talking, Rafael suddenly fell backward off his stool. It was just before dawn after an all-night ceremony. Like Saul on the road to Damascus, he dropped to the ground in awe and amazement. Finally the moment had come where he learned the origin of the great ayahuasca, not from the natives nor his beloved master, but from a wandering Jew, an *amigo gringo*. It happened when I shared the Waorani legend of the origin of miiyabu that Mengatue had told me. Rafael had not yet come down from the purga, and as I spoke he went into a profound trance and saw the legend occurring before his eyes. Thunderstruck, he fell backward. From the floor he cried out joyously, "Yes, that's it, that's how it was, I saw it, I saw it!" He was very happy, knowing with unshakeable certainty the origin of this sacred vine he drank with his master. Don Solon nodded in agreement. He hadn't heard of an origin for ayahuasca, and the story was convincing. (The story is told at the end of Chapter 7.)

Through such experiences our camaraderie grew and we spent some great times together. We visited the rainforest to learn about herbs, prayed in a local Catholic church, and discussed the nature of the universe and the things in it. To me, meeting these men was a great and humbling honor.

Rafael Is Visited by Christ and His Disciples

On my second visit to don Solon's house, I noticed that Rafael didn't drink the ayahuasca. Yet he joined don Solon in the ceremonies, and he would stay up all night with the master as well. During the second ceremony, he sang, though the previous time he had not; and he healed people as well, but why didn't he drink the medicine? I asked Rafael with all my respect what was going on.

He smiled and proceeded to share the following. "My maestro," he said, referring to don Solon, "was invited to accomplish healing work in Argentina, and while he was gone, Christ and all his disciples came to me. They called me 'son,' and they told me that I no longer need to drink the ayahuasca or smoke the mapacho. They also told me that when don Solon returned I was to join him in all his ceremonies, but without drinking or smoking. I was to stay up singing and healing the people, helping don Solon, and they would give me the energy to heal."

Don Solon was listening and he nodded in confirmation. "This happened to him," he said, then added a moment later, "but it didn't happen to me, so I still drink ayahuasca and smoke the mapachos."

Rafael did an amazing blessing for my trail before I left. And he told me, "If you ever have trouble, think of me. Call my name three times and visualize my face, and my spirit will always help you." I accepted this offer. Rafael continued, "So that my energy will pass into you, we must sleep side by side, with our arms interlaced. And here, use my pants rolled up as your pillow." Rafael's pants were old and funky blue jeans, and it was the only pair he had. I complied.

His life was simple. He would awaken at 4 AM and go to the market where he worked as a peanut vendor. Afternoons he spent in casual contemplation with don Solon, watching the people walk by. He had been studying with don Solon for more than forty years, and he sat next to the older man in most of his ayahuasca ceremonies, barely saying a word. Though he no longer drank la purga, Rafael continued to humbly and sincerely help don Solon accomplish his healing work. The example of such a life is beyond opinion or judgment of others.

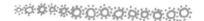

Don Casimiro Mamallacta, Seventh-Generation Keeper of a Sacred Mountain

In 1990 when I was volunteering at Jatun Sacha biological reserve on the Rio Napo, a place that protects a significant stand of Tropical Wet Forest, I met don Casimiro through his daughter Mercedez Mamallacta, who was working there at the time. Mercedez invited me to her home, where don Casimiro and I promptly became great friends. Suddenly and spontaneously, he was taking me on a two-day journey on foot into the wilderness region of Wachiurku and then on to the Pusuno River, at the base of the venerable Napo-Galeras Mountain. It was the first of many treks and epic adventures. This is one of them from 1994.

As described in the previous chapter, in the early 1990s I was working for the Rainforest Information Centre, known in Spanish as the Centro de Investigación de los Bosques Tropicales. This work came to include lobbying the various government institutions, such as the Park Service and the Institute of Cultural Patrimony, to support us in gaining maximum protection for Napo-Galeras by officially designating it a national park. After many visits to the Institute's office in Quito to impress upon the staff the importance of this mountain, we managed to plan a trip to Galeras with one of the Institute's representatives, a man named Lenin Miño, who wanted to see the area firsthand (a requirement for the Institute's involvement). He and I traveled by bus to Archidona, where we arrived at don Casimiro's home. However, because we were a day late, don Casimiro had decided to set out alone. I enlisted Casimiro's son Benjamin and Benjamin's cousin Eduardo to guide us and catch up with him.

That afternoon we reached the spot where Casimiro had camped the previous night; sure enough, he had left that morning. The next morning we set out early, hoping to find him at the Pusuno River camp some eight hours' walk ahead, where he always went to fish and enjoy the solemnity of non-trampled nature. When we reached the effervescent, jade-green Pusuno River, we were sure we'd see him there, but no, the old man had decided to hike all the way to the mountain's summit, as originally planned, with or without us.

Miño, the bureaucrat from Quito, had been complaining since the beginning of the trip. Uncertain of our destination, he kept insisting that we turn back. We just kept saying, "We're on a mission now and won't return until it's rightfully concluded."

Every other time I had come to the Pusuno River, don Casimiro had been with me. In the previous few years I'd made at least a dozen visits to his favorite camp. I too had fallen in love with this sacred place, two full days' trek out of Archidona, where the clear bubbling river flows through chasms and over flat, exposed faces of the mountain's limestone floor. The deep tranquility of the rainforest with all its mysterious nocturnal sounds had me always looking forward to returning. I greatly enjoyed walking softly across this virgin land, soaking up each felt moment of life's original natural glory.

We left don Casimiro's camp by the river and continued on his trail to the summit. Here the magnificent forest has yet to be altered by the hand of people; it flourishes in its original splendor as the Great Spirit made it: towering trees, thick hanging vines, mosses moist from the heavy rainfall and constant mist, life growing upon life growing upon life. We continued to climb up the mountain's increasingly steep, slippery slopes. In places, fragrant blossoms from large trees filled the air with deep aromas carried upon breezes that sifted the fragrance through the canopy. Along high ridges we walked, then down and across steep ravines, to find that don Casimiro had camped the previous night high up on a slope, a most uncomfortable spot. Apparently when night had fallen he simply stopped where he was and slept. We camped there as well. He had left that morning and we arrived late that afternoon.

It rained on us in the night, and we awoke early to ascend even higher up into the wilderness of the sacred mountain. That day we were blessed with good weather. The sun shone through the trees, and shafts of light streaked across the forest floor. Miño finally stopped complaining, stunned by the sheer beauty of the wilderness. Flowering bromeliads splattered globs of light, and it felt as though we were in the painting of a great master. The mosses and leaves here take on tones of lilac, purple, rusty orange, and mustard yellow, and of course many, many shades of green. We arrived at the top of a large ridge, near the mountain's summit, where the trail then dropped steeply into a deep ravine and passed through a cave tunnel.

It was evident that don Casimiro had come down this way, but when we reached the cave, we found that a recent landslide had blocked its mouth with a large boulder, and it seemed impossible to pass. We realized that we needed to climb back up the steep valley slope to take another trail. At this point Miño's exhaustion trumped his exhilaration, and he began to complain again. After about an hour of backtracking and looking for Casimiro's trail, we had to conclude that he must have passed through the cave after all. So we returned. This time we inspected more carefully. Sure enough, where the water flowed out there was a large boulder blocking any possibility of our passage, but to the left, amidst the darkness, there was a tunnel, which we followed. We ducked down, walked into the creek, and squeezed through a low passage where the roof of the cave came only a few feet from the surface of the water. Then we climbed up to a large rock and crept through another opening to find ourselves in a giant cathedral-like cavern that opened out onto the forest. There, at the grand opening of the cave, silhouetted against the darkening twilight, standing upon a large round boulder under an arch that extended some 16 meters high, was don Casimiro.

We were very happy to see him, and he was surprised and happy to see us too. We made camp there on a ledge overlooking the mouth of the huge cave. Screeching oilbirds *(Steatornis caripensis)*, called *tayos* in Spanish and *cacapischku* in Kichwa, went in and out the mouth of the chasm, clumsily flying around some nests low to the ground alongside the wall of the cavern; they are among the only birds known to use echolocation, habitually foraging for palm fruits at night. I watched in mesmerized silence, beholding the tremendous beauty and mystery before me.

Our companion from the institute had seen enough to be thoroughly convinced of the need to conserve Napo-Galeras. He informed us that although he would have to leave the following day, he intended to get the full support of the Institute for Cultural Patrimony to protect this place.

Around the campfire that night, don Casimiro shared legends of the mountain. He told how his grandfather found this cave by following a troupe of monkeys, then returned frequently, using the place for ritual fasting, gaining strength, and clarifying wisdom.

In the morning we visited a waterfall that cascaded down over limestone cliffs, glowing yellow. The colors were most intriguing, completely unlike those in the lower forest. Rare and endemic plants blanket the massif, a unique quality permeates everything, and it is easy to see why indigenous peoples from at least three separate communities, the Kichwa, Secoya, and Waorani, consider Napo-Galeras sacred.

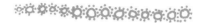

Amazanga Community: Flavio Santi, Taita Rafael, and Mama Lucila

Not long after returning to Ecuador from California in 1990, I was staying at the apartment of the Rainforest Information Centre. One day a fellow arrived there, and he looked at me for a good while. Then he said, "*Disparo.*" This was a nickname I had received many years earlier.

My birth name is actually Sparrow. I started going by Jonathon when I lived in New York and attended a public grade school in the Bronx, where everyone teased me about my name. It is also hard for Ecuadorians to pronounce. When I was a kid growing up in Quito, a lot of friends called me Ésparo, because in Spanish a word beginning with an "s" often automatically acquires an extra "e." *Disparo,* meaning "gunshot," was a variation of this, indicating my inclination to be straightforward and unhesitant.

In those days, my parents were running a vegetarian restaurant, the first of its kind in Quito; it was also a cultural center and a bookstore. The establishment was named Hojas de Hierba after the book *Leaves of Grass* by the great and most forthright poet Walt Whitman (1819–1892), who wrote,

> The armies of those I love engirth me, and I engirth them,
> They will not let me off till I go with them, respond to them,
> And discorrupt them, and charge them full with the charge
>   of the Soul.[2]

So Flavio Santi recognized me from those days, and now I recognized him too. We had both changed a lot in the past eight years. We'd met when I was eleven years old, and then again at age thirteen. Both times my mother had sent me on a journey with a botanist friend of hers. I accompanied him on these two occasions to visit the Santi family when they lived at Rio Chico outside Puyo. I helped the botanist collect plants and played with the kids, including Flavio, who remembered me using the family's long blowgun to pole vault.

Mama Lucila was still a mainstay of the community, with her unconditional devotion as a midwife. The people maintain a community garden of medicinal plants.[3] The family's stories brought me back to my first impressions of the jungle. The botanist and I got there late after a two-day bus ride that we broke up by spending a night in Baños. In those days there weren't the giant tunnels they've now blasted through the rock, and the bus ride from the mountains down to the Amazon was treacherous—so much that the buses in Baños would stop at the church and have the priest put holy water in the radiator! We got to Puyo late and hiked in the gathering dusk toward the village where the Santi family lived. (In those days, they lived at a place called Rio Chico, and later they moved to a new location and began calling the new community Amazanga, after the spiritual protector of the rainforest.)

We had left the asphalt of Quito and the shiny cobblestones of Puyo's rained-on streets for the mud of the trail. It was deep because it had been raining hard. Soon I was covered head to toe in mud. We came to a place where a horse had gotten stuck in the mud, and people were trying to get it out. We helped, digging for a long time to no avail. Then the horse died. This event left a strong impression on me—the presence of the jungle in all its unexposed power, crude and unhindered.

Grandfather Yu Heals Himself from Being Shot by a Stray Bullet

Rafael Santi told me about his father, Virgilio Yu, a Shuar warrior and fully graduated old-school master healer. In his youth, the following occurred. There was an intertribal tiff going on between the Kichwa and Shuar. Yu was standing atop a cliff overlooking a river. Suddenly, out of nowhere, he was hit by a stray bullet on the back of the neck. The force of the shot knocked him over the cliff and he landed in the river, limp. At the bottom of the river he opened his eyes to see many underwater creatures coming to him. There was the anaconda, the river dolphin, the turtle, and large fish of many types, as well as the electric eel and caiman. They started kissing him and moving their lips over his body. He heard gunshots above him and could see the underside of the water.

He reached the rapids. Gasping for air, he pulled himself over to a crevice between the rocks. The gunfire had stopped. Where he lay was a *guanduc* bush, a wild *Brugmansia* growing along the river. Yu drank infusions of it for five days. Then he walked home, basically unharmed. Rafael attests that there was a scar on his neck where Yu had been hit, but it was like an old healed wound. Yu lived for many years after that, to a great age; he was well over a hundred years old when he died, his relatives attest.

Virgilio Yu fought for his people's land rights, being the accomplished shaman that he was. Where the church of Puyo stands today is where his ceremonial lodge once stood. In the cemetery his grave is insignificant, the tombstone's epitaph painted by hand. It reads, "Here rests Virgilio Santi Yu, the founder of the city of Puyo."

Reclaiming Grandfather Yu's Sacred Grounds

Upon being reunited with the Santi family, I was amazed and inspired by this community's self-determination and aspirations to cultural revival and rainforest conservation. Flavio, his younger brothers and sisters, and Taita Rafael and Mama Lucila had organized many cultural gatherings, granting opportunities to youth to be with elders and learn the traditions. I joined the educational effort.

It was and still is a turbulent time for many developing communities. Many local people have simply sold out, colluded, or caved in to Western influences, seeing themselves as powerless to resist and no longer having a viable alternative. They accept jobs carrying out non-sustainable activities—cattle ranching, oil development, logging—and the rainforest becomes a wasteland around them. Some communities, though, are reverting to nonviolent civil disobedience in order to demand that the Ecuadorian government not allow oil prospecting on their land, such as in the victorious case of the Kichwa community of Sarayaku on the Bobonaza River, in Pastaza Province.

In 1991, oil companies were attempting to build a road into the headwaters country of the Amazon extending outward from Puyo. Many communities farther inland wanted the road, and local people were employed in the seismic operations (in which holes are drilled and dynamite then inserted and detonated; the echo that returns is studied because it may reveal the presence of a field of oil underneath). Further in, though, a community on the Bobonaza River called Sarayaku has been using all its intellectual wit and savvy skill to successfully defend themselves against the unwanted intrusion of the oil companies. To date (2013) they have been successful.

Back in 1991, the companies needed permission from the Santi family to enter and cross a ±100,000-acre area to which they had just received title from the progressive government of Ecuadorian president Rodrigo Borja, so the Santis were under a lot of pressure. Rafael had held strong in his family's resistance despite receiving many visits by oil representatives offering goods, money, and assistance; he accepted none of this. His two brothers, in debt and finding no way out, signed and agreed. Rafael did not, and this caused a family feud.

Then a terrible incident happened. At a meeting in a neighboring community, a stranger suddenly walked up to Rafael, lifted a knife, and stabbed him, plunging the blade deep into his chest. Rafael jumped back and the puncture wound missed his lung by a millimeter. His wife was there and helped him, and others intervened as well; the would-be assassin disappeared as mysteriously as he had appeared. Rafael was quickly brought to the local hospital. "Thank God," the doctor said, "he moved out of the way in the nick of time." While Rafael was recovering, the oil companies moved in with the permission of his brothers, who had sold out for a ridiculously low amount. There was nothing Rafael could do. The road went in, and the companies started drilling in their beloved lands of San Virgilio east of where Amazanga is today.

A great portion of their ancestral lands had already been colonized, and land title had proven a double-edged sword. This was, of course, something that the people had no way to know in advance, having been cheated and lied to again and again. By receiving the land title, they had unknowingly forfeited the subsoil rights, which the government maintains for all titled land. On the other hand, land title makes evident at ground level the limits of a particular territory, so the inhabitants can know what is rightfully theirs and defend it against colonization. Given all that has been occurring to these people since the turn of the twentieth century, a land title is for the most part considered a step in the right direction.

After this, Taita Rafael and his family decided to abandon the territory of San Virgilio, and they left, never to return. They dropped all claims to this land—just left it there in the hands of destiny. Flavio told me that was when he was in the process of researching his family roots, and he'd learned that his grandfather Yu had fasted and trained to be a shaman in the hill country above San Virgilio territory. A Shuar relative told him that Yu had fasted in an area where there were two small lakes up on a ridge, and he took him there. It was on the other side of the Pastaza River, overlooking the mighty Llushin River. Flavio saw his grandfather's guayusa tea trees. The land was now owned by a humble colonist who was trying to raise some cattle. The colonist told him if he was interested in buying the land, he wanted to move. His chickens all died and nothing went well for him there, he said. Having now learned some of the history of the land, Flavio was interested. He asked if I'd help raise the money.

I agreed, with the idea of organizing a tour, since I didn't own a large bank account. I thought we could collect the money for the property from the tour proceeds. This was the first Sentient Experientials retreat to the Ecuadorian Amazon (a multifaceted adventure by all standards). The location was a beautiful blackwater lake known in

Paicoca as Puñujaira. The Kichwa call it Pañacocha. Both names mean "piranha lake."

This was 1996 and I had already been working for a year with the Secoya, while continuing to spend time with the Santi family. I invited the Secoya leaders to the retreat because Puñujaira had been part of their ancestral lands. It is now a biological reserve managed by Kichwa people. Sadly, oil prospecting has caused major damage to this beautiful Amazonian ecosystem, but in 1996, the area was still remote wilderness. I also invited Moi and some of his Waorani relatives to the gathering. Taita Rafael and his healer Taita Herbacio Machoa were there. We rented the comfortable Pañacocha Lodge, and a mix of guests from North America and Europe joined to experience the area with newly made Secoya, Waorani, and Kichwa friends.

One afternoon on a forest walk we came across a deer only recently killed by a jaguar. It smelled strongly of urine and was covered in leaves, a habit of cats who plan to return later to eat. We also found abundant large yoco vines, and we rasped some and drank of this powerful energizer. We found the rare and medicinally potent, clove-scented and rubefacient clavohuasca (*Tynanthus panurensis*) and drank an infusion of its bark to enliven the body. Meanwhile, some of the Secoya had been fishing in the lake and shared with us upon our return.

One day after a long walk I realized I had lost my watch. Herbacio offered to find it and backtracked swiftly into the forest alone. Amazingly, he followed our trail back and found it. He sang wonderfully in the ceremonies and healed everyone including the Secoya. It was a grand event. From the modest tuition fees gathered, the Santi family was able to purchase the first property (of many since added) in the Llushin River area that is today maintained as a biological reserve. The Amazanga community calls the purina tambu *El Bosque Eterno de Los Niños*, the Eternal Forest of the Children, currently encompassing 2,800 acres of tropical premontane rainforest from 800 to 1,400 meters in elevation. The reserve can be visited with the Santi family, who are the caretakers. This preserve honors the purina tambu of Grandfather Yu, where he fasted and prayed and learned to be a healer.

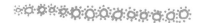

Stories of the Old Waorani Warriors

Putting Down the Spear

The experiences I had while working on the demarcation of the Waorani territory and visiting their communities left indelible memories, as well as profound insights into the nature of existence and our place in this life.

A charismatic Waorani elder and grandfather named Wepe Coba was one of the last to live far downriver, in the heart of the Amazon, and he adopted me as a son. He always called me Ñame, which is just a common Waorani personal name.

As I was editing this chapter in 2013, I received an email from a friend who works with the Waorani: "Wepe died." The old man left to walk along the forest path in the awakened afterlife. In the '90s when I worked with the Waorani on the demarcation lines, I calculated Wepe's age at approximately mid-eighties. His sons would often chant about the "green men"—how they, their father, and the other Waorani defended their territory from Peruvian soldiers in 1942. I figured that if the youngest son was of age to go on spearing raids, about fifteen years old, then Wepe would have been at least thirty-five at the time. This would mean he was at least 105 when he died in 2012.

There could be an entire book written about Wepe. He participated in many spearing raids in the 1960s and killed many people. In about 1973, an evangelist named Toña, who was the first Waorani to become a missionary, was sent into the jungle to talk to Wepe. I got to hear the story firsthand from Wepe himself, who told it laughing with gusto. Here's my retelling:

Toña came to the village, saying, "I've come to speak of the word of God." Wepe said, "I know about Memehuengongi, Grandfather Creator." He tried to tell Toña the Waorani legends of the Creator—insisting that the Waorani already knew everything he was trying so urgently to bring.

"But he didn't want to listen to me," Wepe said. "He just wanted me to listen to him." So Wepe asked Toña, "Where are your ears?"—questioning why he didn't have the holes with balsa plugs in his earlobes like all traditional Waorani. "Just because you can speak Waorani doesn't mean I can trust you, or that what you can teach me is what I can hear."

He said that Toña wore a golden watch, and he asked him, "What's that thing on your wrist?" Toña also had short hair. "I think you're not a Waorani," Wepe concluded. "I'll listen to you only if you can make a good spear, the way the ancestors made spears."

They went out to the forest and chopped down a chonta palm to make a spear. Wepe watched him, and started urgently calling out, "This guy's not making the spear right. That's not the way we make spears! This is the Devil!" He lifted his axe and chopped Toña to pieces. He came back to his family clan hut with Toña's hand, complete with gold watch, saying, "Don't worry, people. I've killed the Devil. We can all go on fine now," and he threw the hand with the watch in the river.

Wepe told me that story laughing and laughing. I sat there quietly just listening. I knew that the village of Toñampare had been named after Toña. Toñampare is where the missionaries from the Summer Institute of Linguistics were based.

Wepe told me that he realized he could not go on killing people like he had. He only wanted to secure safety for his children, to not see their land get ravaged by the destruction of the couode. He made an oath to put his spear down forevermore. He told me his urge to kill was like a spirit grabbing him on the back. He resisted many temptations, many deeply felt urges to run and spear the invading couode, as he had done so many times in the past. He told me he held strong to his oath, and like a gust of wind the spirit that had him crazed lifted off his back. After that Wepe never had the urge to kill anyone. No matter how painful it was to see the loss of his lands and the changes that are upon them, he never again reverted to the old ways of the warrior.

The oldest Waorani I knew, Wepe once said to me, "The only Waorani law is, never get used to anything."

A First Impression Can Only Be Made Once

The Waorani take very seriously first impressions and things that happen immediately upon the arrival of a visitor. I must have been destined to spend a little time with the Waorani, because the first time I walked into Wepe's hut, a strong and robust baby boy was born—the exact moment I walked in, he plopped out. This was taken as a positive sign, and immediately I was like family!

Wepe fed me like a king, bestowed spears on me, and taught me how to make oomae (dart poison). He gave me a protection dance and song to practice, and crafted me armbands with his own hair woven in and a spectacular crown made of the chest feathers of the blue-and-yellow macaw *(Ara ararauna),* backed with an elegant puff of fluffy white harpy eagle chest feathers.

All Life Is Sacred

I'll never forget a particular moment with Grandfather Wepe. He and I went to chop wood at the edge of his garden. A small, somewhat frail butterfly was attempting to land on what was left of a decrepit little flower. Old Wepe found this a hilarious scene and began laughing from the bottom of his gut. The laughter was contagious, and soon I was laughing too. Then when the butterfly managed to land on the flower, we fell on the ground and rolled around, holding our stomachs, we were laughing so hard. After a while it actually became painful, but neither of us could stop laughing. Finally we stumbled back to his hut like a pair of old drunks, arm in arm, drunk on life, holding each other up, unable to stop laughing. Wepe was not teaching, he was just being himself, but to me this was a profound and penetrating teaching. Life is everywhere—even what looks pitiful is infused with it, and all of it is sacred.

Mengatue: An Ant at Times, and Other Times a Jaguar

On my first visit I brought Mengatue a chicken as a gift, and when I handed it to him, it instantly dropped an egg into his hand. It was a funny coincidence—a baby had been born in Wepe's hut when I first went there, and now a chicken laid an egg when I arrived at Mengatue's house.

Mengatue was a shaman, an *iroinga* in Waorani parlance. Traditionally, the *iroinani* (plural) served as communication mediums, transmitting messages to other iroinani in distant villages. They instigated spearing raids when, with the aid of the Jaguar Guardian, they detected the presence of invaders in their territory. The Waorani shamans are strong at every level of their being. They also are the most humble people. Everyone constantly gives them the heaviest loads to carry and the hardest work to do and they do it without thinking, for they can handle immense pressure.

I remember one time a little kid laughed and pointed at Mengatue from behind as he lay in his hammock. "Watch this!" he whispered to me. He crept up with a lighter that he had somehow gotten hold of, and lit the back of Mengatue's hair on fire. A whole bunch of it went up in flames. Mengatue jumped up, laughing his brains out, just splitting his sides laughing, and everyone else started laughing too. Kids are always testing the elders to see if they'll get upset or angry—that's how they help them to maintain their purity. The wise ones never get angry and have to be laughing, rolling around in joy. When he wasn't laughing, Mengatue would lounge around, looking off into space, dreaming.

Coincidence or Synchronicity?
An Urban Encounter with Mengatue

The Waorani elders and friends lived in remote rainforest territories in Napo and Pastaza provinces, in the villages of Queweiriono and Qiwaro—places that can only be accessed via airplane from the jungle town of Shell, or by long treks along narrow rainforest paths, which is how I would get there. Qiwaro, where Wepe lived, is more remote. It took us four days to walk across the territory to arrive. Queweiriono, where Mengatue lived, is two days' foot travel from Yurallpa (on the Napo), or several days' travel up the Shiripuno River, accessed by the Via Auca, the oil road that runs south from Coca.

In 1994 I had almost finished my participation in the demarcation project. I hadn't been to Queweiriono in a long time, but had been working elsewhere, and I'd taken a bus to Archidona to visit don Casimiro. To my great surprise, right there when I got off the bus were Mengatue and his wife Conta. I could not believe that they were here, far from their rainforest territory.

I greeted them in Waorani, "*Waaponi, pomonipa!*"

The shaman was overjoyed and hugged me. "*Buto wawa,*" he said, "*buto wawa,*" "my son, my son," half in Waorani (*buto* means "my") and half in Kichwa (*wawa* is "child"). We laughed and I asked him if he had his penis tied up even under his shorts. He peeled the edge of his shorts down to show me that indeed he was wearing the Waorani *gumi*, the traditional clothing that consisted of a cotton band and nothing more.

Mengatue and Conta said they had been waiting for me but had just arrived a few minutes before my bus. Their daughter was married to a Kichwa, he explained. It had been years since they last saw her and they wanted to see her again.

As mentioned above, in between trips into the forest to demarcate the Waorani territory, I lived at the house of don Casimiro Mamallacta on the outskirts of Archidona. Mengatue had remembered this, and this is where he heard his daughter was living, so they had decided to come look for her and hoped that they would find me so I could help. Their plan was off to a good start, because they had found me immediately.

I brought them to don Casimiro's house, where the family was amazed by these old Waorani and our friendship. Mengatue sang powerfully at don Casimiro's house, and everyone sat perfectly quiet, listening.

Sadly, though, neither don Casimiro nor anyone in his family had heard of a Waorani woman living with a Kichwa man in their region. The next day we left and asked around town at different stores, but no one seemed to know. Mengatue asked me to help him and his wife get back home. He said if I could get them to Yurallpa they would be very thankful.

To avoid paying for a hotel that night, we took a bus to Jatun Sacha biological reserve and education center, where I was friends with the administrators. I had volunteered there and also brought them seeds from the different rainforest places I found myself in. Sure enough, they were happy to give us a cabin to crash in, and they invited us to dinner as well.

A group of students from the United States was visiting the reserve and soon we were all talking. Their instructor could not believe the company I had with me, and our casual relationship. They had many questions for Mengatue and his wife. I translated. Of course my Waorani is basic, but somehow I was able to understand a lot, partly from the energy transmission and partly from the sincerity of their expression and generous use of body language and facial gestures. The other guests asked Mengatue about his life and he responded joyously. I introduced him as a Waorani jaguar shaman at the level of someone like Geronimo or Red Cloud or Black Hawk, explaining some of what this meant. He had fought valiantly against the intrusion, but knew when to surrender, and now you see him today, content and in good health at a ripe old age. At the time he was at least in his late sixties, a number I reached based on his participation in fighting off Peruvian soldiers in 1942.

Mengatue chanted for us, and the students were mesmerized. He spoke to them about his life—how he had two children who were jaguars, who hunted for him. They left meat for him to eat behind certain logs, and when he needed to travel fast they would let him ride on their backs. He himself, he went on, could transform into a jaguar if he liked, or into an ant, when he wanted to walk up close to see something. He was concerned about the last uncontacted clans, hoping they would never give in; it was really sad, he said, to see how people are killing nature.

I asked him to share about healing. Mengatue related how he had transplanted a spider monkey bone into a Waorani youth's leg that had been splintered by a falling tree. I had met this young man, who walked with a limp; he attested that, indeed, he had a monkey bone in his leg. He was given a new name after this operation: Ahuetai, meaning "the tree didn't fall." It seems as though the new name was given in order to nullify the event of the tree falling; or, possibly, though he was injured, perhaps he was symbolically the "tree that never fell." (It is not uncommon for the Waorani to view themselves as trees.)

"The oil companies," Mengatue pronounced, "are very, very bad. The Earth will cave into a deep chasm if this continues. Can't you see it will remain empty underneath? It is like sucking out all of a human's blood."

Then he started to recall an event that had happened at a nearby creek. Not far from where we were, he said, he had speared some of the couode, the outsiders who were invading these lands, which only thirty years earlier had been his. Everyone grew stone cold, and still.

Soon, though, he dispelled the intensity and had everyone laughing.

I explained that all this was part of their ancestral lands and that until the late 1960s they had fiercely defended this south bank of the Napo River. The Waorani wanted everyone to know that south of the Napo River no one was to cross. Brutal stories of spearing raids can be obtained from any of the settlers of this region who moved there between 1950 and 1960, and Mengatue was one of the main jaguar shamans who instigated and led many of these raids.

"We never wanted to kill," he said. "We did it only for our children. We were told to do so by the Jaguar Mother." He was referring to the ancestral protector deity of the Waorani people, the Meñeiriwempo.

He continued, "When we saw it wasn't going to help any more we stopped, and this is one reason the government is respecting us now: we have fought hard to keep what we now have. If the people respect our boundary line we will respect them as well. We want to live in peace."

The following day I rented a canoe from a local settler and brought Mengatue and Conta down to Yurallpa. It was hard to leave them there and return upriver, but there was something I needed to do. I wanted badly to go with them back to their rainforest home along the Shiripuno River, a place that really is like a glimpse of Heaven on the Earth.

The river runs green, the rolling hills are loaded with petohue palms heavy with edible fruits, and hunting is still abundant. We waved to each other as they slipped into the jungle like rocks into a river, and I forged my way back upstream, chilled by low-hanging clouds and the kind of drizzle that just goes on all day.

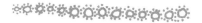

Torchbearers in the Darkness

Shining lights in life like these people show us how the divine immortal essence can appear in human form. By writing about them in this way, I do not mean to over-idealize my friends, since as human beings we all have virtues and flaws. But they have risen to the level of helpers, healers, and guides for humanity. Only when an individual can embody the highest values on a consistent basis can they also enter and strive to master the ultimate realms of celestial knowledge. Thus today while there are many ayahuasqueros, there remain few masters of the ancient spiritual science.

Often living simple and humble lives, lineage holders of these ancient ways tend to teach by their soft-spoken, selfless examples more than anything else, including their ways of experiencing and responding to each moment. Yes, they are experts on the sacred who (like secular professionals) have worked and suffered for the sophisticated knowledge they now possess, but they know that such spiritual knowledge and capability are intrinsic to our original human nature. We are all capable of touching or knowing intimately the other realities alongside this one. And we all must rise to the highest human standards of behavior and relationship, which is the important work and the only path to ultimate happiness, and to greater and greater knowledge, health, creativity, and success. Through their example, these torchbearers have taught me to prioritize service to others and the Earth and to view generosity, service, and an even temperament under any circumstance as golden objectives of human character formation.

To our detriment, many of us tend to assume the superiority of

Western knowledge, despite our science's denial of a spirit world capable of filling human life with meaning and ever-unfolding and ever-deepening mystery. Given the current state of global affairs, we need for our own edification to return to nature and recognize natural wisdom, respect elders and ancient ways, and see nature herself as the teacher. Learning to adapt to the environment and to situations that arise without complaining, always finding the positive solutions and bringing things about in a positive fashion—these are ways of following what nature teaches.

In my opinion, the ancient Chinese teaching of Tao parallels the ancient truth upheld by the original Amazonian torchbearers. The two traditions reflect each other, enabling us to better understand the essence of each. Both teach that it is necessary to perceive truth with the heart, not just the mind. The Taoist tradition and the indigenous scientific method of the Amazon share the same cardinal features of the universal culture of service as a path of spiritual development, as revealed in the oral tradition of Amazonian peoples and the example of their most respected leaders, and in the timeless classics of the Taoist canon. This diverse body of ancient writings offers us a glimpse into original human essence, granting tools for navigating through life in any era, and it illuminates the subtleties of indigenous science and other truth-seeking methodologies. Refining one's energy level and gathering more and more subtle energy is at the root of the indigenous science. In this way one can best serve others.

CONCLUSION

As you may imagine after having read this far, each chapter in *Rainforest Medicine* could be expanded to the length of its own book. I'm able to offer only a small sampling of this profound wisdom tradition, with its aim to know through experience the normally invisible realms of spirit and consciousness that interpenetrate our three-dimensional reality. That's a pretty tall order for any science or path of knowledge, yet the plant sciences of the Amazon may fill it, along with the vast array of already contributed and "proven" (to Western science) health and healing applications of indigenous knowledge such as aspirin, quinine, and curare, to name a few.

What I share in this book is more than just a story or information that I consider relevant to our future on Earth. Contained within these pages are energy designs, intended to offer a form of protection to these sacred medicine ways. I hope the book transmits only the deepest respect this subject deserves, contributing in a small yet significant way to the documenting of the great ancestral sciences of the upper Amazon and to the preservation of traditional Amazonian medicine and the mighty rainforest itself. I have tried to portray a kaleidoscopic panorama of some of the myriad indigenous traditions from northwestern South America, including symbolic myths, intriguing rituals, ancient wisdom, and impressive healing arts. There are so many traditions, and each is distinct. The stories and practices shared in these pages are often specific to a clan or tribe and do not necessarily represent a widespread concensus mythology or way of life of all forest people.

I hope I have made my point about the scientific side of indigenous knowledge. These practices and the historical uses of plants deserve widespread and well-funded investigation for their proven healing ability and potential to grant spiritual insight. It could be said that the most exalted or sacred plant teachers help us humans navigate the space in which knowledge of many types can be obtained. The "truth" or value of experiential knowledge becomes evident in one's own life—whether and how it is enhanced or improved by the knowledge. The value of knowledge is multiplied when it can help or heal others as well.

What I have shared here is but a miniscule fraction of the great body of practical knowledge known to spiritually developed beings, shamans, and wisdom-keepers the world over, who for millennia have conducted experiments to explore altered states of consciousness and gain the help of spirits to address problems of survival. The cross-cultural similarity of many of these techniques lends credence to their universal applicability. They are similar because they work. Curious people everywhere continue to carry out experiments and pass on the results to others, with plants, techniques of hunting and animal husbandry, and working with spirits and the mind. This is the ongoing process of expanding individual and human knowledge.

Don Pablo explained to me how he used ayahuasca as a tool in order to apply rigorous scientific scrutiny to understand the truth of this existence. In *Ayahuasca Visions* he writes, "It is only when the person begins to hear and see as if he were inside the scene, not as something presented to him, that he is able to discover many things. There is nothing that he is not able to find out. I saw how the world was created, how everything is full with life, how great spirits intervene in every aspect of nature and make the universe expand. I was like a tourist, always asking the spirits what is this and that, asking them to take me from one place to the other, demanding explanations for everything. The world is multifaceted, so mysterious and unfathomable that it is beyond imagination. I also understood that human beings will never be happy until they realize their connection with the Creator and the spiritual dimensions."[1]

"Shamanic" experiences are available to all of us, especially once we realize that everything is a spirit. We can tune in to visions, dreams, stories, physical experiences, synchronicities, messages from nature. Tragic, challenging, and unusual circumstances often open doors to new perspectives and knowledge, but opening the mind is the first important step. Anyone can engage and transform the self; we all have wisdom within and a capacity for imagination. We can experience life beyond the confines of enculturation.

Ayahuasca can reveal realms of consciousness and also heal many physical ailments and illness, even so-called terminal ones, but this may not be possible entirely on its own. These cures can be accomplished when the plant medicine is combined with the advanced mastery of the graduated or adept drinker, who as a result of a lifetime of earnest spiritual training and practice, using methods handed down from generations of devoted masters, is able to associate with powerful healing spirits and to direct energy appropriately. This is where our Western pharmacology is often divorced from its energetic origins and the mastery of human healers.

Participants in ayahuasca ceremonies report a wide range of experiences, with a common theme of personal healing, however that occurs for each individual. People might have wracking emotional catharsis, or less intense yet emotionally loaded thoughts and feelings that provide insight into one's tendencies and relationships. They might have beatific and loving thoughts and visions and feelings, reinforcing the unity of all life and all times. It's possible to make new mental connections and to glimpse better ways to live one's life, respecting the natural world around us and the lives of other beings. Often people are motivated to find ways to serve others and important causes. Sometimes they realize how they can best accept a situation, how to be with pain and sadness. The medicine has many times led to healing when Western medicine or therapy proved inadequate. It's a nature-given means of expanding one's consciousness and notion of self, and creating possibility.

With its extension of experience beyond ordinary consciousness, ayahuasca lets us merge the everyday world of human beings with the limitless and profound celestial realms. This gift includes a state of grace that lingers and resonates long after the visionary experience itself. The vision vine is a portal to mortal experiences of the grandeur, power, and mystery of the universe.

The concept of plant communication and even teaching contradicts our established modes of knowledge in the West, and it's unfortunate that we have no cultural placeholder for experiences of this type. Not only are they undervalued, they are denigrated and made illegal. It's past time to expand our belief systems in the West, because beliefs and definitions can limit what's possible.

Maybe we just need to honor and reincorporate older methods of apprehending reality directly. Many writers have theorized that psychotropic plants are an original source of human spiritual experience, and thus of animism, religion, and shamanism. While this may be true, it's important to note that the plant-medicine sciences of the Amazon—like most shamanic practices the world over—were developed as a methodology not a religion. Because time-tested shamanic methods are proven to work for physical and mental healing as well as spiritual development, we in the West have in recent decades exhibited a rise of interest in shamanic practices and the potential for modern applications. While many open questions exist, such as how to proceed with the loss of so much traditional cultural context, and how to guide transmission of the Amazonian science to Western students and patients, people the world over are working with traditional healers to access their wisdom and far-reaching knowledge. Many of us are hungry for it, embracing it both as patients and practitioners. The treatment of illness (both physical and mental) at a spiritual and energetic level continues to deliver its millennia of healing results into the present. The Grandmother Medicine, ayahuasca, is certainly part of this cross-cultural exchange.

Grandmother Medicine is wise and powerful. Perhaps the plants themselves are catalyzing new opportunities for survival of their wisdom as well as their rainforest home, and maybe us too! How? Through ceremonies everywhere that inspire and imprint the experience of oneness and connection on a personal basis—no longer only in a jungle setting but all over the Earth. This ayahuasca experience is currently in fashion but it is sometimes ungrounded in tradition. This book seeks to present some of that tradition as a necessary context for working with the medicine.

We can act as medicine for the rainforest if we grasp ayahuasca's message of oneness and help preserve the great treasures of the Amazon and the Earth. This task is urgent. Industrial globalization threatens the very existence of the forest and the botanical knowledge that could provide so many solutions.

Ayahuasca too is in danger of being integrated into Western consumer patterns and economic laws. Drug tourism is a big new business in the Amazon. Will the medicine become another mass-market item divorced from its traditional origins and incapable of providing the benefits we seek? We can see how the tradition in its contact with Westerners balances precariously on the edge of being a ceremony facilitating true communion with spirit or a foolish form of entertainment and potential thrills, diluting the ritual aspect and missing the entire point. I'd like to quote Kathleen Harrison once again in regard to properly respecting the plant teachers and existing traditions:

> "I encourage those who are certain they want to experience these visionary states to turn to indigenous practices and guidance. The indigenous traditions that have used these plants for generations know how to explore these realms. I also encourage people to read. There's an extensive body of deeply informative literature that can be of great help in preparing for such experiences. Approaching these substances recklessly guarantees that there will be some casualties.
>
> "... There is no doubt that in the indigenous cultures that have dealt with these medicines for a long time, it's not always love and light. Those in our culture who choose to explore these realms need to take great care of the 'set and setting.' It is crucial to be in a place where you feel totally safe so that your consciousness can relax and go inside."[2]

While we cannot embrace Amazonian plant-medicine practices in exactly the same way it has been done for centuries, we can respect these ways and forge a new tradition and cultural synthesis. That is a worthy challenge and great adventure.

Don't forget that as powerful and beautiful as the medicine can be, every great shaman and achieved sage in any culture will agree that a particular substance is not essential in order for one to progress on the spiritual path. Ayahuasca and other sacred plants can reveal many things to us, yet ultimately they are not necessary. The culture of service is the centerpiece and foundation of this path of spiritual development and subtle scientific understanding that we call traditional Amazonian medicine. In the end it's all about getting beyond oneself and being able to help others.

One of the contemporary demands on our energies and an excellent arena for service is to awaken oneself and others to the need to shift to sustainability—to consider not only the needs of people but the needs of nature alike. Now is the time to nudge our dormant yet inherent abilities to trigger the unifying powers of the culture of service to enact positive change, standing ready to serve all of life's creation, in order to enact a life in reciprocity, balance, and harmony among all living beings. This is our planetary mission, and this must become our direction.

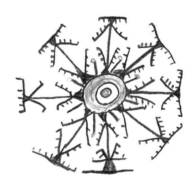

ENDNOTES

Preface

1. About the yutzu *(Calliandra angustifolia): Yacu yutzu* is a rather tortuous woody shrub with long outstretched branches. Its regal, flat-topped crown of slender small dark-green multifolate leaves stretches out over the river, and its thick mat of roots keeps a strong grip in the river's banks. Amid this great tumult of energy, the seeds of yacu yutzu sprout, thrive, and grow into impressive trees, the impenetrable tangle of their roots victoriously maintaining the fragile riverbanks. Sometimes communities of yacu yutzu will even establish themselves on seasonal islands in the river, and when the rainy season comes their trunks can be seen rising straight out of the rapids. This tumultuous environment is part of the "signature" that this plant is associated with and as such is perceived to give the qualities of tenacity and strength to adapt to life circumstances. Metaphorically, the power of a quickly rising river can take the form of illness, calamity, or conflict, and this is when the complementary physics embodied by this plant can help to protect one in the face of these energies. These are the kind of situations in which traditional elders must look to yacu yutzu. A once-common practice, yacu yutzu fasts have been largely uprooted by the process of acculturation to Western values and practices, to which the complex fasting sciences seem to be especially susceptible. Today, yacu yutzu fasts have fallen out of practice almost as swiftly as the flow of rivers on whose banks these hardy trees grow. The illustration shown here depicts a scene from the Kichwa legend of the Juri-juri, starting on page 250.

Chapter 1: Introduction to Indigenous Science in the Upper Amazon

1. Michael Harner, *Cave and Cosmos: Shamanic Encounters with Another Reality* (Berkeley, CA: North Atlantic Books, 2013), p. 199.

2. As a quick summary, human ceremonial use of yagé originates among the Tukanoan speakers of lowland Amazonia. The term "Tukanoan" denotes a language group. According to the Secoya people, the sacred science of yagé was first taught by the Ñañë Siecopai (God's

Multicolored People), progenitors of the Secoya way of life (that also inspired other tribes); it was given as a way by which people could retain their original nature, and thus to mirror heaven on Earth. From the other distinct tradition that can be called "the science of ayahuasca" we learn a different origin of the sacred plant that relates to having sprouted from the grave of the first Inca, Manko Cápac, so that his people would benefit from his knowledge. To learn about the variations of these traditions see Chapter 3, p. 58.

3. Harner, *Cave and Cosmos,* p. 49.

4. There seem to be different perspectives among yagé drinkers about the Pai'joyowatí. In his autobiography *The Yage Drinker,* Fernando Payaguaje describes this spirit as harmful, while Cesareo Piaguaje (also Secoya) explained to me that it is a great ally of the healer, being that it is the commander of the multitude of earthly spirits, collectively referred to as *Watí.* These spirits are considered to be responsible for all illnesses, with each Watí (of which there are thousands) having its own illness. The Pai'joyowatí can, upon request of the shaman, summon the corresponding Watí and request it to remove an illness. In Secoya spiritual science it is believed that all illness has a spiritual counterpart. There are several other powerful spirits that the gradu-ated and advanced drinker of yagé can invoke in order to aid him in accomplishing complex cures. To meet and befriend the Pai'joyowatí is an affair of advanced graduation-level ceremonies accomplished through the drinking of ancestral varieties of pejí (*Brugmansia sua-veolens* var.) carefully prepared according to strict guidelines. The master prepares the powerful pejí through specific incantations. This type of graduation ceremony is administered to only two students at a time. Knowledge of how to accomplish such feats is why many schol-ars have said: "When a shaman dies, so does an entire university of understanding."

5. To gain a deeper and parallel perspective see Ni Hua-Ching, Chapter 8, "The Integral Science of Ethics," in *TAO: The Subtle Universal Law and the Integral Way of Life* (Santa Monica, CA: Seven Star Communica-tions Group, Inc., 1993). From p. 101: "The fortune and misfortune in our lives is self-created and results from our ignorance and violation of the universal law of subtle energy response." On p. 103 Master Ni lays forth the intentions of an integral science: "The reality of ethics and physics are actually the same. The intention of the integral sci-ences is to demonstrate the identicalness of metaphysical and physical

phenomena, the oneness of the reality of spirit and the reality of matter, the oneness of spirituality and ordinariness in our lives. The human mind creates duality, but through integral knowledge and practices, one may reintegrate the apparent dualities in one's life and experience oneness."

6. Matilde Payaguaje, *Ñumine'eo: Mito y Cosmovisión Secoya* (Quito, Ecuador: Imprefepp, 2002), p. 154. Translated to English here by the author (JMW).

7. See Jeremy Narby, *The Cosmic Serpent: DNA and the Origins of Knowledge* (New York: Tarcher/Penguin, 1999).

8. Stellar energy rays are a certain type of energy arrangement that emanates from specific celestial regions and/or starry clusters, which according to the people's own stories, impel alignment with the traditional ways of life of the vastly diverse aboriginal peoples. These energy rays can be viewed as "arranging winds" or as a "celestial trail" and they are responsible for every part of the peoples' traditions—in Secoya they are called *Wiñapai ma'a* ("trail of the celestial immortals") or *toyá ma'a* ("the designs path") or *matëmo tutu* ("celestial winds"). When connection to these subtle energy rays is severed, the traditions are quickly lost. To maintain connection with these energy rays is the very purpose of the ceremonial life of the people, with communion made noticeable, even visible, through song and sacred invocations.

9. Anthropologist Laura Rival, personal communication, 1992. To learn more about the Waorani (also spelled Huaorani), read her works, which are a window into the pulsating heart of this tribe. Book titles include *Hijos del Sol, Padres del Jaguar: Los Huaorani de Ayer y Hoy* (Quito, Ecuador: Ediciones Abya-Yala, 1996); *Trekking Through History: The Huaorani of Amazonian Ecuador* (New York: Columbia University Press, 2002); and *The Social Life of Trees: Anthropological Perspectives on Tree Symbolism* (Oxford, UK: Berg Publishers, 1998). Laura Rival introduced the Waorani to the Rainforest Information Centre (an Australian-based nonprofit working in Ecuador), which subsequently worked with them to demarcate their legally granted homelands during the years 1990–1994. To learn more about the Waorani, other important books, written by Capuchin priest Miguel Angel Cabodevilla, are *Los Huaorani en La Historia de Los Pueblos del Oriente* (Coca, Ecuador: CICAME, 1994); *El Exterminio de los Pueblos Ocultos,* (Quito, Ecuador: Vicariato Apostólico de Aguarico, 2004); and with Randy Smith and Alex Rivas Toledo, *Tiempos de Guerra:*

Waorani Contra Taromenane (Quito, Ecuador, Ediciones Abya-Yala, 2004). Padre Alejandro Labaca, whose life was taken by a splinter group of Waorani in 1986, wrote *Crónica Huaorani*, published after his death by CICAME, Vicariato Apostólico de Aguarico, Quito, Ecuador, 1988). An English-language chronicling of the stark reality of the clash between industry and the rainforest people is Joe Kane, *Savages* (New York: Knopf, 1995).

10. *Jessenia bataua* is a primary rainforest palm; from its fruits a rich oily purplish drink is made. This highly nutritious palm is an important food source for indigenous peoples all over the Amazon. The Waorani believe it is the reincarnated soul of a woman who loved her people so much that she returned in the form of this palm in order to continue nourishing her grandchildren. Thus the drink made from its fruit is known as *badagone,* "grandmother's milk."

11. Personal communication with don Cesareo Piaguaje, one of my main informants. I lived in his home during my time among the Secoya between 1995 and 2000.

12. At the core of this enigmatic indigenous science is the quest for ways to assist people and oneself (i.e., the dedication to service). This is central to most spiritual traditions and can be practiced by anyone at any time. Being helpful, working to heal others and the planet, and being gentle with oneself are good places to start aligning oneself with a universal way of life.

13. There is no way to comprehend how this can happen, other than the possibility that the light these elders emit, in their selfless devotion to service at any hour of the day or night, is too bright for the darkness of these times—as if malicious spirits continue to repeat the tragedy of the erasure of traditional ways of life. Don Esteban Lucitante was a great-spirited man, always dedicated to service, and always laughing—one could say he was truly selfless! He would be the first to rise to the occasion and help, and set the standard for such behavior. Then he would drink yagé and sing all the night long and heal as many people as would come to him. I wrote the following short song to commemorate our friendship:

> "Taita Esteban, I will never forget you
> Green green feathered crowns and mañapë*
> You're the beaded master of healing songs
> You have returned to the universe"

*Mañapë is the Secoya emetic of choice, used for purifying the blood and overcoming laziness (*Callichlamys latifolia*, Bignoneaceae).

14. These are first six lines of the "Spiritual Harmonization with Great Nature" from Taoist Master Ni Hua-Ching, *The Golden Collection of Spiritual Practices, Part I: Workbook for Spiritual Development of All People* (Santa Monica, CA: Seven Star Communications Group, 1995), p. 106. I make reference to the great works of the Taoist canon for three principal reasons. 1. There are many cross-cultural similarities between the Amazonian worldview and the traditions of Tao. 2. Indigenous science of the forest people is an oral tradition, with truths and spiritual instruction often passed through wordless teachings; it is elusive and thus can be easily lost, misinterpreted, and diluted, as we see happening. The teachings of Taoism and various commentaries have been available in written form for centuries, enabling their study outside the inner circles of master and student. They remain useful today as a spiritual foundation for all sincere students of any life path. 3. Given the increased interest in ayahuasca use among Westerners, I personally believe that the study of Taoism can greatly assist in spiritual growth and the necessary auspicious progress on the path, and it gives a valuable perspective from which to better understand the original Amazonian way of thought. Yagé and/or ayahuasca then becomes a tool to cultivate Tao. The ancient teachings of Tao are such a valuable perspective that to not refer to this traditional time-tested perspective would be a great omission. Master Ni's books are highly recommended for any sincere student of life.

15. This is an epic book about the life of a Secoya shaman, Fernando Payaguaje, published in Spanish by CICAME Books in Ecuador, 1994. The book, an important testament to the plant-medicine tradition of yagé, was translated to English in 2008 by a friend of the Secoya, Nathan *"Toanké"* Horowitz, who lived among them for over a year in 1996–97, allowing him to offer this superb English rendition. (Note: This book did not use the accent on "yage" and thus it is reproduced that way when quoting from it here.) In a stroke of auspicious good fortune, Nathan was available to help edit this manuscript *(Rainforest Medicine)*.

16. The matipë is a decorated ceremonial scepter used in the drinking of yagé. An ancient legend calls it the *matiyai* ("heaven jaguar") and relates how the use of the scepter came to be (see Chapter 4). The matipë plays an important role in traditional Secoya yagé drinking.

When the ceremonial leader is in deep concentration singing, invoking the presence of the celestial spirits, the Wiñapai see the matipë. One might say it acts as an antenna of sorts, along which the celestial energies and patternings can descend and enter the ceremonial space and fill all the drinkers, not just the maestro. (The divine energy always comes first to the maestro, then to the cooks, then to the other elders, and then it goes spreading out into the room to fill the rest of the drinkers.) There are many references to the pivotal place the matipë holds among the celestial immortals.

Often, as a pre-ceremony ritual, the master will request that a student take the matipë and go around to all the people gathered there to drink and ask each one, "Do you want to drink yagé?" as the trainee places the scepter on their shoulders or top of the head. Each person is to affirm his or her intention by answering "yes." This is so the energetic emanations of the yagé can come out of the medicine and reach them without delay. Consequently at the onset of the ceremony, after the effects of the medicine have begun to take charge, a student, relative, or the individual who called the ceremony will hand the scepter and the leafy broom rattle to the ceremonial guide, as a form of requesting that the ceremony be enacted. At dawn, no one is to walk around or talk until the ceremonial guide has returned the scepter and leafy broom rattle to the same person who handed it to him at the onset, thus marking the closure of the ceremony. After this people are free to walk around, talk, or depart.

17. Yai José was a true master of the many spiritual arts. He was a selfless and accomplished guide, healer, and friend who is remembered with fondness as the generous and upright man he was. His life was devoted to healing and to service. He was a great drinker of yagé, who interestingly enough never smoked tobacco. Cesareo (his grandson) told me that upon his death, Yai José was heard to call out for his family after his body had been laid to rest in a hammock in a traditional pit covered only with palm fronds. His body disappeared, as if Yai José left his grave, and his hammock was hung back up in the kitchen. This occurred in Lagarto Cocha wilderness area where Cesareo was raised.

18. The Secoya cultivate several varieties of the cyperaceous plant nuní, a Secoya word used to designate a group of plants in the genus Cyperus. There is *watí nuní,* "spirit nuní" (with a fragrant tuber no larger than 2 cm in diameter, the plant consists of a sedge-like cluster of long, thin, smooth, tubular-shaped leaves); *yiyó nuní,* "glass-bead nuní" (it has

abundant fragrant tubers 5–10 cm long); *aña nuní,* "snake nuní" (used to heal snakebite, it is similar in appearance to yiyó nuní but the sedge is slightly smaller); and *pai'saye nuní,* "good-bye people nuní" (which I have never seen). The potency and healing efficaciousness of these plants may be related to the presence of a white fungal mycorrhiza that this plant has a symbiotic relationship with. These plants are not found in the wild—they are fragile heirloom treasures. It is possible that they may have been collected in times of old from certain wilderness places such as savannahs or isolated ridge tops that contain locally endemic plants. For example, yiyó nuní looks similar to *Cyperus odoratus,* a plant found near the edges of certain lagoons at Pëquë'yá.

19. Fernando Payaguaje, *The Yage Drinker,* pp. 175–176.

20. Ibid., p. 176.

21. One of these plants obtained from spiritual realms is the ancestrally cultivated varieties of pejí (*Brugmansia suaveolens*—Solanaceae family). The Secoya, unlike any other indigenous group, have mastered the science of drinking pejí. After the fourth flowering of the pejí grown in a remote garden, forty entire pejí plants—roots, stalks, flowers, and leaves—are all yanked and used. These are pounded well and cooked in a pot. Some of it is baked or roasted on a hot clay plate, and this baked pejí is added to the pot as well. These graduation ceremonies occur with one or two students and the master. The master will be drinking yagé to guide the students, who each drink a full gourd of pejí: about one liter of a thick, almost gelatinous substance that must be drunk without thinking. The elders attest that if one vomits, one must vomit into the gourd and then slam it back down. Only by drinking the entire amount can the spirit leave one's body to learn; otherwise one's spirit stays trapped in the body, playing out all one's impulses and habits. The following day, extra-thick ëo yagé is drunk—in order to come down! From what I understand, this is really what brings the ceremony together and allows one to make a little sense of the pejí experience. It is a serious thing to drink pejí, something that is approached with reverence. This is something no one should attempt unless under the strict supervision of a trained master.

22. Patricio Fernández-Salvador, *The Amazon, Shamans, God and Ayahuasca* (published by author in English in Quito, Ecuador, in 2006), p. 115. On the previous page of the same book there is a photo of the necklace. The author was a friend of Esteban Lucitante. The "People of Yagé" referred to at the end of the quote (known as the Yagémopai in

Paicoca, the Secoya people's language) is a term used for all the different kinds of spirits and immortals revealed to the drinker by the yagé.

23. Gerardo Reichel-Dolmatoff, *The Forest Within: The World View of the
Tukano Amazonian Indians* (Devon, UK: Themis Books, an imprint
of Green Books Ltd., 1996), p. 186. Similarly, Manuel Cordova-Ríos
describes ayahuasca use among the Huni Kui as a way to see and learn
about all the forest animals, their most intimate traits and singular
peculiarities. In this way the medicine serves as an investigative agent
allowing the people to achieve piercing knowledge of rainforest ecology, biodiversity, and evolutionary biology. (With this in mind, the
question can again be asked, is this not an advanced form of science?)
The Huni Kui today are still largely a non-contacted people living in
voluntary isolation in the remote Peruvian Amazon. For a fantastic
glimpse into their life and use of ayahuasca, read *Wizard of the Upper
Amazon: The Story of Manuel Córdova-Rios* by F. Bruce Lamb and
Manuel Córdova-Rios (Berkeley, CA: North Atlantic Books, 1974).
Manuel Córdova-Rios (1887–1978) was a renowned herbalist and
healer from Iquitos, Peru, who lived among the Huni Kui as a young
man and learned their medicine.

24. Gerardo Reichel-Dolmatoff, *The Forest Within.* The quotes are from
pages 88, 92, and 171. As for the word *maloca,* this is a widespread term
for the traditional Amazonian long house, called among the Secoya
tui'quë'wïi'e, or among the Waorani *uncu.* Both refer to a large lodge
where traditionally many generations and many families lived together.
These houses have become increasingly rare in the past 50 years. Over
the past decade my friends and I have been influential in supporting the
building of three of these ancestral long houses among the Secoya community in Ecuador. The traditional way of life is intimately associated
with the type of house they live in, and the loss of the long house and
the adoption of the individual small house represents the leaning away
of a collective society and the adopting of a more individually focused
society. The lodge's central area is always left open, with this spacious-
ness representing the cosmos. On page 49 of *The Forest Within* Reichel-
Dolmatoff writes about the maloca: "The choice of raw materials, such
as house posts, beams, rafters and struts, together with a roof thatch
and vines for fastening the parts together, follow traditional rules which
are controlled by shamans and elders during the process of construction.... The individual parts are associated with cosmological models,
astronomical phenomena, anatomical and physiological functions,

kinship notions, ritual dimensions, and landscape features, in short, with all spheres and scenarios of human experience." With the loss of the maloca we see yet another separation of Heaven from Earth, and the disintegration of the original order of things.

25. The following account occurred in the Secoya territory of Peru in the late 1930s, at a place where different family clans would gather to drink yagé. The account was told to me by Rogelio Piaguaje. A Spaniard named Ligerio lived among the Secoya and began drinking abundant yagé. He was learning well and progressing in a good way, but he became anxious before leaving for home and wanted to learn more. His Secoya friends, fond of him, didn't want to show him too quickly because they were aware of the perils of rushing the process. At one of these gatherings Ligerio was most impressed with a certain yagé drinker who had come from the Putumayo River. He was from a family clan called the Cantëyapai. Ligerio told him that he wasn't learning quickly enough and that he had to return soon to Spain. Before leaving he wanted to prove the ancient science. The Cantëyapai, who ultimately wasn't concerned with what the outcome might be, agreed to give him powers. In three ceremonies the Cantëyapai showed Ligerio everything. In the morning after one such ceremony Ligerio walked toward the riverbank and entered the river. From under the water his songs could still be heard. Not long afterward he came out bringing with him dry cloth (from the Camiyai) that he generously gave those participating in the ceremony, and everyone was impressed. But knowing that when one learns too quickly, one can also begin killing people, they became wary. Sure enough, it wasn't long before Ligerio started killing upstart disciples—he would use sorcery on a spiritual level to take their lives, and it would happen so quickly that he was not even aware of what he was doing. In one of the ceremonies Ligerio passed his powers to a Siona man named Catáë, and it wasn't long before Catáë, with his recently acquired powers, started doing wrong deeds and killing people as well. As a result Catáë was soon killed.

In another ceremony Ligerio announced he was going back to the store of the Camiyai to obtain more cloth. After sunrise he walked singing toward the banks of the river, when a baby appeared floating in the air before him. He took the baby and placed it in the canoe, and as soon as it was placed there it mysteriously disappeared. The others had placed a spiritual trap on him so he would lose the powers he had obtained, and that if indeed it was Ligerio who was killing people through sorcery, then the same magic he was using would return to him and as a consequence take his life. If he had not killed people, then nothing would happen to him. Young disciples were dying, but the people could not outright prove if it was something that Ligerio was doing. It wasn't long after this occasion that Ligerio was killed. Interestingly enough, the name Ligerio sounds a lot like the Spanish word *ligero* that means "casual" or "to take one's time." The Secoya believe that in the development of one's spiritual abilities it is customary to progress slowly, to remain humble and proceed one solid step at a time, and that it can be dangerous to learn too quickly, where one runs the risk of being corrupted by the powers received.

26. Francisco de Orellana was a barbaric Spanish conquistador who in 1541 first "found" the Amazon River from the city of Quito, giving Ecuador its claim (that it lost in 1942) over a vast territory stretching to the Amazon from the west. On a return voyage he arrived to the Brazilian coast in December 1545 and proceeded into the Amazon delta. After much tragedy and the loss of his crew to hostile natives, Orellana was never again seen.

Chapter 2: Degradation of the Spiritual Science—Sorcery and Superstition

1. Bessie Head, *A Question of Power* (London: Heinemann, 1974).

2. Don Solon Tello (1918–2010) was a master ayahuasquero from Iquitos, Peru. He was firmly dedicated to healing and loved by many people. Some of his epic icaros can be heard on YouTube. I had the great fortune of meeting him and participating in his ceremonies in 1997 and 1998. His complete sincerity and love for humanity deeply moved me. A glimpse into his life is provided in Chapter 9.

3. Pablo Amaringo (1943–2009), personal communication at Guaria de Osa Ecolodge, Costa Rica, January 2004. Pablo's life story and tremendous contribution to deepening humanity's understanding are elucidated in two books, *Ayahuasca Visions: The Religious Iconography of a Peruvian Shaman* and *The Ayahuasca Visions of Pablo Amaringo* (please see the bibliography under lead authors "Charing" and "Luna"). I was fortunate over several visits to Peru between 1996 and 1999 to spend time with don Pablo, from whom I learned so much, and in these same years he accompanied me, with some of his students, on three visits to Secoya territory in the Ecuadorian Amazon. Later on two occasions I accompanied him as translator to the Unites States. Pablo signed a copy of his book *Ayahuasca Visions* for me. At the end of his note, he

added (translated here to English), "With plenty of happiness and full of empathy, our friendship is a sign of perfection." Though he had discontinued his practice as a vegetalista (ayahuasquero), he never surrendered the culture of service. Pablo Amaringo was one of the most service-oriented and heartfelt people I have ever met. To have received his encouragement when I first began this project is a great and deeply humbling honor, and it is he who insisted I feature samples of his paintings in this book, including the cover art.

4. Excerpt from my journal entries of personal communication with Cesareo Piaguaje, at his home in the Secoya community of Sewaya, Aguarico River, Amazonian Ecuador, August 2006.

5. Fernando Payaguaje, *El Bebedor de Yage* (Quito, Ecuador: CICAME, 1994, in Spanish). First English edition 2008, *The Yage Drinker*, translated by Nathan Horowitz, quote on p. 119.

6. Ibid., pp. 120–121. The mawaho people that Fernando refers to are commonly spoken of among Secoya elders versed in the traditions of yagé. The term means "butterfly people," as *mawaho* is the Secoya name for the elegant blue morpho, a large rainforest butterfly with satiny sky-blue-colored wings. Cesareo in 2009 at his home explained it to me like this: He was concentrating on a cure for his nephew who was gravely ill. He concentrated all his energies and prayers on this sole act of healing his nephew. Cesareo was fasting to drink yagé that evening in order to accomplish the cure. Suddenly that afternoon, with no invitation, the Mawahopai came. (They are never called since it is they who know when to come.) One appeared on each side and they took hold of his arms. They lifted him up and took him for a ride. In the case of a healer who has a solid relationship among the celestial people and the doctor people, the Mawahopai bring him to their abode. This was where Cesareo journeyed. "There they had a basket up high tied to a pole with *aun* [dried tortillas made of yuca flower]. They were eating from it, and the sound of their bites was loud; piercing, snapping sounds were reverberating all over. They offered me some aun and I only lifted my hand in indication that I would not take any. By offering things they try to get healers to downgrade. One must never accept anything from the Mawahopai, and then they forget about that and they think about what you are thinking about. They see that you want to heal a patient, then they want to help you." They informed him how he was to heal his nephew. He was to cure the water of a specific root for the boy to drink, and he would recuperate.

Then they flew him back over the forest to his home. He went to get the root they had recommended. His nephew drank it and quickly recuperated.

7. Cesareo Piaguaje, personal communication, 2006. See note 4.

8. Cesareo Piaguaje, personal communication, 1996.

9. Related to me in a personal communication with Secoya educator Celestino Piaguaje in the year 1997 at his home in Sewaya village, Aguarico River, Sucumbios Province in Amazonian Ecuador.

10. Fernando Payaguaje in *The Yage Drinker*, p. 120.

11. The Demon King, known in Paicoca, the Secoya language, as the Pai'joyowatí (which translates literally as "people soul/heart spirit"), is the spirit of an ancient shaman that once lived upon the Earth. This spirit can be invoked by the master drinkers, who use it to aid them in accomplishing advanced healings. This spirit is an authority among all lower spirits and can request that they remove the damage they have caused. See Chapter 1, p. 8.

12. Personal communication from Secoya cultural historian and educator Celestino Piaguaje, at his home on the Aguarico River in August 1996.

13. This is a generalization related to the work of US-based evangelical bible translators such as the Summer Institute of Linguistics, among others. Knowingly or not, their work paves the way for local acceptance and collusion with (some would say addiction to) the modern economic motives of profit-focused corporations that erode biological and cultural diversity.

14. I am referring in particular to the work of Miguel Angel Cabodevilla, a Capuchin priest, who has been a strong and outspoken voice in favor of life in the Ecuadorian Amazon, the peoples' ability for self-determination, and enhanced government protection of the remaining hidden peoples. For some of his publications see Chapter 1, endnote 9.

15. See the writings of Sir Roger Casement of the United Kingdom Foreign Office, and Peruvian Amazon Company. "Correspondence Respecting the Treatment of British Colonial Subjects and Native Indians Employed in the Collection of Rubber in the Putumayo District" (United Kingdom: National Government Publication, 1912).

16. The Shuar are an authentic nation of the Amazon, but along the Aguarico River they are considered colonists, since they are originally from the southern province of Morona Santiago and arrived on the Aguarico as part of the expanding colonization frontier. Colonists

include mestizo settlers as well as members of Ecuador's indigenous majorities such as the Shuar and the Kichwa, who have skillfully colonized large tracts of the ethnic minorities' lands such as those of the Cofán, Siona, Secoya, Waorani, and Záparo peoples. In Ecuador a colonist is considered anyone who was born in one province and lives in another province, but the colonial frontier in many regards is coming to an end. Today there are no more *tierras valdías*, "free lands," and IERAC (Ecuadorian Institute for Agrarian Reform and Colonization) has been abolished. All lands have now been adjudicated to communities or are held by the government as conservation areas. Despite this, the upper Amazon is a region of complex land tenure issues.

Chapter 3: The Gift of Ayahuasca

1. Richard Evans Schultes, Albert Hofmann, and Christian Rätsch, *Plants of the Gods* (Healing Arts Press, Rochester, VT, 2001), p. 124.

2. According to anthropologist Michael Harner in *Cave and Cosmos* (Berkeley, CA: North Atlantic Books, 2013, p. 47): "Based on archaeological and comparative ethnological evidence, shamanism is believed by many scholars to be at least 30,000 years old, and quite possibly is more ancient."

    On the back cover of Don José Campos, Alberto Roman, and Geraldine Overton, *The Shaman and Ayahuasca: Journeys to Sacred Realms* (Studio City, CA: Divine Arts, 2011), it says in reference to the sacred vine, "according to the latest finds, has been used for healing by Amazonian shamans for as long as 70,000 years." The source of such a statement is not verified in the text yet given the scholarly approach of its authors, I cite this estimate nonetheless.

3. Richard Evans Schultes et al., *Plants of the Gods*, pp. 126–127.

4. Luis Eduardo Luna and Steven F. White, eds., *Ayahuasca Reader: Encounters with the Amazon's Sacred Vine* (Santa Fe, NM: Synergetic Press, 2000), p. 1.

5. The Kichwa name *chacruna* (*Psychotria viridis)* incorporates *chak,* referring to the rung of a ladder, or to a bridge or the ladder itself, and *runa,* a word of extensive symbolism and meaning that evokes a state of being. *Runa* can be translated as "an integral and spiritually developed person"; in the high Andes the word refers to a married couple. The implication is that the bridge or ladder joining the physical and spiritual realms (and thereby conveying the wisdom and visions of the

latter) can only be accessed by being *runa,* a person who leads an integrated, balanced life of virtue, upholding all the standards conveyed by the word. Chacruna—a term used mainly in Peru—is a shrub related to coffee called *amiruka panga* or *samairuku panga* by the Kichwa-speaking people in Ecuador's Napo Province. *Amiruka* or *samairuku* can be translated as "sleepy old wisdom," and *panga* means "leaf": thus "sleepy old wisdom leaf."

6. Richard Evans Schultes and Robert F. Raffauf, "El Bejuco del Alma: Los medicos tradicionales de la Amazonia Colombiana, sus plantas y sus rituals," traducción de Alberto Uribe Tobón (Bogotá: El Áncora Editores y Ediciones Fondo de Cultura Económica, 2004), pp. 38–39.

7. Jim DeKorne, *Psychedelic Shamanism* (Berkeley, CA: North Atlantic Books, 2011), p. 155.

8. Kichwa is also the name of the Incan language, which they call *Runa Shimi,* meaning "the people's tongue." Until recently, scholars wrote the name of this language as heard among lowland peoples as "Quichua," whereas the language of highland dwellers was spelled "Quechua."

9. Personal communication from Pablo Amaringo, 1997, 2002.

10. Personal communication with Secoya traditional elder and cultural historian Basilio Piaguaje, 2012.

11. Irene Bellier, *El Temblor y La Luna: Ensayo Sobre Las Relaciones Entre Las Mujeres y Los Hombres Mai Huna,* (Quito, Ecuador: CICAME, 1991), p. 48, listing some of the Western Tukanoan-speaking clans of the eighteenth century found along the Caqueta and Putumayo rivers in the southern Colombian Amazon near the modern-day border region with Ecuador.

12. Personal communication, 2009.

13. Richard Evans Schultes, "An Overview of Hallucinogens in the Western Hemisphere" in *Flesh of the Gods: The Ritual Use of Hallucinogens,* Peter T. Furst, editor (New York: Praeger, 1972), pp. 38-39.

14. Terence McKenna, *The Archaic Revival* (HarperSanFrancisco: 1991), p. 78.

Chapter 4: Elements of the Experience

1. F. Bruce Lamb, *Rio Tigre and Beyond: The Amazon Jungle Medicine of Manuel Córdova* (Berkeley, CA: North Atlantic Books, 1985), p. 136.

2. From a 1997 Bioneers Conference presentation, "Women, Plants, and Culture," recorded in *Visionary Plant Consciousness: The Shamanic*

Teachings of the Plant World, J. P. Harpignies, editor (Rochester, VT: Park Street Press, 2007), p. 103.

3. This can be compared to the study necessary to open the spiritual eyes on one's forehead. The Secoya tradition includes the opening of five eyes—two to each side of the "third eye" in the center between the brows—in order to see the truth of the spiritual realms and the divine immortals. For this matter, one must open the heavenly ear as well in order to hear the heavenly songs. Cesareo explained to me that a pressure is felt building in oneself that culminates with a loud popping sound. Suddenly and most unexpectedly you hear the exquisite celestial medicine songs of the Wiñapai.

4. When I first arrived to grandfather Wepe's home in the forest outside the remote Waorani village of Qhiwaro, the very moment I walked into the door a baby was born. It was May 1994. He took me by the arm and we danced together, back and forth, back and forth, while he sang this song in traditional Waorani style. Afterwards he told me I should dance like this and sing this song often, and that "all negativity is dispelled by this song."

5. The name Yasuni comes from Tsuníyá, the Secoya name for this river, meaning River of the Tsuní *(Caryodendron orinocense),* an oil- and protein-rich nut-bearing tree. Not far upriver from its mouth is the lagoon of Garzacocha, where in the past the Secoya lived. Today Kichwa speakers have settled the mouth of this river. The upper areas have always been part of the Waorani people's territory, who call the river Dicaron (River of Stones) because when it is low many stones are exposed. Its various tributaries carry Waorani names such as Pañono ("River of Bamboo"), Cahuimenco ("where grows *caguimenca,*" a vine with an edible nut: *Cayaponia ophthalmica*) and the Ahuemuro ("River of Tall Trees"). The Yasuni River flows into the Napo just upriver from the border of Ecuador and Peru. Today this area is at the forefront of a great international debate, called the Yasuni ITT initiative, where Ecuador is asking the world to be compensated for the price of the oil lying beneath this priceless wilderness rainforest area that is home to Waorani communities and wandering, still-hidden deep-forest clans such as Wiñetare. The big question of to drill or not to drill is being put to the decision-makers of the world.

6. See the story of Mengatue becoming an iroinga (one who embodies all experiences) in Chapter 7.

7. I heard don Pablo's account of his experience with the divinity known as Altos Cielos ("High Heaven") in 1997 at his home in the jungle city of Pucallpa, Peru, at the Usko Ayar School of Amazonian Painting.

8. This boat is illustrated in many of Pablo's visionary masterpieces. Vision 20 in the book *Ayahuasca Visions* shows the *Aceropunta*. The text reads, "This vision shows the great steamer *Aceropunta*. It is a truly esoteric ship that can only be seen under a strong *mareación,* when it is called by a well-sung *icaró.* This is how it appears and it is surprising to see how it comes from a great distance, producing an electrifying sound as it reaches us. Its mission is to travel round the world paying visits to all those that call it."

9. The Secoya speak of this phenomenon as well, especially when a healer is first learning. When he has learned only a part of the secret invocations, the inconvenient side effects can be seen as snakes appearing near the shaman's house. Once the complete invocations are learned, the snakes disappear. Sometimes during a healing the snakes will appear while the energy of the song is unraveling, then disappear when the song is complete. The only way to learn how to use these songs, and how to complete the song's mission—like a perfect ring, a bead, a crown, the Secoya attest—is by upholding the dieta and through copious drinking of extra-strong yagé.

10. Inside the high hill called Jaicunti, which is the isolated limestone massif of the cordillera Napo-Galeras, live the Jaicuntipai, the Secoya elders attest. Among these spiritual immortals of pure medicine and total integrity there is no sorcery because they are devoted purely to healing. The truth of the existence of the Jaicuntipai is one of the foundations of the Secoya people's spiritual science. Elders claim they have married there and have spiritual wives with whom they have children, who grow quickly to look as though they are forty years of age, remaining like this for generations without further aging. When the shaman's body physically perishes, he or she opens their eyes in that immortal abode and *is* that spiritual child, an immortal in the immortal realms.

11. Masaru Emoto is a Japanese author and doctor of alternative medicine who has carried out extensive experiments with water and its ability to record positive and/or negative frequencies. Dr. Emoto's pioneering work offers provocative demonstration of water's ability to hold positive intentions and auspicious energetic emanations that can be effectively used to enhance people's well-being.

12. The Waorani, who have neither linguistic affiliation nor intercultural exchange with the Secoya despite living in relative proximity, have a strikingly similar legend. Mengatue shared this legend with me in 1992, translated to Spanish by Nihua Enomenga and paraphrased to English by me. In ancient times, the land of the living and the land of the dead were separated only by a narrow creek. A simple wooden log served as a footbridge to cross over, and relatives who were alive would frequently visit relatives who were dead, and vice versa. Essentially there was no separation between the land of the living and land of the dead. An old brother died and his younger brother came to visit, to whom he gave a killing stick, saying to not overuse it, to share the meat and be generous. He advised not falling asleep with the killing stick exposed, to only sleep at home when the stick is in a clay pot covered by a leaf, and never shall it be used to kill people. The younger brother did as instructed. One afternoon some Waorani were following a troupe of monkeys. The younger brother was tired and took a nap next to a large tree. The monkeys the other Waorani were following ran into that tree. Next to him, leaning against the tree, was the killing stick. A Waorani climbed into the tree to dislodge a monkey he had shot with a poisoned dart that got stuck on a branch. At that moment the other Waorani appeared and the brother awoke, but one of them had already lifted the stick, saying, "What is this?" when the man in the tree fell dead.

 The next morning there was a hole broken open in the side of the pot and the stick was gone. He ran to the bridge to cross over and tell his brother. The bridge had fallen into the water that was no longer a stream but rather a widening torrent. The dead brother was on the other side and called out, "My brother, there is nothing I can do!" Today the world of the living and the world of the dead are no longer close together but very far apart, and the fluid intercommunion that once was, is for the most part gone now as well.

13. These words of Pablo Amaringo's clearly depict the association of the pinta—the designs, the energetic emanations of universal powers, divinities, and spirits—with the drinking of ayahuasca, quoted from page 45 of *The Ayahuasca Visions of Pablo Amaringo*. Huairamama ("Air Mother") is considered to be one of the three primal powers of the universe by the Kichwa and mestizo ayahuasqueros, depicted as a giant multicolored and intricately designed serpent. Spiritual masters and advanced shamans can be seen riding on its back.

To have powerful visions one must have a clear mind, and Pablo had many techniques to cleanse and balance the mind. Here is a method he shared with me in 2008 at his home above the art school. Paint a board (approx. 9 x 45 cm in size) with horizontal bands of five colors—green, red, yellow, white, and blue, each 9 cm wide. Look at these colors rapidly, jumping with your gaze from one color to the next color to the next. Move from left to right, then from right to left, following with your sight the bands of color. The sizes mentioned are only approximate dimensions. Most important is looking at each color back and forth as a means to clarify the mind. Another method is to scribble along a piece of paper from right to left, then left to right, using your right hand, then using your left hand. Using both hands helps you develop both sides of the brain. Scribble quickly the letters of the alphabet and any other symbols you can. This simple practice helps one achieve balance in all aspects of life, enhancing intelligence, determination, and ability to discern. This is especially helpful for children and youth. Pablo also strongly believed in the therapeutic qualities of music to balance the brain. In order to play an instrument, one must use both hands in coordination. Here is a tip for memorizing poems, songs, or literature: Read something you want to memorize over and over. Then recite it in pitch darkness. The mind is more receptive in the dark. To gain the benefits of these simple exercises, practice them daily. Once an icaro or invocation is learned, it must be practiced continually in this manner.

14. In *The Ayahuasca Visions of Pablo Amaringo,* page 32, in the vision called Jehua Supai, the cloak is described: "He is wearing a *manto de fuego* (cloak of fire). To win this honor he must rigorously follow a dieta to learn from sublime teachers and gain spirit allies: anacondas, parrots, *guacamayos* (*Ara arauna*), black dolphins, red dolphins, and the *anguilamama* (mother of the *cocha brava,* which is a wild mystical lake where few people dare to venture)."

15. See the story of Yai Yoí in Chapter 6.

16. Personal communication, Pucallpa, 1997.

17. Personal communication at Guaria de Osa Ecolodge in Costa Rica, 2002.

18. This type of tobacco log is used for spiritual learning as well as healing a wide array of ailments. Drinking black tobacco water obtained from the soaked pulp from these tobacco logs is a necessary accomplishment in Kichwa culture when becoming a healer, as it is believed that this process not only teaches how to heal but also "seals" one's body and energy

through purification and strengthening in order to make it less suscep-tible to sorcery. The traditional elders who adhered to this custom as part of their initiation would drink six to twelve of these tobacco logs. Every morning a sliver several centimeters thick is chopped up finely and soaked in a gourd with about a cup of water. This is mashed up well and left to "cook" in the sun. After sundown, the liquid is drunk through one's nose. This practice is most effective when accomplished alone in the forest. Casimiro shared with me that in his youth he drank a full twelve taucumasu logs while living in the deep forest of Galeras with his grandmother. He followed a zasina of mainly green plantains and dry fish. He was very thin while he underwent this process, and says this is when he learned the sacred arts of healing.

Casimiro's grandfather related that when you are hunting and an animal suddenly appears nearby, in the spirit land it has drunk too much tobacco juice and has now accidentally stumbled into this world before you. In the spirit land there is a lake of tobacco where all the animals come to drink. Sometimes one drinks too much and gets very drunk. Similarly, when we drink tobacco, we get drunk and stumble into other worlds, realms governed by spirits.

In the book *Samay, La Herencia del Espíritu,* on page 161, author José Miguel Goldaráz writes, "Tobacco, according to *runa* wisdom, was made by the brothers Lucero and Kuyllur, the great *kurakas*—cultural heroes. The first people carried tobacco during the struggle against the destructive monsters of humanity in the beginning times, the times of *kunan pacha.* Without tobacco they would not have been able to sur-vive. It protects against all dangers. It is blown onto the forest to dispel malignant spirits, and to not be affected by the invisible darts of the *sagras.* It is blown towards the clouds to liberate the environment of threatening storms."

Tobacco, as we all know, is a powerful plant, and like all plants of power it can be used for good as well as harm. Wilbert Johannes quotes the late anthropologist Alfred Métrux: "In Pilagá mythology a cannibal-woman is killed by the cultural hero (and burned) and from her ashes the first tobacco grows." From Johannes Wilbert, *Tobacco and Shamanism in South America* (New Haven: Yale University Press, 1987), p. 151.

19. Tzicta (*Tabernaemontana sananho*) of the Apocynaceae family is a small, latex-producing, understory rainforest shrub or small tree with white flowers. This is a most appreciated and revered plant known as *tzicta* among the Kichwa, *paisu'u witó* among the Secoya, *pengunkowe*

among the Waorani, and *lobo sanango* among the mestizo vegetalistas in the Iquitos and Pucallpa area of the Peruvian Amazon. The use of the powerful ibogaine-containing entheogenic bark of the tzicta was at one time a highly respected plant-medicine tradition of the Kichwa people of upper Napo, although today this tradition for the most part is waning. I learned about it with don Casimiro on several occasions between 1991 and 1994 at his Pusuno River wilderness retreat. Early in the morning after having only drank guayusa tea, one walks through the rainforest to locate the tzicta trees. After leaving an offering of tobacco and prayers, the gatherer rasps a wad of bark from the base of ten mature plants, always from the eastern side, where the bark is believed to be the most potent. (One must not rasp too deeply or it harms the tree, which will otherwise regrow the bark.) The bark is boiled in a small pot with a thick piece of taucumasu from a cured tobacco mace. Once cool, the liquid is strained and drunk after it has been blown on by the maestro. This is very strong, the gripping effects of which last all night and well into the next day. All one can do is remain still and quiet, and shiver until the effects pass. The tzicta builds one's energy level and ability to withstand the zasina, the diet one needs to follow afterward that consists of five, seven, or nine days of eating pure green bananas. It is taken to sharpen the senses and improves one's ability to concentrate.

At Amazanga village among the Santi family in Pastaza Province, tzicta is used as an emetic, in a much less intense application. The emetic is employed eight days after a baby is born. A large wad of tzicta bark is cooked in an extra-large pot with a few pieces of the bark of the powerful *piton* tree *(Grias neuberthii)*. Everyone, starting with the mother, drinks from a large gourd. The elder grandmother or grandfather of the village passes the gourd three times in front of the person about to drink, who stands with their arms held open to the sides and palms facing forward. This ritual is believed to "tune" the medicine to each person's body, allowing it to "see" the person who is about to drink. The large gourd is drunk only after the entire family has drunk guayusa tea from another pot. The drink soon sends those consuming it onto the patio to puke deeply.

The Waorani use this plant for pain in and above the eye. The leaves are steamed and applied over the eye. For healing cataracts, the white sap of the tree is placed daily in the eye, for three to nine days, and a small seed of the basil bush may also be placed in the eye. This is only kept in there for 30 minutes or so while one rolls the eye around in circles underneath the eyelids. The basil seed goes around accumulating the cataract, which eventually can be pulled off with a piece of cotton. The sap is also used to remove tropical botfly.

20. Hua-Ching Ni, *Workbook for Spiritual Development of All People* (Santa Monica, CA: Seven Star Communications Group, 1995), pp. 51–52. Near the opening of this powerful book we read, "The Subtle Essence that is sought by all sciences and all religions transcends all attempts to reach it by means of thought, belief or experiment. The Universal Way leads directly to it and guides you to reach it yourself by uniting with the integral nature of the universe." Anyone on a spiritual path will greatly benefit from reading Master Ni's books. See www.taostar.com.

21. Hua-Ching Ni, *Uncharted Voyage Toward the Subtle Light* (Santa Monica, CA: Seven Star Communications Group, 2008), p. 236.

22. Quoted in Michael Harner, *Cave and Cosmos* (Berkeley, CA: North Atlantic Books, 2013), p. 195. Original source given as George Quasha, "Speech by Essie Parrish, recorded March 14, 1972," *Alcheringa: Ethnopoetics 1* (1975), pp. 27–29.

23. *Pistia stratiotes* in the Rosaceae family is not your average rose. This one is a floating pan-neotropical aquatic plant, found in the blackwater *igapó* lagoons of Pëquë'yá. I heard about this enigmatic use of the plant on a visit there in August 1996.

Chapter 5: Preparing a Proper Brew

1. William Burroughs, *The Yage Letters* (San Francisco: City Lights Books, 2006; originally published 1963), p. 99.

2. Specifically for addictions: Takiwasi, Center for the Rehabilitation of Drug Addicts and for Research on Traditional Medicines, facilitates dietas and healing; it is located in the outskirts of Tarapoto, Peruvian Amazon, and produces a newsletter. For more information, www.takiwasi.com. Many other centers have sprouted up.

3. From a 1992 Bioneers Conference panel discussion entitled "Visionary Plants Across Cultures" in *Visionary Plant Consciousness: The Shamanic Teachings of the Plant World,* J. P. Harpignies, editor (Rochester, VT: Park Street Press, 2007), p. 116.

4. Ibid., pp. 131–132. This quote is from a different Bioneers Conference, in the year 2000, during a discussion between Kat Harrison and mycologist Paul Stamets.

5. Yoco is a stimulating drink obtained from the rasped bark of the rainforest vine *Paullinia yoco* of the Sapindaceae family. It is used by the Secoya to begin the day's work and beat inertia.

6. There are many birds associated with the sacred culture of yagé. Among the most appreciated and esteemed by the Secoya are: *jëesaipë*, the masked tanager *(Tangara nigrocincta)*, which has an iridescent blue neck; *pisasá*, the paradise tanager *(Tangara chilensis)*, which has five colors, a light-green head, sky-blue underparts, and carbon-black upper-body plumage with a yellow and red rump; and *mapia*, the scarlet tanager *(Piranga olivacea)*, which is brilliant red with black wings. Certain legions of Wiñapai are seen as wearing long hanging necklaces made of these birds, along which colorful lights are seen swirling. Other sacred birds are the *yai jëesaipë*, the blue dacnis *(Dacnis cayana)*, chiefly turquoise blue with black turquoise-edged wings and tail; and the *mapeka*, the hepatic tanager *(Piranga flava)*, cardinal red, brightest on its forehead and throat, with a dark eye streak. These birds and the other tanagers previously mentioned are believed to be messenger birds who carry the prayers of the shaman to the realms of the celestial beings. *Toama*, the scarlet macaw *(Ara macao)*, *kënjepë*, the Salvin's curassow *(Mitu salvini)*, and *ñantse*, the white-throated toucan *(Ramphastos tucanus)* once played an important part in the Secoya peoples' ceremonial attire. The long red tail feathers of the scarlet macaw are employed in crafting the matipë (ceremonial scepter). The fluffy white crissum feathers of the curassow (which is hunted for food) are used to decorate the long hanging yagé-drinking necklaces. The bright yellow rump and red crissum feathers of the toucan are employed in crafting the traditional yagé drinking crown, as are the brilliant azure-blue neck feathers of the masked tanager and the scarlet-red chest feathers of the scarlet tanager. Today, though, the elders see that these birds are getting scarce and have decided to craft their ceremonial objects using colorful yarn. The *payotinque*, the squirrel cuckoo *(Piaya cayana)*, is believed to be a messenger bird of the spiritual owner of the yagé. When yagé is to be harvested, this bird can appear. If it stays still and is calm, it is a good day to harvest, but if it is in a flurry, jumps about, and passes by quickly, it is best to refrain and wait until another day to harvest.

7. During a visit to his home in 2004, I heard the following from Secoya elder Delfin Payaguaje. There was a master of old who kept honeybees.

One day he ate too much honey and entered a trance. He met a celestial being from the heavenly realms who gifted him a variety of yagé. Honey is highly revered among many indigenous peoples not only for its sweetness, but also for its symbolic place in spiritual life. The old master said, when you dream of mobs of happy children running and jumping, their outstretched arms and fingers reaching toward long strands of honey hanging down like vines from a blue sky, when you see a pool of honey, you dive in and swim through to the other side . . . and drink only one sip, then you know you're getting close to touching the celestial energies!

8. These are the guidelines by which the Secoya grow their yage: The plants are grown where few people walk, especially where people with overly active sexual lives and or woman who may be menstruating or pregnant will approach or touch them. The vines are grown in a humid tropical setting where they receive plenty of sunlight and plenty of water, while not being overexposed, such that there are other plants growing near them and the vegetation is left to overgrow and conceal them. They are visited only in the early hours of the morning or in the afternoon, when they are sung to and offerings of natural tobacco are left at their base.

9. Luis Eduardo Luna and Pablo Amaringo, *Ayahuasca Visions: The Religious Iconography of a Peruvian Shaman* (Berkeley, CA: North Atlantic Books, 1991), page 48, Vision 1, "Preparation of Ayahuasca."

10. During the inebriation of the yagé the elders and the yagé itself teach, wordlessly, many types of spiritual practices that one must undertake in order to progress on the path of self-development, of awakening and purifying one's inner energies, in the energy centers of the body. The first of these is a profound state of inner self-reflection, where one considers many aspects of one's life or lives, many of which have been invisible to one for much too long. One learns to become still, very still, like a rock in the river. To have visions you have to slow the breath down, until it becomes very very still, until it seems as if you are not even breathing. After sustaining this for a given time one can achieves osmosis and begin breathing out of one's pores; one can purify the organs, and enter into alternate dimensions, such as inside the water where the doctor spirits abide.

11. Cesareo explained two ways to drink. The first is to dish out an extra-large gourd at the onset. Often, though, this will make one vomit; for

this method the drinkers must have undergone prior purification and be able to handle the large doses. Another stiff dose is repeated at midnight, and then another at three in the morning, for a total of three strong doses. The other method taught by the Wiñapai is to drink first one healthy sip, an hour later drink two healthy sips, another hour later drink three healthy sips, then after midnight, drink two healthy sips and near dawn one healthy sip, for a total of nine healthy sips, in five servings. A healthy sip is a decent-sized gulp, not a small tip-of-the-mouth-type sip. He also said that these are guidelines, not rules. The Secoya believe it is important to drink stiff doses, and that the yagé must always be strongly prepared. They say if one gets accustomed to drinking only weak brews and small doses, one can become a sorcerer. One is unable to break through the cortex of the ego, necessary to see the Wiñapai, and gets caught in self-importance. For this reason the Secoya, when initiating their youth for the first time, give them very strong yagé, which makes them scream most of the night!

Chapter 6: The Celestial Summer of the Cicadas

1. Fernando Payaguaje, *The Yage Drinker* (Quito, Ecuador: CICAME, 1994), p. 81.

2. In Spanish, this period is called *Veranito de San Juan* by local Ecuadorian mestizo settlers. The proper dry season comes later, from the end of December up to February; it is called *Ome'tëkahuë*, "summer season." That is when the ceremonial drinking of ancestrally cultivated varieties of pejí *(Brugmansia suaveolens)* would traditionally occur so drinkers could become acquainted with the Omepai, the "summer people," celestial spirits who are an important element of Secoya cosmology.

3. From Irene Bellier, *El Temblor y La Luna: Ensayo Sobre Las Relaciones Entre Las Mujeres y Los Hombres Mai Huna*, (Quito, Ecuador: CICAME, 1991), p. 48, quoting E. Jean Matteson Langdon, *The Siona Medical System: Beliefs and Behavior* (Ann Arbor, MI: Xerox Univ. Microfilms, 1974, pp. 145–147), who mentions: ". . . different types of people from the spiritual realms, occupants of cosmic strata, divine immortals: oko bai – 'people of the rainy season' or 'water people,' gina bai – 'people of the metal,' *insi hʷina bai* – 'people of the young sun,' *hʷina bai* – 'young or new people' or 'people of *yagé*,' *kako bai* – 'people of the August month,' the 'cicada people,' *tutu bai* – 'people of

the wind' or 'people of strength,' *yaya bai* – 'people of the moon.'"

4. Personal communication, 2011. When I asked the significance of the white or purple clothing, Miguel explained that according to his grandfather (Fernando Payaguaje) there are different heavenly realms: "When they wear many colors, it's easier to learn from them. They are from a heaven closer to the Earth and their wisdom can be more easily perceived. Wearing all white is symbolic of their purity. Heavenly beings who wear all one color are much more difficult to see. Since their energy levels are more refined, they are more sublime."

5. Again Taoism can provide a reference point from which to understand these indigenous perspectives: Lao Tzu wrote, "All my friends and disciples should attune their minds to all life and hold no antagonism towards any living thing, whether it is born of womb, egg, moisture or any other kind of transformation; whether it can think or is unable to think; whether it has form or is formless. You should dissolve all discriminations of individuality and absorb all things into a harmonious oneness. All lives are one life that can be called the One Great Universal Life." Hua-Ching Ni, *The Complete Works of Lao Tzu—Tao Teh Ching and Hua Hu Ching*, p. 110. Though the two philosophies arose in different parts of the globe, they come to similar conclusions about the human being's true nature.

6. An important part of learning the yagé phenomena is seeing the posá. These appear in the visions of yagé as various types of symbols. They are vibrational patterns representing trans-dimensional energy portals through which Wiñapai can pass in order to enter the ceremony; one goes through them to learn about other realms as well. A familiar posá is the plus sign, representing the balance inside one's being of heaven and earth; the plus sign also represents the sun. "And it reminds us to be like the sun," happily explained Esteban Lucitante.

7. *Bixa orellana* (Bixaceae) is known as *manduru* to the Kichwa, *bonsa* to the Secoya, *kakahue* to the Waorani, and *achiote* to Spanish speakers. This plant is used as a medicine and as a pigment for the face and body. There are several varieties; the most medicinal is one the Secoya call *katobonsa,* which in Costa Rican Spanish dialect is called *achiote criollo.* This variety does not have the bristly hairs on its fruit, and when it is mature it is green, unlike the common achiote, which is bright red when mature. Some strips of the bark of katobonsa are peeled and boiled and consumed in sips to stop someone who is

vomiting. The leaves are boiled and drunk to stop menstrual hemorrhage. The seeds are dried and nine are taken like little pills in the early hours of the morning for nine days to treat stomach ulcers. The leaves and stems are boiled and used to treat pains in the eye and for bruises on the eye. The seeds are mashed in a cup of water and strained, and the red drink is taken to control epileptic seizures, the drink being taken immediately after the seizure.

The Kichwa have a variety of this type of achiote that grows no taller than one meter called *paju manduru,* "power achiote." In times of drought, shamans of old would cover their bodies with its red pigment and swim in the river to make it rain. Also, when there is a storm just above the house, the green leaves and fruits are placed on the hot embers of the fire. The sizzling smoke that is released rises into the clouds and makes the storm pass.

The Waorani use the achiote tree to start their fires. The trunk is split and dried and a straight branch is dried as well. The branch is spun between the palms of both hands until it pops through the board, dropping a hot ember on a soft dry bed of cotton and leaves. This is blown on and soon it will burst into flame.

Pablo Amaringo shared a cure he used often to heal sorcery and spiritual damage, a cure he learned in an ayahuasca-induced vision using *Bixa orellana.* This cure can be effective for a wide array of conditions that can be called "spiritual imbalances" or "spiritual damages" (as would the copal cure in endnote 9, below). This could potentially include dyslexia and even autism (especially if the patient is still young), since these are considered in many indigenous medicine systems to be spirit attachments. The cure must be carried out on four consecutive days, without interruption, as follows: Young achiote branches some 40 cm long, complete with leaves and young shoots, are tied together in a bundle to form a leafy broom. The patient faces east, the direction of recovery, growth, and health. The healer stands in the east facing the patient. The strong black tobacco is lit. This is preferably rolled in dried plantain leaves. The cigar has to be large, so that enough smoke can be blown. The leafy broom is passed in sweeping motions over the front of the body first, from the head to the feet, then from the feet back up the body to the head, and finally again from the head back down to the ground. This way the leaves and smoke are passed over the front of the body three times. Then the patient faces west and the process is repeated. Afterward, the leftover stub of the tobacco must be rolled up in an achiote leaf and tied together as a little bundle. This leaf bundle is given to the patient, who puts this under his or her pillow and keeps it there overnight. The following morning the bundle needs to be untied and thrown into the bushes. This will allow one to see in dreams the cause of illness; it also helps in the visualization of one's recovery. These dreams should not be divulged to anyone; if one needs help interpreting them, they can be discussed with someone of confidence after a week's time has passed. Another important aspect of this cure is that every day after the healing, the achiote bundle is tied up onto one of the four main corner posts of the patient's home, until the fourth bundle has been tied to the fourth and final post, and all four posts now have achiote bundles tied onto them. It is important to not take the bundle down; the leaves must be left to dry and fall to the ground on their own accord, over time.

8. *Ocomaña* in the Secoya language means "water fragrance." This beautiful ground plant is grown near the houses of traditional families and is used as a ceremonial perfume. The ocomaña of the Secoya has large, greener leaves than the small-leafed yellow variety cultivated among the Kichwa called *piripiri,* a name that refers to an "enchantment" of sorts. When working toward the creation of Napo-Galeras National Park, don Casimiro would blow the fragrance of these leaves onto the documents to be delivered to the government so that no malicious energies would intervene in the portrayal of the authentic message, and it worked! The plants are grown near the houses as heirloom treasures, except for wirisaka, which grows wild in the hill country rainforest.

   There are several varieties of *Justicia pectoralis.* One called *hewë-maña,* "river otter perfume," is a wild variety found growing along the river, to a height of over a meter, whereas cultivated ocomaña grows no taller than 30 cm. Another variety is *remolino* or "whirlpool" piripiri. This uncommon variety of *Justicia pectoralis* has leaves that spiral outward (thus the name whirlpool); it's used to strengthen babies, as well as children's elbow and knee articulations as they grow; it's also used to reduce growing pains. I have seen this plant only at the Amazanga community in Pastaza Province.

9. Copal: *Dacryodes peruviana* (Burseraceae) is known as *kënje* to the Secoya and *wiñimunca* to the Waorani. The resin from this tree is considered sacred and is highly prized as a ceremonial incense. Copal is also used effectively to treat ailments of the lungs. The resin is heated

up and poured onto a piece of newspaper. When it cools this is placed over the lungs on the front and back of the chest and wrapped on with a cloth. For this same effect, honey works as well: the honey is poured onto the chest and back and the body covered with newspaper for quick relief of lung inflammation and heavy coughing. For broken bones, the sap is heated in a small pot and then a cloth is placed in the melted resin; once it cools, this cloth is wrapped around the broken limb and then a splint is added. Other trees carry aromatic resin or wood used for clearing negative energies, including *Bursera graveolens* from the dry rainforests of coastal Ecuador, known as *palo santo* and burned in the churches of the high Andes to invoke religious piety.

Following is one of don Pablo Amaringo's cures using copal, which he called "an empire of spirits." This cure is especially effective for people undergoing spiritual crisis or suffering from nervous disorders, for children who are restless and suffer from insomnia, for spirit possessions, and for illnesses that are not responding to treatments. It can work well for people who are good-hearted and sincere yet seem to be struck with misfortune. To accomplish this cure, the following must be undertaken, preferably in an outdoor area protected from wind: Some copal resin is ground up to a fine powder and placed in the sun to dry. Just after nightfall, a small fire is built on the ground and allowed to settle until it becomes glowing embers. The patient stands in front of the coals, ideally facing east. The healer must be "well-kept," meaning a person who is sincere and who lives a life of poise and self-discipline—necessary attributes in order to invoke an appropriate response. Prayers should be made for recovery of the person who is ill, imbalanced, or going through crisis. The incense powder is placed on the embers before the patient, and the fragrant smoke rises up toward his or her body. It should rise straight up one's body, into the air above like a column. If the person is not that ill, and if he or she is virtuous and kind, this can happen readily. However, sometimes it doesn't happen this way. Sometimes the patient is so ill that the smoke rejects him or her; the smoke drifts upward and off to one side or in a direction that does not go onto the person's body. If this occurs after several attempts, the following can be done. The patient and the healer face each other, holding hands with the fire in between. Then, facing each other, they walk around the fire three times in one direction, repeated by the same movement in the opposite direction. After this, more incense powder is placed on the coals, more prayers can be made as well, and then the smoke will eventually rise up toward the patient, enveloping his or her body, rising straight up into the air above. This can happen even if there is a gentle breeze. If the smoke rises up straight like a column and is not deflected by the breeze, this is a sure sign that the healing will be effective. Then the process is repeated on the patient's backside.

That night the patient is likely to have a lucid dream; this should not be told to anyone until at least a few days have passed. Also, the fact that one has undergone this cure should not be rapidly divulged either; it is best to keep this a secret for a while, at least until one is healthy again. Then one can then share this cure with others who may be in need.

Vital for the effectiveness of this cure is the following: the patient must remain out of sight of all people until two in the afternoon. If they leave their room before 2 PM, the patient will lose the energy and not be healed. For this reason food is brought into their room the night before or it can be placed at the patient's door, but retrieved without being seen, once the helper has left. At two in the afternoon, the patient must leave the house or place where he or she has been and go to a public place, greet people and shake their hands. He or she must hug a family member or friend and greet them in a cheerful manner, and everyone is enhanced by the life-affirming energy.

10. Wansoka is a close relative of *Macoubea witotorum,* an edible fruit known among the Witoto as *amapa.* Two other related trees with edible fruits and sap are *Lacmellea edulis* and *Lacmellea lactescens,* both known among the Waorani as *depemoncamo,* and in Kichwa as *chilcemuyu,* whose edible fruits are appreciated by the children and are high in vitamins concentrated in its edible oily sap. In Spanish it is known as *chicle,* but it is not the chicle that made world fame for its latex used in making of bubble gum. That is *Manilkara chicle* of the Sapotaceae family, found in the Central America tropical rainforest.

11. Visited by the Macuripai—an experience of don Cesareo: "Years ago when I lived at the Cuyabeno lakes, I had a small lodge that was a distance removed from the other villagers. Once, the Macuripai came right into my lodge to visit. They wore red tunics. They had beautiful maña on their arms and wrists. And their faces and legs were beautifully painted with intricate designs." He explained that these immortal celestial beings rarely visit the Earth, and when they do it is in the wilderness where things are pristine and non-contaminated, far from

the stench of human settlements, hypocrisy, and corruption. "When I was a child," he went on, "my grandfather brought me a small black palm nut charm from their world. It was my first necklace." Cesareo went on to explain that when his grandfather died, the palm nut charm necklace was no longer where he had left it. He looked all over and then asked his grandmother if she had seen it, who told him solemnly that she had burned it. As ancient custom mandates, she had burned it along with the rest of his grandfather's spiritual belongings, artifacts, and ceremonial utensils. It is believed that if these artifacts, such as his yagé drinking scepter, tunic, necklaces, and crown or other sacred items are passed along to a descendent, the person who wears them may fail to accomplish their own spiritual development. Some of these items may be passed along while the master is living. But upon his death, it's especially important to burn anything he received from the sky, such as a magic charm like a palm nut or an instrument like a flute.

12. Just upriver from its mouth, Wajo Sará lured the Portuguese colonists toward a high hill where the defenders had built a straight and steep trail to its summit. When the hostile invaders followed them up this trail, Wajo Sará and other Secoya rolled down heavy logs that they had hauled into place. This crushed the intruders. The cultural hero Wajo Sará was to the Secoya like Samson was to the Israelites. It is believed that if it weren't for Wajo Sará the Secoya would have died out. He was a great drinker of yagé, a leader of mighty ceremonies. On several occasions he was seen transforming before the drinkers into a harpy eagle, claws grabbing into the ground, tremendous wings outstretched. He led his ceremonies strictly according to the ancient guidelines in all respects.

13. The city of Coca is also known as Puerto Francisco de Orellana, after the Spanish conquistador of that name. Then in 1998 the entire eastern portion of what was Napo Province was divided and made into a two provinces with the new one called, of all names, Provincia de Orellana, showing that sadly Orellana's undeserved legacy as a great man lives on in the corrupted historical memory. It always amazes me how, despite Ecuador's having achieved independence from Spain in 1822, and despite its 2007 constitution that declares the country a pluri-cultural country founded on respect and recognition of all its citizens' intrinsic rights including those of nature, the country still chooses to honor a ruthless barbarian such as Orellana.

14. Secoya elders attest that the modern name of this town, Pantoja, is

derived from the name of a Secoya clan that lived there, the Pioje clan, in a large village called Quacosariyá. This was the home of another cultural hero and master of the heavenly tradition—a great yagé drinker of old by the name of Wao Sutú, a source of inspiration to Cesareo in his youth when his grandmother told him stories. One story involved Wao Sutú through his song bringing down a giant celestial turtle, a Matëmo Cou. Many villagers saw the hands of the Matëmopai holding it and were able to eat a piece of the meat when it was butchered. Wao Sutú breakfasted on turtle fat dipped in yagé. On another occasion Wao Sutú made two large clay pots and covered them, and the next day they were filled to the rim with turtle eggs. In the village of Quacosariyá around the same time lived Yai'wankeo, a powerful woman yagé drinker and healer who would transform into a jaguar and would summon wild boar.

15. In the early 1990s, under the presidency of Rodrigo Borja, the Secoya received legal recognition to an area of land along the Aguarico River (known in Paicoca as the Jaiyá) that was 39,414 hectares in size (152 square miles). This may seem like a lot, but it is important to recognize that this represents a mere 2.5% of their ancestral homelands in modern-day Ecuador. While writing this book, I received great news. Here are some excerpts from SERNANP, *Servicio Nacional de Areas Naturales Protegidas por el Estado* (the Peruvian government institute for the country's natural protected areas) official website (translated from Spanish): "Great news for conservation of our natural patrimony on behalf of supreme government decree No. 006-2012-MINAM, published in the Bulletin of Legal Happenings of the Peruvian newspaper *El Peruano*, the status conversion from Reserved Area to that of The Güeppí-Sekime National Park on October 10, 2012, as well as the Huemeki and Airo Pai community reserves, constitute the creation of three new Natural Protected Areas by the Peruvian State. This declaration will protect and maintain in a pristine state for perpetuity and lower human impact on the area 592,749 hectares of rainforest lands (that's 2,289 square miles) where reside Secoya, Kichwa, Huitoto, and mestizo settlements."

16. This is from an estimation of the sum of all the family clans to have existed, their names remembered by the elders as part of the oral tradition.

17. Black Hawk (1767–1838), of the Sauk American Indian tribe whose life story is portrayed in *The Life of Black Hawk,* by Black Hawk, edited

by Milo Milton Quaife (New York: Dover, 1916), said: "Let us reflect how many animal tribes we ourselves have destroyed, maybe our time has come like the melting of the snow."

18. These cultigens include *paiwea*, "people's corn," a type of corn that is planted only when Orion's belt is seen at zenith at sunset. A number of crops are cultivated, such as *pi'ré* (*Xanthosoma* sp.), which has edible tubers; *uncuisí* (*Renealmia alpinia*), a nutritious oily fruit pulp used for flavoring fish soup; *se'ú* (*Calathea allouia*), a rare plant cultivated for its edible tubers; *yají* (*Ipomoea batatas*), sweet potato; *cantë* (*Saccharum officinarum*), sugar cane; and *ëné* (*Bactris gasipaes*), the peach palm fruit, among many others.

19. San Pablo is located on the Aguarico River in Sucumbios Province. It is reached from the oil boomtown of Shushufindi. In 2011 the road was pushed all the way to the village, an act that has begun to powerfully transform the society.

20. Pëquë'yá (Black-Caiman Lagoons) is a classic igapó ecosystem type, characterized by blackwater lagoons and firm soil ridges. If you have been trying to learn the Paicoca words, you might have noticed that the suffix *–ya* means "river" and thus this name would read "Black-Caiman River" in a strict translation. But along this river are found several lagoons, so I have translated it more appropriately as "Black-Caiman Lagoons." Pëquë'yá is characterized by the presence of *ocobeto* palms (*Astrocaryum jauari*). Growing along the lagoons' edges can also be found *ocha'sá* (*Myrciaria dubia*), which has an edible fruit high in ascorbic acid. Other notable native species include *ma'yëi* (*Pseudobombax mungupa*), a tree whose bark is peeled and used to make a kitchen utensil for squeezing the juice from grated yuca tubers, and *ható* trees (*Macrolobium acaciifolium*), whose sunny exposed branches are favored by a calm-natured hairy monkey with a long hanging tail that the Secoya call *waosutu*—saki monkeys (*Pithecia aequatorialis*). In these lagoons can be found the *mawëwë* or pink Amazonian dolphin (*Inia geoffrensis*), the *quaheyo* or giant river otter (*Pteronura brasiliensis*), the *mañumi* or green anaconda (*Eunectes murinus*), and the infamous man-eating *neapë'e* or black caiman (*Melanosuchus niger*), after which the area is named. All these species are emblematic of the igapó areas, not found along the Aguarico River where the Secoya live today.

The Secoya have many legends related to this region. When we returned there on the first visits decades after they had had to abandon the area, it was as if they had never left. The youth knew every river's bend and the name of all the lakes solely from listening to the elders.

21. Igapó and Varsea ecosystem types: *Igapó* is a Brazilian term used to describe areas where blackwater lakes and flooded forest are found. In Paicoca the term is *daiawë yejá,* "flooded land." Along the upper reaches of Pëquë'yá there are firm ridges and solid riverbanks where mature canopy rainforest thick in palms can be found. In Ecuador, igapó areas are not common, as the majority of the forests are of the varsea type, still being relatively close to the base of the Andes. Varsea ecosystems are areas where firm soil meets brown-water rivers. Nearly all the rivers that run east off the Andes are brown-water rivers, and the lowland rainforest that they wind through is considered to be varsea. The Secoya call this area *sewá yejá,* "sewá land," due to the prevalence of sewá palms *(Phytelephas microcarpa),* a palm known as *tagua* in Ecuadorian Spanish, the source of vegetable ivory.

22. The Rio de Janeiro Treaty of 1942 resolved the Ecuadorian-Peruvian War of 1941. This was a territorial dispute between the two countries, over the course of which Ecuador lost to Peru nearly all of what is today the Peruvian province of Maynas.

23. Marshall B. Rosenberg, *Nonviolent Communication: A Language of Life* (Encinitas, CA: PuddleDancer Press, 2003).

24. Alfredo Payaguaje became friends with Pablo Yépez, a biologist from Ecuador's Universidad Católica. The two worked together to found an ethnobotanical teaching center along the Shushufindi River. Pablo oversaw the publication of three compilations dedicated to Secoya culture. Celestino Piaguaje learned to read and write and taught the younger Secoya this valuable skill in order to interface with the 20th century. I helped him edit a small book, *Siecoya Pai Panihueositorepa, Secoya Origins* (1996).

25. Toyáyai, "designs jaguar," was a humorous nickname the kids gave me in Secoya territory, one that always had the kids laughing.

26. Here Cesareo is referring to different energy realms. The Ñamase proper lives in a high-vibrational energy realm, above that of humans, where as the Ñamase Watí lives in the realms of the Watí, a lower-vibrational realm, below that of humans. This denser energy realm is easier to access from the human realm than are the higher realms. This is why students on the path must have a clear understanding of what they are embarking upon in order to not mistake the lower levels for the higher.

27. Here is an excerpt from the legend of Repao and Rutayo, and the battle between Muhu (Thunder) and Paina (the creator, a synonym for Ñañë). Muhu was finding it impossible to build a good house. The posts were loose and the beams kept falling in. Paina knew how to build a house and Muhu asked him to help make a structure secure. At night Muhu would sleep with his two wives, Rutayo and Repao. By day Paina appeared as a ragged dirty old man, but at night he appeared as a handsome young man. Muhu's younger wife Repao took a liking to him and began serving him food. Muhu saw what was happening and arranged for a fight. He asked his wives to make chicha and he himself made a bamboo spear. Paina took the bamboo that was left over and made a spear himself. Muhu's spear was sharp and charged with lightning, while Paina's was simple. When Muhu went to take a piss, Paina switched the spears and made his look like Muhu's. At that point, Paina called on the Starry Beings and the Heaven Beings to watch. Paina jumped up and held onto a roof beam of the half-built house. Hanging there, he said to Muhu, "You go first." Muhu swung his weapon. Just as Muhu swung at him, Ñañë said "I am rubber." Struck, his belly stretched far out behind him, then snapped back to its original form. Then he said to Muhu, "Your turn." Muhu jumped and hung from the same roof beam. Paina using Muhu's own sword swung and chopped Muhu in half. Blood spilling from his body, Muhu transformed in midair into *quauquiyo* birds, screaming *pihas (Lipaugus vociferans)*, that flew away into the air. The rest of his body dissolved into thunder and lightning. Rutayo, Muhu's older wife, outraged broke the bowls of chicha that spilled over the ground. In that moment she became the goddess of the water world, and the chicha turned to water and covered the Earth. Only right where Paina was standing was there still some land, which disappeared as he ascended. Some bubbles rose up from the water. Paina addressed them silently, "Come forth." Up comes the *Insi Jamu,* the "Pineapple Armadillo." "Bring up the land," thinks Paina, and the Pineapple Armadillo brings up the land, which is why the American continent is called *Insi Jamu Yejá,* "Pineapple Armadillo Land." Paina transformed Repao, Muhu's younger wife who had taken a liking to him, into a comb, put her into his hair, and ascended to Heaven. Upon reaching Heaven he transformed her back into Repao. The two live as husband and wife now. Repao appears in the story of Quequero, elsewhere in this book, which explains how the Secoya received the matipë, the ceremonial scepter.

Chapter 7: The Deep-Forest Perspective of the Waorani

1. Laura Rival, *Trekking Through History: The Huaorani of Amazonian Ecuador* (New York: Columbia University Press, 2002), p. 1.

2. To see a list of her publications, view The Institute of Social and Cultural Anthropology at Oxford University's web site.

3. When asked to heal someone, the iroinga will laugh and respond something along the lines of, "You got yourself sick, you have to heal yourself." If a Waorani heals someone, he is essentially admitting to having caused the illness. The Waorani value independence above all, and the iroinga, more than any of the other Waorani, is the most independent. For this reason, the iroinga is always given the heaviest load to carry, which he does without complaining; he does this laughing. Anyone can come to an iroinga's house and be fed. Every visit I made to Mengatue's house, he would give me a valuable gift. He gave me several 11-foot-long traditional palm-wood spears wound with colorful feathers, a hammock, and an *omena*, a 12-foot-long blowpipe complete with a quiver full of smoked darts dipped in jet-black *oomae* (curare) hunting poison, a piranha jaw to notch the darts, and a gourd with a small hole packed with cotton.

4. The *azulejo* (blue tanager, also called the masked tanager, *Tangara nigrocincta*) is a symbol of the Wiñetare, a remote non-contacted group of Waorani living in deep isolation. Laura Rival writes: "Huaorani culture and society is shaped by their will to self-isolation. Very little is known about their past, except that they have for centuries constituted nomadic and autarkic enclaves fiercely refusing contact, trade and exchange with their powerful neighbors, be they indigenous or white-mestizo colonists." Quoted from her article "Ecuador: The Huaorani People of the Amazon, self-isolation and forced contact," World Rainforest Movement bulletin #87, October 2004.

5. James S. Boster, James Yost, and Catherine Peeke, "Rage, Revenge, and Religion: Honest Signaling of Aggression and Nonaggression in Waorani Coalitional Violence," *Ethos 31*(4): 471–494, American Anthropological Association, 2004.

6. William S. Burroughs, Allen Ginsberg, and Oliver Harris, *The Yage Letters Redux* (San Francisco: City Lights, 2006), p. 35.

7. Norman E. Whitten, Jr., book review, "Trekking Through History: The Huaorani of Amazonia," Tipití USA: *Journal of the Society for the Anthropology of Lowland South America*, Vol. 1, Issue 2, Article 4, 2003.

8. Laura Rival, "Ecuador: The Huaorani People of the Amazonia, self-isolation and forced contact," see note 4 above.

9. *El Comercio* (Ecuadorian newspaper), April 14, 2013, interview with Miguel Angel Cabodevilla, translated by the author. *Interviewer:* Why do you not share the use of the definition "people in voluntary isolation" to refer to Taromenane? *Cabodevilla:* I prefer to call them hidden people, although it is not a good term either. But I oppose calling them "people in voluntary isolation" because it can sustain unnecessary taboos in people's minds. Society often identifies these sorts of tribes as people living happily in the jungle. On the contrary, the signs that we have collected do not indicate they necessarily want to be isolated, nor do they want to be in close contact with Ecuadorian people. This is because they need a number of tools that they do not have.

Interviewer: Why did the Taromenane spear Ompure and his wife Buganey, both members of the Huaorani tribe, two months ago? What does their death mean?

Cabodevilla: Some say it is absolutely absurd that Ompure was attacked because they [the Taromenane] were afraid of the noise coming from the oil wells. Two hundred meters from Buganey and Ompure's hut there was a small group of unarmed Repsol workers, going about their day [Repsol is the Argentinian oil company operating various oil-drilling bases in the Ecuadorian Amazon], and they were not attacked. Ompure used to walk for four or six hours into the depths of the jungle alone, and shared hunting grounds with the Taromenane. He [Ompure] did not want to live in a Huaorani village, he dressed with gumi [traditional Huaorani waist strap], he was the closest thing to them, they had continuous encounters with him.

Interviewer: Why was he killed?

Cabodevilla: I do not know if Ompure had done acts of violence against them. Ompure was perhaps killed just because he could not deliver the things they asked of him: machetes, axes, cooking pots. He distributed too few, and the people inside the Taromenane probably fought for the novel things that were scarce. This is a hypothesis that should not be ruled out.

Interviewer: On March 29, [2013] a Huaroani group took revenge for Ompure's death and, according to the Huarani leaders, killed 30 members of the Taromenane tribe. Why did so many die if they attacked only one house?

Cabodevilla: We have our own information. The Taromenane live in fairly large village houses. One of the things we know is that the Huaorani attacked the Taromenane at a time when they were having some sort of celebration. Perhaps there were several families gathered, because in that area there are three or four Taromenane village houses. If a Huaorani leader says there were 30 and another says there were only 10, we may not know for sure, but we fear that the number of victims is closer to 30.

Interviewer: On Saturday, April 6, the President of Ecuador, Rafael Correa, said that this incident was due to a fight between clans. What do you think?

Cabodevilla: It is evident that this situation is due to a clash between clans. The question is, why are they fighting? After the 2009 attack [on a small settlement called Los Reyes] when Taromenane tribesmen killed a colonist woman and two children, the government lost track of the Taromenane. This contact would have helped to prevent further deaths such as Ompure and Buganey's. When some deaths occur, why do people from the government never arrive? Advanced precautionary measures are not taken and even rejected by the Huaorani. The Taromenane are protected by the state. If the state's protected people cause any damage, the state must cover the cost of such damage. The state was not ready, they had no plan, no rules, nothing. Why has the government not prepared any plan for compensation for victims of its protégés after four years? After the death of Ompure, I told some acquaintances, "Go right away, make a fair and generous proposal to the Huaorani, and say that you will make it happen immediately. But if they will instead take vengeance, then such compensation will not be given." But nothing was done. The people [Huaorani] made three search missions into the depths of the jungle to reach the Taromenane; the first and second failed, and the third one was successful. How can you say it's just a fight between clans? Especially when there is a specialized commission for the protection of these people, why is it not working? There is no plan; if they fail then what are they there for?

10. A fabulous video on the Waorani life in peace can be seen on YouTube: "Nomads of the Rainforest," produced by PBS (1984). To learn more about the intangible zone: www.huaoraniintangiblezone.wordpress. com. And for yet more Waorani culture: In May 1991, friends and I produced an album called *Waorani Waaponi,* showcasing a cappella chanting in the Amazon. The recording can be obtained through the

album's producer, Tumi Music Co. in Bath, England: www.tumimusic.com/Waorani_Waaponi/tumi043/albums/music/

11. Wepe showed me the type of termite nest used for healing wounds, especially the smaller nests that are found near the ground. These nests are quickly repaired when disturbed or poked. Thus the Waorani use a heated poultice of the termites and nest material to heal stubborn wounds. Likewise, from observing the bark of the *dohi*, the *Spondias mombin* tree, the Secoya saw that when marred it heals itself quickly and completely. When the bark juice is topically applied to human wounds, it heals them expertly as well. As with many traditional medical sciences elsewhere, native Amazonian dwellers read nature through the "doctrine of signatures." This approach to nature was once common in Europe, widely promoted in the late sixteenth century by the Swiss botanist Theophrastus Paracelsus. See *The Doctrine of Signatures* (Whitefish, MT: Kessinger Publishing, 2010) and *The Language of Plants: A Guide to the Doctrine of Signatures* by Julia Graves (Great Barrington, MA: SteinerBooks, 2012). The doctrine of signatures has taught for millennia that every aspect of a living being contains an insight about the intrinsic nature of the whole. In any one genetic fingerprint of a species, the entire species can be studied and understood. It offers a pathway to heighten one's awareness of nature and feel more connected to the web of life that we are an inseparable part of.

12. This narration is written as told by Mengatue Baihua on February 29, 1992, at a small hunting camp on the banks of the Gueyemonpare Creek, in the headwaters of the Shiripuno River, Napo Province, Amazonian Ecuador. It was translated from Waorani to Spanish by Jonas Kahuitipe Cohue. The same myth was told by Wepe Orengo Coba at the Waorani village of Quihuaro in Pastaza Province on April 6, 1993. Another aspect of this myth was told by Ohue Coba on May 3, 1995, in Quehueiriono, a village at the headwaters of the Shiripuno River. These recordings were translated from Waorani to Spanish by Namonka, Niwa, and Nenquerei Enomenga. The accounts were recorded on audio-cassette, and translated from Spanish to English by Jonathon SMW. The version appearing in these pages is an abbreviated version of the myth as rendered in English for publication in *Ayahuasca Reader: Encounters with the Sacred Vine* (Santa Fe: Synergetic Press, 2000).

Chapter 8: The Eyebrows of the Andes

1. F. Bruce Lamb, *Rio Tigre and Beyond: The Amazon Jungle Medicine of Manuel Córdova* (Berkeley, CA: North Atlantic Books, 1985), p. 17.

2. The life and ways of the highland Puruwa Kichwa of this region can be considered the mother culture of northwestern South America, much as the ancient Olmec culture is the mother culture of Central America. Everyone respects the highland Kichwas for their unequalled work ethic as farmers and weavers. For the most part the people of this region adhere to a disciplined way of life they call the Sumak Kausai. This phrase has now become a national adage under Ecuador's new constitution, which respects indigenous cultures as an integral part of the country's heritage. *Sumak* is "beautiful" and *kausai* means "life."

   Diushun, "may God repay you," is a phrase commonly heard, expressing these people's ingrained gratitude. They dedicate long hours to agriculture and raising livestock such as sheep and guinea pigs. They supply much of Ecuador's grains and vegetables.

   Among the highland Kichwa, indigenous spirituality, Catholicism, and the mountains have been synonymous for a long time. This veneration of mountains can be seen in the annual pilgrimage of the Puruwa Kichwa to Mount Alacahuán. This occurs in the province of Chimborazo each year in March to conclude the festivities of the Warmi Pascua, Woman's Easter, which celebrates the sprouting of the grains. During this festival, thousands of people from many different communities meet to pray and to give thanks at the mountain's summit. The Ecuadorian Andes is a land rich in many kinds of festivals, all of which commemorate a life close to Pachamama, "Mother Earth." In the Intiraimi, the summer solstice festival, costumed characters teach morality through chaos. One of these iconic characters is the diablouma, "devil head," who wears a mask made of cloth and felt; colorful protrusions of wound cloth rise above his head. The diablouma always wears chaps made of thick fur. He carries a whip, a small tube filled with chili pepper paste, and a little wooden wand; to protect the festival dancers from harassment, he uses the whip, and with the wand he smears chili pepper paste on the lips of rowdy drunks. He dances gleefully, skipping through the colorfully dressed dancing crowds. He is a force of good at the festivals and demonstrates how spirit protects, but it also punishes those who step out of bounds. Another pair of characters is a child leading a gorilla. In one hand the child holds a shield (often a garbage can lid) and in the other hand a leash that controls an adult dressed as a gorilla. The gorilla goes swinging his arms wildly through the crowd trying to grab people, making everyone run and laugh, because he never grabs anyone, just scares them off. Meanwhile the child has him firmly leashed and prevents him from escaping and causing harm. This represents how through the innocence of the inner child we control our inner "gorilla," the impulse within us that wants to grab ahold of all it sees.

3. Personal communication in 1994, while I was collaborating on the physical demarcation of Waorani territory. To learn more about Moi and the struggle of the Waorani, read *Savages* by Joe Kane (Knopf, 1995).

4. Edward O. Wilson, *The Diversity of Life* (New York: W.W. Norton, 1993), page 353.

5. BioMed Central Limited, "New biodiversity map of Andes shows species in dire need of protection," ScienceDaily, 29 Jan. 2012. Another article in ScienceDaily from two days earlier was headlined, "80 Percent of 'Irreplaceable' Habitats in Andes Unprotected." The article relates that "Hundreds of rare, endemic species in the Central Andes remain unprotected and are increasingly under threat from development and climate change, according to a new Duke University-led international study."

A personal note on biological extinction: When I was a child growing up in Ecuador, my friend's father would take often take him and me rabbit hunting on the tundra-like slopes of Mount Cayambe and in the high country near the village of Papallacta. There were hundreds of sluggish carbon-black frogs with bright orange underparts called *jambato (Atelopus ignescens)*. We had to watch where we walked in order to not step on them. Today these frogs are extinct, possibly from a combination of fungal disease and climate change.

6. According to the Holdridge Life Zone system, which classifies ecosystem types based principally on temperature and moisture levels. To clarify, the Tropical Andes is the region extending from the Tropical Wet Forest up the forest-covered slopes of the Andes. Conservation International calls the Tropical Andes the most species-rich region on the planet, the number-one "hotspot" in terms of biological diversity. In 2010, in a personal communication with Paul Malo, coordinator for the *Red de Amigos del Corredor Biológico Llanganati-Sangay,* an organization located in Puyo dedicated to local sustainable development, I learned that although Ecuador contains a mere 1.6–2% of

the Amazon basin, the country contains an impressive 69% of the Tropical Andes bioregion. Ecuador—nestled at the center of north-western South America and snug along the equator—is considered to be among the most species-rich regions on Earth. Regardless of its small geographical size (283,560 sq. kilometers = 109,483 sq. miles), the country is extremely high in biodiversity. Until not long ago, all of Ecuador was one big botanical garden and zoo. Today this beautiful country is teeter-tottering, like many countries, between the potential of a sustainable future of productive ecosystems and people and ecofriendly industries and a dysfunctional developing-world scenario of poverty, overpopulation, corporate takeover, rampant deforestation, and other ruthless and inappropriate activities. This harsh reality promises to push many species of plants and animals beyond the point of no return, as well as to increase the suffering of the country's people. In 2007 Ecuador adopted a new constitution, called *El Plan del Buen Vivir* (The Plan of Good Life), granting constitutional rights to Nature and recognizing indigenous cultures as an essential part of the national heritage. Yet the gap is wide between these new progressive laws and the reality at ground level, and the future of many species is uncertain. On the scale of the global economy and the huge industry of tourism, the only thing that Ecuador has to compete with on an international level is biodiversity. Biodiversity is the only category that places Ecuador in a league of its own.

7. Walter Palacios, *Cuatro especies nuevas de árboles del Ecuador* (Four new tree species from Ecuador). Herbario Nacional del Ecuador (QCNE), Universidad Técnica del Norte, Ibarra, Ecuador. *Caldasia*, Vol. 34, No. 1 (2012): 75–85.

8. Missouri Botanical Garden's Alwyn Gentry (1945–1993) determined that endemism and biological diversity increase directly proportional to the level of rainfall. His field guide, *The Woody Plants of Northwest South America (Colombia, Ecuador, Peru), with Supplementary Notes on Herbaceous Taxa* (Chicago: University of Chicago Press, 1996) reveals his tremendous skill and mastery of tropical botany. Gentry wrote many remarkable articles about biodiversity. One of them, co-authored with Calaway Dodson (a leading orchid expert), "Biological Extinction in Western Ecuador" (*Annals of the Missouri Botanical Garden*, Vol. 78, No. 2 (1991): 273–295), states, "within western Ecuador there are loci of much narrower endemism, especially on isolated ridge tops. Some of these patches of high local endemism may consist of habitat islands

no more than .5-10 km^2. That such extreme local endemism is typical of certain tropical forest has only recently been realized. . . . Thus, from a conservation perspective, to avoid massive extinction it is not only important to conserve patches of the major forest types, but also to conserve individual or semi-isolated habitat islands."

9. The SNAP *(Sistema Nacional de Áreas Protegidas)* is Ecuador's National System of Protected Areas, under the administration of the Ministry of the Environment. A forestry conservation incentive called "Plan Socio Bosque" is proving effective in offering campesinos and indigenous peoples' communities the opportunity to place their land holding under a conservation easement whereby they receive a certain amount of money per hectare per year for the land set aside in conservation. This plan is protecting small and large patches of various types of rainforest all over the country.

10. While I was studying at Humboldt State University, a professor of mine spoke to me of Jatun Sacha, a Tropical Wet Forest biological reserve and research station on the upper Napo River co-founded by a student from HSU and colleagues from the Missouri Botanical Garden. This is where my ten-year Amazonian sojourn began. In 1990 I volunteered there for some months on the creation of a botanical garden. I met Mercedes Mamallacta and Angel Alvarado, Kichwa ethnobotanists active in recuperating their people's plant lore. The reserve can be visited and they accept volunteers.

   According to biological inventories carried out by the Missouri Botanical Garden, the neo-tropics have been found to contain more than 90,000 species of plants (Central and South American tropical regions), with ±35,000 of these found in Ecuador. Compare these figures with those of Africa (including Madagascar) with ±30,000 species, and the Malaysian archipelago with ±35,000. Undeniably this abundance of plant life in the neo-tropics is related to the dramatic altitudinal and climatic transitions. Nowhere else do you find glaciers on the equator, on snow-capped peaks over 19,000 feet high. Their slopes drop into lowland tropical rainforest. According to the Holdridge Life Zone system, which identifies 116 life zones on Earth, Ecuador has about two dozen of these. It is important to note that within each of these life zones many distinct habitat types exist.

11. The main body of the Curaray River, known among the Waorani as the Ëhuengono (River of the Scarlet Macaws) is their southern territorial limit.

12. To accomplish this work and formalize the responsibilities, we forged an agreement with the Ecuadorian park service. This was Agreement #87, signed August 25, 1993, by the CIBT (*Centro de Investigación de los Bosque Tropicales,* the foundation I worked with on the demarcation of the Waorani territory, which agreed to help take on this project); the Mamallacta family, represented by the three elders, Casimiro, Vicente, and Cesar Mamallacta, and their descendents; and INEFAN, the Ecuadorian Park Service (today this institution is known as the *Ministerio del Ambiente,* the Ministry of the Environment).

13. In the village of Agua Santa near Mount Chimborazo lives my *compadre,* Juan Pilco, and his family. His eldest son, Juan Patricio, has been dedicated since 1994 to "Dressing the Mountains in Green," as he has dubbed the community project that he initiated and oversees. Thanks to his ardent devotion, he and his friends and neighbors have planted more than 90,000 native trees. He hopes to help stabilize the region's weather patterns, help recuperate the dwindling water supply, and allow the native birds that once populated the region to return. Other aspects of the project that friends and I have been able to support have been building water catchment systems, improving the water quality of the villagers, and assisting the reforestation and restoration of the degraded landscape. For more information on this project, please visit, www.4biodiversity.org or www.livingbridgesfoundation.org.

14. In 2010, to commemorate UNESCO's declaration of the International Year for Biodiversity, I presented a petition to the park service, together with another report that demonstrated even more clearly the work we had accomplished on behalf of Wairachina Sacha, including negotiation of a biological corridor with the Kichwa community of Santa Rosa de Arapino. The report, *Criterios Técnicos y Científicos para la ampliación del Parque Nacional Sumaco Napo Galeras y Diseños para el Desarrollo local Sostenible en sus Zonas Periféricas,* "Technical and Scientific Criteria for the Enlargement of the Sumaco Napo-Galeras National Park and Designs for Local Sustainable Development in its Periphery Zones," was successful in re-establishing the original status of Wairachina Sacha as a forest protectorate area. The fact that it had been given this status was almost forgotten and was not reflected on conservation maps; today, thanks to this effort, it is at least back on the map as a *Patrimonio Forestal.* PDFs of this report and others I have written regarding the Sumaco and Napo-Galeras areas can be found online at www.4biodiversity.org.

15. Here in the headwaters of this creek, up the mountain's southeastern slope, there is said to be a cave. There, in times of old, the yachac (sages and spiritual masters) would enter and be transported to the high mountains, where they would emerge out of other cave mouths and walk into the central valley of the high Andes to visit and enjoy the festivals occurring there.

16. To support the creation of the necessary intercultural bridge, I started a company called Guayusa Tea House (www.guayusateahouse.com). Until recently, guayusa tea was rarely found outside Ecuador. Today the Guayusa Tea House has created a market-driven rainforest conservation and restoration project in order to link conscientious people worldwide in a fair trade swap: rainforest conservation for good health. Customers pay above-market-value prices directly to indigenous growers who are protecting the most biodiverse ecosystems in the world and supplying high-quality guayusa tea and other rainforest products. The initiative aims to contribute to the preservation of the sacred mountain of Napo-Galeras and its beautiful rainforest through an attempt to create sustainable economic alternatives for forest-dwelling people.

Chapter 9: Lineage Holders of the Traditions, Deep Forest and Urban

1. Hua-Ching Ni, *The Golden Collection of Spiritual Practices, Part I: Workbook for Spiritual Development of All People* (Santa Monica, CA: Seven Star Communications Group, 1995), p. 54.

2. Lines 2–4 of the poem "I Sing the Body Electric" from *Leaves of Grass* (1855).

3. At Amazanga village the drum can be heard at 3 AM. Taita Rafael, Mama Lucila, their eldest son Flavio, and other family members and friends all begin to arise and gather to participate in the morning ritual of guayusa. This is *Ilex guayusa* of the Aquifoleaceae or holly family, a rather nondescript tree, with simple coriaceous leaves with serrate margins, often with faint black tracing below. While drinking tea they share that night's dreams, plan the activities of the coming day, and oftentimes discuss the vast topics and lore that compose the oral tradition of the people.

   Drinking guayusa has been found to balance the body's pH and blood sugar levels, detoxify the blood, improve the functioning of the kidneys and urinary tract, improve digestion and elimination while strengthening the lungs, and to remove cholesterol and balance blood pressure. Many people find drinking guayusa both relaxing and stimulating at the same time. It is sometimes referred to as "dream tea" for its effect of helping promote lucid dreaming and better dream recall.

Many teas are known to contain antioxidants, which fend off cancer-causing "free radicals" in our bodies. In studies of guayusa, this tea has been found to contain twice the level of antioxidants in green tea and to have one of the highest antioxidant levels known in any food or supplement, second only to raw cacao powder, obtained from the dried and ground seeds of the cacao tree (*Theobroma cacao*). Guayusa tea offers a unique synergistic blend of theobromine, theophyline, guanidine (an amino acid), and caffeine, producing smooth, sustained energy.

Among the forest-dwelling Kichwa people of the upper Napo, the tea is known as known as waísa or waísamama, a word that conveys the concept of a certain kind of power or energy found in nature—that of medium-sized rivers that run crystal clear. This same subtle energy can be cultivated and accumulated over time in a human body, and the results make one strong, happy, and wise. In order to accumulate this subtle and sacred power or energy of the river, guayusa tea is drunk every day, very early in the morning, at the wee hours of pre-dawn. Then one bathes in the river shortly after, before the first bird sings, most specifically before the hummingbird bathes. Waísamama is *waísa* combined with *mama*, meaning "mother, power, authority, or protector." To drink waísamama and gain the river's waísa is the Kichwa health-insurance policy, as one who embodies the waísa will not easily become ill; on the contrary, this person enjoys good health, laughter, and vitality. Once the hummingbird bathes, it is believed in the science of the people that it takes the river's waísa away for that day. After the stillness of the night it is restored while the hummingbird sleeps. This is why if one can bathe before the hummingbird, then the river's energy is available to be absorbed into one's being at that time of morning. The hummingbird is representative of perfection: its feathers always gleaming, its energy vibrations high. It is believed to be like this because it gathers the waísa from the river. Also, the fact that the guayusa tree is strong and resistant to wind-throw is another reason the people grant it such powerful attributes of bestowing longevity and strength to those who drink the tea of its leaves.

Conclusion

1. Luis Eduardo Luna and Pablo Amaringo, *Ayahuasca Visions: The Religious Iconography of a Peruvian Shaman* (Berkeley, CA: North Atlantic Books, 1991), p. 27.

2. Kathleen Harrison in *Visionary Plant Consciousness,* J. P. Harpignies, ed. (Rochester, VT: Park Street Press, 2007).

GLOSSARY

Key to language abbreviations

Achuar = Spoken in the Ecuadorian and Peruvian Amazon
Ai = name of the Cofán people's language
Cañari = an pre-Incan confederacy of tribes from southern Ecuador and
   northern Peru
K. = Amazonian lowland Kichwa (Runashimi)
K.-Highland = Kichwa from central Andes highlands (Quechua)
K.-Napo = Kichwa from Napo Province
K.-Pastaza = Kichwa from Pastaza Province
K.-Peru = Kichwa dialect from the Peruvian Amazon
Quitus = an extinct language once spoken in the north-central Andes
S. = Secoya (Paicoca)
Sh. = Shuar, spoken mainly in the Ecuadorian Amazon, and in the
   Peruvian upper Amazon as well
Sp. Mestizo = mestizo Spanish (mixed ancestry)
Sp. = Spanish; Ecuadorian and Peruvian dialects
Tucano = spoken in the Colombian Amazon
W. = Waorani (Wao Terero), spoken in the Ecuadorian Amazon

Aceropunta (Sp. Mestizo) Steel Point, phantom boat (barco fantasma)
Achuar (Sp.) an Amazonian community of some 18,500 individuals along
   either side of the border of Ecuador and Peru
Airo Pai (S.) means "forest people," a name the Peruvian Secoya go by
Airoyai (S.) the spotted forest jaguar *(Panthera onca)*, also referred to as
   toyáyai
Ajenjo (Sp.) *Artemisia absinthium*—medicinal plant from Andes
Ajuswaska (K.) *Mansoa alliaceae*—a medicinal vine with garlic-scented
   leaves
Albahaca (Sp.) *Ocimum campechianum*—an aromatic herb, basil
Altamisa (Sp.) *Ambrosia peruviana*—medicinal plant from the Andes
Amiruka panga (K.-Napo) *Psychotria viridis*—ayahuasca admixture plant
Amotamini (W.) Waorani traditional chanting
Aña (S.) snake
Añapëquë (S.) a mythical fish of exaggerated proportions

Antisana (Quitus) most sacred heights or beacon. It is a mighty snow-capped volcano along the eastern range, 5,704 m (18,714 ft)

Arcanas (Sp.-Mestizo) spiritual protection chants

Arutam (Sh.) spirit of the forest

Atacapie (K.-Napo) the mythical seven-headed anaconda

A'pó (S.) *Ammandra natalia,* a palm from whose young shoots are made ceremonial maña

Auca (K.) the term used by outsiders to refer to the Waorani. It means "savage," and/or deep-forest "uncivilized" tribal folk

Aun (S.) Large tortillas of grated and then squeezed yuca tubers

Aunghue (W.) *Inga edulis,* a cultivated tree with edible fruits

Awacolla (Cañari) *Trichocereus pachanoi*—sacred cactus of the high Andes

Ayahuasquero (Sp.-Mestizo) practitioner of the ayahuasca drinking tradition

Azulejo (Sp.) any one of a variety of small blue birds

Baane (W.) tomorrow, the future

Badagone (W.) a drink made from the fruits of the petohue palm (*Jessenia bataua*) mashed with miiyabu *(Banisteriopsis caapi)* leaves; translates to "grandmothers' milk"

Bogá (Tucano) organizing principle of the universe, the life force

Bonsa (S.) *Bixa orellana,* a medicinal plant called *achiote* in Spanish, *manduru* in Kichwa, and *kakahue* in Waorani

Bonsáwito (S.) *Brosimum utile,* Moraceae family, a latex-bearing tree

Brujo (Sp.-Mestizo) a witch or sorcerer, someone who enacts harm on a spiritual level

Bubeka (W.) *Ceiba pentandra,* represents the tree of life, also called gemenebe

Buyu kakahue (W.) *Bixa platycarpa,* a tree whose name means "stingray achiote," used by the Waorani to start fires

Caanda (W.) a palm-wood machete, symbolic of Wood Age cosmology and way of life

Camiyai (S.) the Crab Jaguar, mythic elemental water power

Campo yariwá (S.) "where the sun is at 9 AM" (a type of spiritual trap placed on sorcerers)

Camporazá (S.) Fragrant Medicine Bark (traditional elder's name)

Caña agria (Sp.-Mestizo) *Costus guianensis,* a wild cane employed in treating kidney ailments

Canco'tëkahuë (S.) translating literally as "cicada season," considered to be the most auspicious time for drinking yagé

Cancopai (S.) cicada people, a type of Wiñapai

Cancowitoyai (S.) the "Downy Cicada Jaguar," Deity of the Southern Cross

Cantsë (S.) *Grias neuberthii,* a medicinal tree, called *piton* in Kichwa

Capirona (K.) *Calycophyllum spruceanum,* a tree with peeling bark, called *soco* in Secoya

Carihuairazo (K.) Volcano neighboring Chimborazo, 5,020 m (16,470 ft), translates to "Eternal-master-of-the-icy-wind"

Cayambe (Quitus, Sp.) on its summit exists the only glacier along Earth's equator; the peak is 5,790 m (18,996 ft), and the name translates to "origin of youthfulness" or "origin of life" in the ancient Quitus language

Cedron (Sp.) *Aloysia triphylla,* an aromatic tea from the Andes

Cejas de la montaña (Sp.) "eyebrows of the mountains," refers to the Tropical Wet Forest areas at the base of the Andes

Cerro Hermoso (Sp.-Ecuador) located in the Llanganati wilderness, the peak is 4,571 m high (14,997 ft); the name translates to "beautiful mountain"

Chacruna (K.-Peru) *Psychotria viridis,* an ayahuasca admixture plant

Chagropanga (K.-Peru) *Diplopterys cabrerana,* ayahuasca admixture plant

Chali panga (K.-Napo) *Diplopterys cabrerana,* ayahuasca admixture plant

Chapo verde (Sp.-Mestizo) green plantain mashed in water, used for dietas

Chicha (Sp.-Mestizo) nourishing gruel made from starchy fruits and tubers

Chilcemuyu (K.) *Lacmellea lactescens,* tree with edible fruits and sap

Chiri (K.) adjective meaning cold or penetrating like the cold

Chiriguayusa (K.-Napo) *Brunfelsia grandiflora,* cultivated medicinal plant

Chisparumi (K.-Napo) quartz sparking-rocks nicked together to start fires

Chucula (K., Sp.-Mestizo) gruel of boiled ripe plantains, called *peneme* in Waorani and *noncagono* in Secoya

Cocawasi (S.) *Xylopia benthamii,* a flexible wood used in making yagé drinking crowns

Cofán (Ai Cofán) an indigenous group of people native to Sucumbios Province of northeast Ecuador and to southern Colombia, autonym: Ai

Cotopaxi (Quitus) the second most active volcano on Earth at 5,897 m (19,347 ft); the name translates to "song of the moon"

Cou pinzi (S.) *Bauhinia guianensis,* turtle vine, medicinal for kidney ailments

Couode (W.) the Waorani term means "those who ate their father, the cannibals, maggots, or those that cut everything to pieces," the name for all two-legged creatures, including other Waorani who have strayed from the celestial moral order

Cruzcaspi (K.) *Brownea grandiceps,* a rainforest tree that plays an important role in women's medicine

Cubacarehue (W.) *Minquartia guianensis,* medicinal and toxic tree with wood that does not rot, called *yajisiu* in Secoya and *wambula* in Kichwa

Cuchi (K.) domestic pig

Cunti cou (S.) the land tortoise, *Chelonoidis denticulata*

Curarina (K., Sp.-Mestizo) *Potalia amara,* an understory rainforest plant with extremely bitter leaves used for healing snakebite and venereal diseases

Curirumi (K.) rocks to which are attributed powers for healing; name means "golden stones"

Cushilla (K.-Highland) "May the entire universe be filled with God's joy"

Cushillucambiac (K.) *Theobroma subincanum,* wild cacao relative

Daiawë yejá (S.) meaning "flooded land," this is the Secoya term for the igapó forest type

Degihue (W.) *Tabebuia serratifolia,* a canopy tree with yellow flowers, representative of the tree of life, known in Spanish as *guayacan amarillo*

Depemoncamo (W.) *Lacmellea lactescens,* tree with edible fruits and sap

Diablouma (K.- Highland) a character from the highland festivals, translates as "devil head"

Diente de Leon: (Sp.) *Taraxacum officinale*—dandelion flower, used for the liver

Dieta (Sp.-Mestizo) a practice for gaining spiritual power

Dius Churimi (K.-Highland) "We are children of the living God"

Dius Samaymi (K.-Highland) "God is life, breath, wisdom, spirit"

Dius Taitaku (K.-Highland) "God the progenitor of all"

Diushun (K.-Highland) "May God repay you," in Spanish commonly heard as *Dios le Pague* or *Dios se lo pague* or simply *Pagi*

Dohi (S.) *Spondias mombin,* a tree also known as *hobo,* used for healing cuts and abrasions

Dunduma (K.-Napo) a medicinal sedge in the Cyperaceae family that the Secoya call *yiyiyo nuní*

Duranibai (W.) the way of the ancestors

Dube (W.) the past—antiquity to five minutes ago

E'jé (S.) a lagoon frog employed in the traditions of yagé to help students stop shitting and better hold high doses

El Altar (Sp.-Ecuador) 5,319 m (17,451 ft); known among the Puruwa peoples of central Ecuador as Kápac Urku, meaning authoritative mountain, an Apu

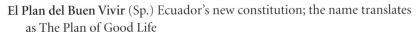

El Plan del Buen Vivir (Sp.) Ecuador's new constitution; the name translates as The Plan of Good Life

Emuyái (S.) aquatic elemental power; the name translates as howler-monkey-jaguar

Encabellados (Sp.) early name given to the Secoya by the first settlers, meaning "long hair"

Encanto (Sp.) an enchantment

Ëné (S.) *Bactris gasipaes,* a food palm known as *chonta, chonta duro,* in Kichwa and *dagenka* by the Waorani

Ënsë Yowë (S.) the Sun Canoe, a cosmic phenomenon of the world of yagé

Gemenebe (W.) *Ceiba pentandra,* represents the tree of life, also called *somona* or *uchuputu* in Kichwa and *imigëi* among the Secoya

Gonewarehue (W.) *Cedrela odorata,* Spanish cedar, medicinal bark, sacred tree, *mëa* in Secoya

Gonomaña (S.) *Ocimum micranthum,* a cultivated rainforest basil

Gran alimento (Sp.) "great food," relating to the drink of yagé

Granadilla (Sp.-Mestizo) *Passiflora* spp.—besides its edible fruit, this vine's leaves are used to purify the blood

Guacamaya manilata (Sp.) *Orthopsittaca manilata,* red-bellied macaw

Guanabana (Sp.) *Annona muricata,* a cultivated fruit tree and medicine

Guanchaca (Sp.-Mestizo) high-proof sugar cane moonshine, also called *puro*

Guanduc (K.) a wild species of *Brugmansia,* also spelled *wantú*

Guanta (Sp.) a.k.a. *paca,* ground-dwelling, herbivorous rodents in South and Central America

Guarumo (Sp.-Mestizo) any of a variety of secondary forest trees pertaining to the genus Cecropia

Hakë (S.) "father" in Paicoca (hako means "mother")

Ható (S.) *Macrolobium acaciifolium,* tree from blackwater lake country of Pëquë'ya (Lagarto Cocha)

Hewëmaña (S.) *Justicia pectoralis*—an aromatic plant that grows on river banks; its name translates to "river otter fragrance"

Hierba Luisa (Sp.) *Cymbopogon citratus,* lemon grass

Hierba mate (Sp.) *Ilex paraguaensis,* "herb for drinking from a gourd"

Hookasayepë (S.) leafy broom rattle made of a cluster of the rainforest grass called mamecocó (*Pariana radiciflora*)

Huambula (K.) *Minquartia guianensis,* medicinal and toxic tree with wood that does not rot

Huiká (S.) tunic, the Secoya men's garment, also called *kushma* or *tunica*

Icaro (Sp.-Mestizo) sacred song of the ayahuasca tradition

Igapó (Portuguese) a Brazilian term used to describe areas where blackwater lakes and flooded forest are found

Imigëï (S.) *Ceiba pentandra,* towering canopy tree, also called *ceibo*

Ingandu (K.-Napo) an old, possibly pre-Kichwa name for ayahuasca

Ingaru Supai (K.-Napo) a spirit that protects the primary rainforest

Insi Jamu (S.) Pineapple Armadillo, from Secoya mythology

Insi Jamu Yejá (S.) "Pineapple Armadillo Land," the Secoya name for the American continent

Inuito (W.) a Waorani iroinga of old who is known for having participated in the creation of the first miiyabu vine (ayahuasca)

Iroinga (W.) a Waorani spiritual master, who embodies all experiences

Iru (K.) a sugar cane variety that grew from Shiu-amarun's heart

Ishpingu (K.) Amazonian cinnamon *(Ocotea quixos)*

Izhu Mangallpa Urcu (K.) meaning literally, "end of the world jaguar mountain," the name of Napo-Galeras

Jaicuntipai (S.) spiritual immortals of the high hills, believed to inhabit an alternate dimension inside the mountain of Napo-Galeras

Jaicunti (S.) the cordillera Napo-Galeras, today an Ecuadorian National Park

Jatun manila warmi (K.-Napo) Sugar cane moonshine; the name translates as "big rope woman"

Jatun Sumak Kangui (K.-Highland) "God, you are the greatest and most beautiful"

Jayawáska (K.) pronunciation of the word *ayahuasca* in Pastaza Province

Jëesaipë (S.) blue-necked tanager, sacred bird of the yagé traditions *(Tangara cyanicollis)*

Jejebonsa (S.) a sticky aromatic body paint that merges texture with aroma and color, used for yagé drinking

Jiñocuado (Boruka) *Bursera simaruba,* a copal relative from the coastal provinces used to treat urinary tract infections

Juju (S.) to heal

Jujupai (S.) spiritual immortals who heal, "doctor people," also called Ujápai

Jujupai toyá (S.) the designs of the doctor people

Jurema (Brazilian P) *Mimosa hostilis,* medicinal plant containing DMT

Kachi (K.) salt

Kana (Barasana) *Sabicea amazonensis,* a vine of symbolic importance, with consecutive fruits representing the united hearts of generations

Kápac Urku (K.-Puruwa) the most majestic authority, the truthful representative of God upon the Earth, Altar Mountain: 5,319 m (17,451 ft)

Kausai (K.) life or alive; "sumak kausai" means beautiful life

Kayahue (W.) refers to the eternal continuum, what transcends all apocalypses

Kayu Runa (K.) Lightning Man, mythic being who lives in the waterfalls; one of his ribs and a testicle are preserved in stone at Galeras

Këhna (S.) a type of celestial metal not found on the Earth

Këhna'curipiarazá (S.) "Golden sky-metal bird," name of a traditional elder

Kënjé (S.) *Dacryodes peruviana,* a sacred tree, source of copal incense resin

Kichwa (K.) term for several indigenous ethnic groups in South America who speak a Quechua language. The Quechua of Ecuador call themselves as well as their language Kichwa, Quichua, or Runa. In the area near Napo-Galeras their autonym is Napo Runa; in Pastaza Province it's Puyuc Runa, meaning "cloud people." In the highlands of Ecuador are other dialects, such as the Otavalo, Puruwa, Salasaca, and Cañari. In Colombia, the Kichwa-speaking group call themselves the Inga. Other Quechua speakers call themselves Runakuna. The Kichwa language, called Runashimi, is believed to have descended from the Incan forefathers, Manko Cápac and Mama Uqllu.

Kuilluruguna (K-Napo) Kuilluru and Duceru, known as the Kuilluruguna, are hero twins of antiquity from the Napo Runa ethnopoetic saga of humanity

Kutipa (K.) negative consequences invoked when not adhering appropriately to a dieta

La purga (K.-Mestizo) term used for ayahuasca brew, meaning "the purge"

Llushtinda muyu (K.) *Couroupita guianensis,* a tree highly revered in ethno medicine, its bark is believed to heal tuberculosis; known among the Waorani as *pankabukabu* and among the Secoya as *watisansá*

Ma'curipai (S.) literally, "red-gold people," a group of celestial immortals

Makëhna yowë (S.) Red heaven boat (there is also the white heaven boat, pokëhna yowë)

Ma'tsimayai (S.) red-poison jaguar, a type of dangerous galactic primal power

Ma'yëï (S.) *Pseudobombax mungupa,* a tree whose bark is peeled and used to make a kitchen utensil for squeezing the juice from grated yuca tubers

Macawá (S.) the laughing falcon *(Herpetotheres cachinnans),* from the legend of the creation of the food plant uncuisí *(Renealmia alpinia)*

Machakui wishuk (K.) snakebite root, an ancestral cultigen whose roots are effective in curing snakebite

Macuri (S.) aromatic face paint, literally translates as "red gold"

Maiangi (K.) a fine soil obtained from the decomposed heart of the Ingaru Supai

Maloca (Sp.-Mestizo) the traditional Amazonian long house

Mama Tungurahua (K.) an active volcano on the royal eastern Andes range, said to be the wife of Taita Chimborazo, 5,023 m (16,480 ft); its name means "Throat-of-Fire"

Mamecocó (S.) *Pariana radiciflora,* a plant used to make a leafy broom rattle for the ceremony of yagé, called *surupanga* in Kichwa

Maña (S.) fragrant herbal ornaments tied to the arms and wrists

Mañapë (S.) *Callichlamys latifolia,* an emetic and medicinal plant from the hilly forests used by the Secoya to eliminate laziness

Manko Cápac (K.-Highland) Incan forefather, from whose grave grew the first ayahuasca vine

Mañoko Wiñapai (S.) starry beings, starry immortals

Mañumi (S.) *Eunectes murinus,* the green anaconda, known as *amarun* in Kichwa, and *obe* among the Waorani

Manzanilla (Sp.) *Matricaria chamomilla,* an aromatic herb, chamomile

Mapacho (Sp.-Mestizo) a cured strong native tobacco

Mapia (S.) scarlet tanager *(Piranga olivacea)*

Mareación (Sp.-Mestizo) the reverie of inebriation brought by ayahuasca

Matëmo Cou (S.) the Sky Turtle of Secoya cosmology

Matëmo qiro (S.) heavenly islands, realms, or celestial abodes

Matëmo tsiaya (S.) river in heaven or Sky River, a branch of the Sariweco'tsiaya

Matëmopai (S.) heaven people, heaven immortals, or heavenly beings

Matimuyu (K.) *Clavija weberbaueri,* a medicinal rainforest understory plant with extremely fragrant flowers

Matipë (S.) the ceremonial scepter

Matiyai (S.) heaven jaguar, an older name for the ceremonial scepter, from the Secoya legend of Quequero

Mawahopai (S.) the morpho butterfly people, terrestrial spirits who help shamans to heal and sorcerers to perpetuate harm

Mawëwë (S.) *Inia geoffrensis,* pink Amazonian dolphin

Mazamora (K.) green banana boiled and mashed in water, see Chapo verde

Medico (Sp.-Mestizo) traditional practitioner of healing arts

Meñeiriwempo (W.) the ancestral protector deity of the Waorani people; "jaguar guardian"

Menka (W.) the olive oropendola bird *(Psarocolius bifasciatus)*, from the Waorani legend of the creation of the first miiyabu

Menkoyiyi (S.) Electric-eel Water-dragon, mythic elemental power of the water

Mestizo (Sp.-Mestizo) a term used to refer to people of mixed European and indigenous heritage

Mëto (S.) *Nicotiana tabacum* and *N. rustica,* tobacco; *taucu* in Kichwa

Miiyabu (W.) *Banisteriopsis muricata,* wild ayahuasca variety found along the rivers, has white pubescence on underleaf

Mishqui panga (K.) *Coussarea dulcifolia,* rare plant of the Napo Valley watershed, used as a natural sweetener; the name means "sweet leaf"

Monakageiri (W.) the Earth's first people, said to be shorter than people today, the ancestors of the present-day Waorani

Mönse (S.) *Cedrelinga cateniformis,* a giant towering rainforest tree, used in Secoya and Cofán ethno-medicine, known in Kichwa as *chunchu*

Mundupuma (K.) the "World Puma" or end-of-the-world mountain lion trapped inside Napo-Galeras Mountain

Ñacoma'sirá (S.) the One-Eye Lagoon, found at Lagarto Cocha

Nairoe (W.) *Brunfelsia chiricaspi,* nightshade relative, known about by the Waorani but not used

Nairoeñai (W.) *Brugmansia suaveolens;* the Waorani are aware of the powerful psychotropic qualities of this plant but do not use it

Ñamase (S.) a spirit used by the shamans to heal; it looks like a deer with no feet and has a long tongue

Namokapoweiri (W.) a triangular-shaped constellation that can be found near Orion's Belt, the Waorani people's starry origin

Ñañë (S.) God, the creator, synonym for Paina, a.k.a. Mai Hakë

Ñañë Siecopai (S.) God's Multicolored People, who taught the Secoya the tradition of yagé

Ñañë Siecopai yagé (S.) God's Multicolored People yagé, a variety of yagé today lost

Ñañëpai hueko (S.) the messenger parrots of Ñañë believed to inhabit the region of Jupo

Naranja Agrio (Sp.) *Citrus aurantium,* bitter orange, used to heal sinusitis

Natem (Shuar, Achuar) tribal name of ayahuasca

Neatañë yai (S.) the black-shadow jaguar, a type of universal primal power, used by shamans to prevent sorcerers from causing harm

Neayai (S.) the black forest jaguar *(Panthera onca),* a rare morph of the spotted forest jaguar

Ne'e (S.) *Mauritia flexuosa,* a food palm of the wetlands, whose young shoots are used to make maña

Ñeñco (S.) grandmother; Ñeñquë is grandfather

Ñe'ñé (S.) woven cotton bracelet used for binding maña onto one's wrist

Nonginka (W.) *Gustavia longifolia,* wild fruit of the forest, a highly revered tree among the Waorani

Ñumí (S.) *Piper* sp.—medicinal plant thought to have been brought from heaven

Ñuñerepá paiye (S.) the Secoya code of upright living

Nuní (S.) a sedge in the Cyperaceae family

Oboye (W.) *Pseudolmedia laevis,* a small red edible fruit; the Secoya call this *yají*

Ocha'sá (S.) *Myrciaria dubia,* bears a fruit high in vitamin c, found in the igapó regions

Ocobeto (S.) *Astrocaryum jauari,* a palm found in the igapó forest type

Ocomaña (S.) *Justicia pectoralis,* used for making maña

Ocopai (S.) water people, immortals of the water world and of the rainy season

Ocoraca jujuyë (S.) the songs employed for making ocoraca, cured water

Ocoyai (S.) the Water Jaguar, the Jaguar Mother's sister

Okaeini (W.) *Nicotiana rustica,* wild tobacco that grows in the territory; though the Waorani are well aware of its stimulating effects, tobacco is not used in traditional Waorani culture

Omepai (S.) summer people, immortals who once inhabited the Earth; now they appear close to the Earth in January, during the dry season

Ometsiapai (S.) eternally-young people of the summer, related to the Omepai

Ontokabe (W.) *Garcinia macrophylla,* wild tree with edible fruit, called *pungara* in Kichwa

Oomae (W.) curare, dart poison

Oonta (W.) *Curarea tecunarum,* a vine that is the principal source of the Waorani people's hunting poison

Oré'o (S.) *Myrmecophaga tridactyla,* the giant anteater

Ocoraca (S.) cured water prepared with ceremonial invocations

Pachamama (K.-Highland) Mother Earth

Pagundu (Sp.-Mestizo) *Iochroma fuchsioides,* nightshade relative, also called *flor del quinde* (Sp.), the hummingbird's flower

Pai (S.) both singular and plural, referring to a person and/or people, it also refers to the godlike divinities and immortal beings of the universe

Pai pitayari (S.) checkpoint on the spiritual bridge to heaven, or the time of midnight; refers to spiritual traps that skilled shamans place on sorcerers to stop them from accomplishing malice

Pai saye nuní (S.) people-departure nuní, *Cyperus* sp.

Pai'joyowatí (S.) People-soul/heart-spirit, the Demon King, a spirit used by the shamans for healing

Pai'puñu (S.) *Colossoma macropomum,* a relative of the piranha but much larger, known in Spanish as *gamitana*

Paico (K.-Highland) *Dysphania ambrosioides,* medicinal herb

Paicoca (S.) the Secoya people's language

Paisuku (S.) protector spirits with dark black skin who smoke extremely strong tobacco

Paitiñia (S.) meaning "river of naked people," this is the Secoya name for the Tiputini River

Paiwea (S.) "people's corn," an ancestral species of *Zea mays*

Paiyai (S.) the people jaguar, an auspicious spirit ally of the novice drinkers

Paju (K.) a power related to the use of medicinal plants for healing

Paju manduru (K.) *Bixa orellana* variety; the name translates as "power achiote"

Pajujinjibri (K.-Napo) a potent variety of ginger that grew from Shiu-amarun's heart

Pakipanga (K.-Pastaza) *Disocactus amazonicus,* a wild cactus used to treat sprains and bruises as well as kidney pains

Palanda (K.-Napo) a banana variety that doesn't perish in abandoned overgrown garden sites; it grew from Shiu-amarun's heart

Paracoco (S.) *Bufo typhonius,* a leafy litter toad that has one stripe straight down its back

Payaguaje (S.) a Secoya family name

Payo tututeh (S.) "filling the liquid with supreme spiritual strength," part of a healing song

Pë'metó (S.) *Pistia stratiotes,* caiman's tobacco

Pë'e (S.) *Melanosuchus niger,* black caiman, can be spelled *pë*

Pejí (S.) an ancestral variety of *Brugmansia suaveolens*

Pëné (S.) *Inga edulis,* a tree with edible fruits, whose delicate flowers are said to represent the Wiñapai

Pengunka (W.) *Tabernaemontana sananho,* a medicinal tree used for pain in the eye; the sap is also used for removing tropical bot fly

Pëpërí (S.) *Sarcoramphus papa,* the king vulture

Pëquë'yá (S.) Black-caiman Lagoons, part of the Secoya ancestral homeland on the Peruvian/Ecuadorian border

Petohue (W.) *Jessenia bataua,* a tropical palm from which a valuable and nutritious oil is obtained from its fruits, used for food and to benefit the hair; known as *shiwa* in Kichwa, *gonza* in Secoya, and *ungurahua* in Ecuadorian Spanish

Piaguaje (S.) Bird Clan, a Secoya family name

Piedras vivas (Sp.-Mestizo) rocks to which healing powers are attributed; see Curi rumi

Pilchi (K.) *Crescentia cujete,* the gourd tree, which has deep ethno-medical and historical implications among all indigenous people of the upper Amazon

Piñon Negro (Sp.) *Jatropha gossypifolia,* a powerful medicinal plant

Pinta (Sp.-Mestizo), Spanish word for the designs of yagé

Pisasá (S.) *Tangara chilensis,* the paradise tanager, a sacred bird of the yagé tradition

Pishkuri (K.) *Teliostachya lanceolata,* mysterious medicinal plant of the Kichwa

Pitajaya (K.) *Hylocereus* sp., an epiphytical rainforest cactus with edible fruit

Pokëhna yowë (S.) White heaven boat (there is also the red heaven boat: makëhna yowë)

Posá (S.) elaborate designs that the Secoya use for painting faces and decorating pottery and cloth

Pumallullu (K.) (*Piper* sp.) a powerful and mysterious cultivated medicinal plant of the Kichwa, used for jaguar transformation

Pungara (K.) *Garcinia macrophylla,* a tree with edible fruits, called *ontokabe* in Waorani

Purina tambu (K.) "a place that's walked to," a biological reserve

Quaheyo (S.) *Pteronura brasiliensis,* giant river otter, *ompore* in Waorani

Retama (Sp.-Mestizo) *Senna alata,* medicinal plant used for skin infections

Reventador (Sp.-Ecuador) an active volcano on the royal eastern range, 3,562 m (11,686 ft); the name means "Exploder" or "Troublemaker"

Rivereños: (Sp.-Mestizo) the people who live along the river banks

Romero (Sp.) *Rosmarinus officinalis,* rosemary

Ruda (Sp.) *Ruta graveolens,* a powerful aromatic medicinal plant used to expel negativity

Runashimi (K.) the language of the Kichwa people; translates as "people's idiom"

Sacha Runa (K.) the spiritual owner of the rainforest, master spirit of the rainforest, represented by the sacha runa lizard (Amazon wood lizard, *Enyalioides laticeps*)

Sacha Warmi (K.) the spirit goddess of the rainforest, represented by the plant chiricaspi *(Brunfelsia chiricaspi)* as well as *Cephaelis tomentosa*

Salvia (Sp.) *Salvia officinalis,* a variety of sage

Samai (K.) breath, life wisdom

Sangay (Sh.) an active volcano in Amazonian Ecuador, 5,300 m (17,388 ft), whose name refers to a tyrant of sorts, someone without shame

Sariweco tsiaya (S.) the celestial river of Secoya cosmology

Sëamëyai (S.) "enthrallment jaguar," a type of dangerous galactic primal energy that kills without pity

Secoya (S.) the Siecopai, an indigenous people living in the Ecuadorian and Peruvian Amazon. They speak the Secoya language Paicoca, which is part of the Western Tukanoan language group. In Ecuador the Secoya number about 600 people who for the most part are located in three settlements: Eno, San Pablo de Cantesiaya, and Siecoya Remolino, all found on the banks of the Aguarico River. In Peru they are called the Airo Pai and number about 1,200 individuals living in Maynas Province near the Ecuadorian border.

Sehué (S.) yagé drinker's necklace, named after the constellation Sehuéwë

Sehuéwë (S.) a Secoya name for a constellation

Sen (Sp.-Mestizo) *Caesalpinia pulcherrima,* also called *flor del niño,* its leaves are employed for intestinal cleansing

Sënorí (S.) A large mesh-like strainer

Sëo (S.) *Psarocolius decumanus,* the crested oropendola bird

Sëra Wiñapai (S.) swallow-tailed-kite immortals

Sera wiwé (S.) *Elanoides forficatus,* swallow-tailed kite hawk

Shiu-amarun (K.) glistening silver-scaled fertility boa of Kichwa mythology

Shuar (Shuar) an indigenous people of Ecuador and Peru considered an ethnic majority numbering about 40,000 in Ecuador

Sidá (S.) *Astrocaryum murumuru*—a palm of the blackwater Lagoon country

Siecoyá (S.) river name in Peru at the heart of the Secoya ancestral homelands

Sincholagua (K.) dormant volcano, 4,893m (16,053 ft); name translates to "power of the heights"

Siripë (S.) *Iguana iguana,* green iguana

Socó (S.) *Calycophyllum spruceanum,* a tree with peeling bark, called *capirona* in Kichwa

Socorá (S.) meaning "sunken lake," called Zancudo Cocha in Kichwa

Sohó (S.) *Hymenea courbaril,* a sacred tree with medicinal bark and aromatic resin

Sohómanë (S.) a ceremonial incense smudge made of multiple ingredients

Sucre (Sp.-Ecuador) the original Ecuadorian currency before the country was dollarized in the year 2000, named after Antonio José de Sucre (1795–1830), one of Simon Bolivar's closest friends

Sumaco (K., Sp.-Mestizo) dormant volcano on the royal eastern range in Napo Province, 3,990 m (13,091 ft); name translates to "the most beautiful one"

Sumak (K.-Highland) the most beautiful or the flawless, the most pristine glory

Sumak Kausai (K.-Highland) a proverb meaning "beautiful life" and referring to a life of integrity and high values

Supai (S.) terrestrial spirits, *Watí* in Secoya

Supai Lancha (Sp.-Mestizo) spirit vessel seen by the medicos in their visions

Taita (K.) father, authority figure; also Taitiku

Taita Chimborazo (K.) Ecuador's tallest peak at 6,268 m (20,564 ft), an Apu, the husband of Mama Tungurahua

Tamia yura (K.) *Leonia crassa,* the rain tree

Tamia Yura, Jardin Etnobotanico (K., Sp.) an indigenous ethnobotanical garden and visitor center located near Tena

Taucu (K.) *Nicotiana rustica* and/or *N. tabacum,* tobacco plant

Taucumasu (K.) tobacco mace, strongly cured tobacco in a log shape

Tepahue (W.) *Iryartea deltoidea,* a palm from the base of the Andes

Tiasnacachun (K.-Highland) "May it be commanded and confirmed"

Toa'tsá (S.) ceramic hourglass-shaped pot stands; three are used for cooking. Secoya cosmology sees them as the three legs that hold up the cauldron that is the universe.

Toama (S.) *Ara macao,* scarlet macaw

Tokawa (S.) large round wooden mortar used for mashing tubers

Toowë (S.) long wooden trough used in conjunction with the tokawa

Toyá (S.) the designs and visual language revealed by the yagé

Toyá ma'a (S.) designs trail, the path that spiritual masters use to travel under the influence of yagé

Toyá Uncucui (S.) a supernatural snake that initiates students into the world of yagé, called Wairamama or Huairamama in Kichwa

Toyákä (S.) the yagé drinkers' cloak, of which there are many different kinds

Toyáyai (S.) the designs jaguar; the term can relate to ally visionary jaguars as well as modest-natured forest cats

Tsantsa (Shuar) shrunken heads of slain enemies

Tui'kuh wü'e (S.) the traditional Secoya long house

Uchu (K.) chili peppers

Ujá (S.) to heal utilizing spiritual influences

Ujájái (S.) *Brunfelsia grandiflora,* cultivated medicinal plant; the name means "great healer"

Ujápai (S.) Healing immortals like the Jujupai, spiritual doctors

Ujáye (S.) sacred healing songs

Ujuangu (K.) *Tovomita weddelliana,* a medicinal plant from the base of the Andes used for sinusitis

Umu (S.) *Psarocolius bifasciatus,* the olive oropendola bird

Uña de gato (Sp.-Mestizo) *Uncaria guianensis,* a rainforest vine that is highly appreciated in local ethno medicine

Uncuisí (S.) *Renealmia alpinia,* used to make soup flavoring

Unkiyabe (W.) "the longhouse mountain," Waorani name of Napo-Galeras

Unku (W.) Waorani pole and leaf hut

Urcu sacha guayusa (K.-Napo) *Ilex inundata,* mountain forest guayusa

Urcu shínchi guayusa (K.-Napo) *Calyptranthes ishoaquinicca,* mountain powerful guayusa

Usepopai (S.) people from the Pleiades

Vaí mashë (Tucano) the master of the animals

Vegetalista (Sp.-Mestizo) a healer specialized in the use of plants

Virote (Sp.-Mestizo) the harmful spiritual projectile or dart, also called *chontapala*

Wabeca Waorani (W.) a term used by the Waorani to relate to people from another place, people who are not Waorani but who abide to celestial moral order

Wairachina (K.) leafy broom rattle used for cleansing and also ritually for healing and relating to spirits; see Hookasayepë

Wairachina Sacha (K.) a significant stand of Tropical Wet Forest east of Napo-Galeras

Waísamama (K.-Napo) a traditional name for the guayusa tea *(Ilex guayusa)*

Wajo Sará (S.) cultural hero of the Secoya people

Wajoya (S.) the "River of War," located in Peru (on the map as Río Santamaria)

Wakara Wiñapai (S.) white ibis immortals

Wansoka (S.) *Couma macrocarpa,* a tree valued for its aromatic white sap

Wanteanco (S.) the Jaguar Mother, also called Yaipai Hako

Wantú (K.) *Brugmansia aurea,* a nightshade relative

Wao (W.) singular for Waorani

Waorani (W.) Native Amerindians from the Amazonian region of Ecuador (Napo, Orellana, and Pastaza provinces) who have marked differences from other ethnic groups from Ecuador

Wao Terero (W.) the language of the Waorani

Waponi (W.) "all that is good," similar to Hebrew "Shalom," Hawaiian "Aloha," and Costa Rican "Pura Vida"

Waosutu (S.) a great Secoya yagé drinker of old; also *Pithecia aequatorialis,* equatorial saki monkey

Warmi Pascua (K.-Highland) A festival celebrating the first fruiting of the grain, celebrated near the spring equinox

Watí (S.) terrestrial spirits; also means spirit generally

Watí gonzá (S.) *Jessenia bataua,* a variety of this palm with low-hanging fruits

Watí nuní (S.) a medicinal sedge in the Cyperaceae family

Watí ujá (S.) invocations to ward off negative spirits

Wecó (S.) *Amazona farinosa,* the mealy Amazon parrot

Wecówiñapai (S.) the green-parrot always-new people

Weku yariwá (S.) "where the sun is at midday," a type of spiritual trap placed on sorcerers, in order to stop them from doing harm

Wí'watí (S.) Growth Spirit, known as a hairy spirit with two faces

Wigagen (W.) *Mansoa standleyi,* the garlic vine used for arthritic pains, also planted around homes to ward off snakes

Wigonza yariwá (S.) "where the sun is at 3 PM," a type of spiritual trap placed on sorcerers

Wiña (S.) young, tender, or new

Wiña caye (S.) sacred ceremonial songs

Wiñapai (S.) the always-new people, always-new immortals

Wiñapai maro (S.) heaven-people crown

Wiñapai ñamero (S.) always-new people's bumblebee

Wiñapai toyá ma'a (S.) always-new divine immortals designs path

Wiñapai toyákä (S.) always-new-people designs cloak

Wiñatsi'bonsë (S.) always-young-and-fresh celestial children

Wiñawai (S.) general term given to all legions of divine immortals, supernal, angelic, godly and/or celestial beings

Wiñetare (W.) a remote non-contacted group of Waorani living in deep isolation

Wira (K.) grease or oil

Wirisaka (S.) *Iryanthera hostmanni,* a tree with aromatic bark

Wito'sawí (S.) *Phyllanthus caroliniensis,* medicinal plant for urinary tract infections

Yachac (K.) sage, a person with deep spiritual knowledge

Yacu yutzu (K.) *Calliandra angustifolia,* a powerful planta maestra that grows along the rivers and a sacred plant used for gaining strength; called *bobinsana* in the Peruvian Amazon

Yagé (S.) *Banisteriopsis caapi,* the vine, and an entheogenic ceremonial brew; this is the Secoya name for ayahuasca

> **Yagé, ëo yagé** (S.) extra thick and strong, honey-like yagé; also refered to as weasiko yagé
>
> **Yagé, jëesaipë yagé** (S.) the "iridescent azure blue" variety of yagé
>
> **Yagé, nea yagé** (S.) the black variety of yagé
>
> **Yagé, sëño yagé** (S.) the yellow variety of yagé
>
> **Yagé, sense yagé** (S.) a wild yagé variety believed to be connected to the peccaries
>
> **Yagé, tara yagé** (S.) "bone" variety of yagé with soft bark
>
> **Yagé, tutu yagé** (S.) a very strong variety of yagé
>
> **Yagé, tzinca yagé** (S.) a variety of yagé with swollen nodes, known as *mucutulluwaska* among the Kichwa
>
> **Yagé, usepopai yagé** (S.) the "people from the Pleiades" variety of yagé
>
> **Yagé, wai yagé** (S.) "animal" yagé, a variety that grows small, with a sub-species that has yellow splotches on its leaves
>
> **Yagé, weasiko yagé** (S.) thickly prepared yagé with a corn gruel-like consistency, a.k.a. ëo yagé
>
> **Yagé, yai yagé** (S.) the "jaguar" variety of yagé

Yagé hë'hë'ñé (S.) Secoya ceremonial songs

Yagé ocó (S.) *Diplopterys cabrerana*—yagé admixture plant, known as *chalipanga* among the Kichwa; *yají* among the Shiwiar, and *wambiza chacruna* and *chagropanga* among mestizo vegetalistas in Peru

Yagé toyá (S.) "designs of yagé" or "visual patterning revealed by the yagé"

Yagé uncucui (S.) a seasoned drinker of yagé and master of the ceremony

Yagémopai (S.) "people of the yagé," spirits directly related to the yagé vine

Yai (S.) jaguar, referring both to actual forest cats, and to primal energy

Yai sinaneñá (S.) *Geogenanthus ciliates,* a medicinal plant whose name means "jaguar's mirror"; its Kichwa name is *supi panga,* "fart leaf"

Yaiujájái (S.) *Brunfelsia chiricaspi,* a wild variety of ujájái, "jaguar ujájái"

Yai Yoí (S.) Jaguar Grunge, a character seen in yagé visions as a jaguar with a human face

Yajisiu (S.) *Minquartia guianensis,* a medicinal and toxic tree with wood that does not rot

Yape (S.) *Spigelia humboldtiana,* an aromatic herb for making maña

Yaupon (Catawban) *Ilex vomitoria,* a caffeinated North American guayusa relative

Yoco (S.) *Paullinia yoco,* a caffeinated jungle vine used by the Secoya

Yuca (Sp.) *Manihot esculenta,* a cultivated plant with edible tubers

Zancudo Cocha (K.) The Kichwa name for Socorá, the sunken lake, part of the Secoya ancestral territory

Zasina (K.) methods to refine one's personal energy followed in order to embody powers given by a shaman, known also as *dieta*

BIBLIOGRAPHY

Andrade, Juan Fernando. "Juicio a Texaco," *Ecuador Terra Incognita,* No. 55 (2008): 8–21.

Anhalzer, Jorge, and Emily Walmsley. *Ecuador: Panoramas.* Quito, Ecuador: Imprenta Mariscal, 2007.

Arvigo, Rosita, and Michael J. Balick. *Rainforest Remedies: One Hundred Healing Herbs of Belize.* Twin Lakes, WI: Lotus Press, 1993.

Balick, Michael J., and Paul Alan Cox. *Plants, People, and Culture: The Science of Ethnobotany.* New York: Scientific American Library, 1996.

Belaunde, Luisa Elvira, and Juan Alvaro Echeverri. "El yoco del cielo es cultivado: perspectivas sobre Paullinia yoco en el chamanismo airo-pai (secoya-tucano occidental)," *Anthropologica,* Vol. 26, No. 26 (2008): 87–111.

Bellier, Irène. *El Temblor y La Luna: Ensayo Sobre Las Relaciones Entre Las Mujeres y Los Hombres Mai Huna.* Quito, Ecuador: CICAME, 1991.

Bernhardt, Ed. *Medicinal Plants of Costa Rica.* Costa Rica: Zona Tropical, 2008.

Black Hawk and Milo Milton Quaife (editor). *The Life of Black Hawk.* New York: Dover Publications, Inc., 1916.

Bolton, Brett L. *The Secret Powers of Plants.* London: Abacus, 1975.

Buhner, Stephen Harrod. *The Lost Language of Plants: The Ecological Importance of Plant Medicines to Life on Earth.* White River Junction, VT: Chelsea Green Pub., 2002.

Burroughs, Stanley. *La Dieta de Sirope de Arce y Zumo de Limón.* Barcelona, Spain: Obelisco, 1999.

Burroughs, William S., Oliver Harris, and Allen Ginsberg. *The Yage Letters Redux.* 4th ed. San Francisco: City Lights Books, 2006.

Cabodevilla, Miguel Angel. *Los Huaorani en La Historia de Los Pueblos del Oriente.* Coca, Ecuador: CICAME, 1994.

Cabodevilla, Miguel Angel, and Randy Smith. *Tiempos de Guerra: Waorani Contra Taromenane.* Quito, Ecuador: Abya-Yala, 2004.

Calvo, César. *The Three Halves of Ino Moxo: Teachings of the Wizard of the Upper Amazon.* Rochester, VT: Inner Traditions International, 1995.

Campos, Don José, Alberto Roman, and Geraldine Overton. *The Shaman and Ayahuasca: Journeys to Sacred Realms.* Studio City, CA: Divine Arts, 2011.

Campos, Rogelio de los. "Huaorani," *Ecuador Terra Incognita,* No. 3 (1999): 4–12.

Capra, Fritjof. *The Tao of Physics: An Exploration of the Parallels Between Modern Physics and Eastern Mysticism.* Berkeley, CA: Shambhala, 1975.

Carus, Paul. *T'ai-shang Kan-ying P'ien: Treatise of the Exalted One on Response and Retribution.* Chicago: Open Court Publishing Co., 1906.

Cerón, Carlos E. *Etnobotánica del Ecuador: Estudios Regionales.* Quito, Ecuador: Ediciones Abya-Yala, 1993.

Cerón, Carlos E., and Consuelo Ayala. *Etnobotánica de Los Huaorani de Quehueiri-Ono, Napo-Ecuador.* Quito, Ecuador: Abya-Yala, 1998.

Cipolletti, María Susana, and Fernando Payaguaje. *La Fascinación Del Mal: Historia de Vida de un Shamán Secoya de la Amazonía Ecuatoriana.* Quito, Ecuador: Abya-Yala, 2008.

Cipolletti, María Susana. *Aipë Koka, La Palabra de Los Antiguos: Tradición Oral Siona-Secoya.* Quito, Ecuador: Abya-Yala, 1988.

Cooper, Murray, and Rudy Gelis. *Plumas.* Quito, Ecuador: Latinweb, 2006.

Casement, Roger. *Correspondence Respecting the Treatment of British Colonial Subjects and Native Indians Employed in the Collection of Rubber in the Putumayo District.* United Kingdom: National Government Publication, 1912.

Castillo, Bernal, and J. M. Cohen. *The Conquest of New Spain.* Baltimore: Penguin Books, 1963.

Caufield, Catherine. *In the Rainforest: Report from a Strange, Beautiful, Imperiled World.* Chicago: University of Chicago Press, 1984.

Cech, Richo. *Making Plant Medicine.* Williams, OR: Horizon Herbs, LLC, 2000.

Cech, Richo. *The Medicinal Herb Grower: A Guide for Cultivating Plants that Heal.* Williams, OR: Horizon Herbs, 2009.

Charing, Howard G., Peter Cloudsley, and Pablo Amaringo. *The Ayahuasca Visions of Pablo Amaringo.* Rochester, VT: Inner Traditions, 2011.

Chirali, Ilkay Zihni. *Traditional Chinese Medicine: Cupping Therapy.* Edinburgh, Scotland: Churchill Livingstone, 1999.

Cowan, Eliot. *Plant Spirit Medicine.* Newberg, OR: Swan-Raven, 1995.

Davis, Wade. *One River: Explorations and Discoveries in the Amazon Rain Forest.* New York: Touchstone, 1997.

Davis, Wade. *The Wayfinders: Why Ancient Wisdom Matters in the Modern World.* Toronto, Ontario: House of Anansi Press, 2009.

DeKorne, Jim. *Psychedelic Shamanism: The Cultivation, Preparation, and Shamanic Use of Psychotropic Plants.* Berkeley, CA: North Atlantic Books, 2011.

Devall, Bill, and George Sessions. *Deep Ecology.* Salt Lake City, UT: G. M. Smith, 1985.

Dodson, C. H., and A. H. Gentry. "Biological Extinction in Western Ecuador," *Annals of the Missouri Botanical Garden,* Vol. 78, No. 2 (1991): 273–295.

Duke, James A., and Rodolfo Vásquez. *Amazonian Ethnobotanical Dictionary.* Boca Raton, FL: CRC Press, 1994.

Emmons, Louise. *Neotropical Rainforest Mammals: A Field Guide.* Chicago: University of Chicago Press, 1990.

Emoto, Masaru. *Messages from Water,* Vol. 1 (Hado Publishing, 1999) and Vol. 2 (Sunmark Pub., 2001).

Emoto, Masaru. *Water Crystal Healing: Music and Images to Restore Your Well-Being.* New York: Atria Books, 2006.

Escohotado, Antonio. *A Brief History of Drugs: From the Stone Age to the Stoned Age.* Rochester, VT: Park Street Press, 1999.

Evans, W. C., and J. F. Lampard. "Alkaloids of *Datura suaveolens,*" *Phytochemistry,* Vol. 11, No. 11 (1972): 3293–3298.

Fife, Bruce. *The Coconut Oil Miracle.* New York: Avery, 2004.

Fleweger, Mary Ellen. *Es un Monstruo Grande y Pisa Fuerte: La Minería en el Ecuador y el Mundo.* Quito, Ecuador: DECOIN, 1998.

Forsyth, Adrian, and Kenneth Miyata. *Tropical Nature: Life and Death in the Rainforests of Central and South America.* New York: Scribner, 1984.

Freire, Paulo. *Pedagogy of the Oppressed.* New York: Continuum, 1988.

Galeano, Eduardo H. *Open Veins of Latin America: Five Centuries of the Pillage of a Continent.* New York: Monthly Review Press, 1973.

García, Hernán, Antonio Sierra, and Gilberto Pereira. *Wind in the Blood: Mayan Healing and Chinese Medicine.* Berkeley, CA: North Atlantic Books, 1999.

Gartelmann, K. D. *Las Huellas del Jaguar: Culturas Antiguas en el Ecuador.* Quito, Ecuador: Trama, 2006.

Gentry, Alwyn H., and C. L. Blaney. "Alternatives to Destruction: Using the Biodiversity of Tropical Forests," *Western Wildlands,* Vol. 16 (1990): 2–7.

Gentry, Alwyn H. *A Field Guide to the Families and Genera of Woody Plants of Northwest South America (Colombia, Ecuador, Peru), with Supplementary Notes on Herbaceous Taxa.* Chicago: University of Chicago Press, 1996.

George, Elder. *Dear Brothers and Sisters: Gender and Its Responsibility.* Baltimore: Publishamerica Inc., 1992.

Gheerbrant, Alain. *The Amazon: Past, Present and Future.* London: Thames and Hudson, 1992.

Gibran, Kahlil. *The Prophet.* New York: Alfred A. Knopf, 1976.

Giesso, Martin. *Historical Dictionary of Ancient South America*. Lanham, MD: Scarecrow Press, 2008.

Goldáraz, José Miguel, and Shirma Guayasamín. *Samay, La Herencia del Espíritu: Cosmovisión y Ética Naporunas*. Quito, Ecuador: CICAME, 2005.

Graves, Julia. *The Language of Plants: A Guide to the Doctrine of Signatures*. Great Barrington, MA: Steiner Books, 2012.

Greco, Thomas H. *Money: Understanding and Creating Alternatives to Legal Tender*. White River Junction, VT: Chelsea Green Publishing, 2001.

Grossinger, Richard. *Planet Medicine: From Stone Age Shamanism to Post-Industrial Healing*. Berkeley, CA: North Atlantic Books, 1990.

Guliayev, Valeri, and Iván Cevallos Calderón. *Viajes Precolombinos a las Américas: Mitos y Realidades*. Quito, Ecuador: Abya-Yala, 1992.

Hanh, Thích Nhát. *Going Home: Jesus and Buddha as Brothers*. New York: Riverhead Books, 1999.

Harner, Michael J. *Cave and Cosmos: Shamanic Encounters with Another Reality*. Berkeley, CA: North Atlantic Books, 2013.

Harner, Michael J. *The Jívaro, People of the Sacred Waterfalls*. Berkeley, CA: University of California Press, 1972.

Harner, Michael. *The Way of the Shaman*. New York: HarperCollins, 1980.

Harpignies, J. P. (ed.). *Visionary Plant Consciousness: The Shamanic Teachings of the Plant World*. Rochester, VT: Park Street Press, 2007.

Harris, James G., and Melinda Woolf Harris. *Plant Identification Terminology: An Illustrated Glossary*. Spring Lake, UT: Spring Lake Publishing, 1994.

Head, Suzanne, and Robert Heinzman. *Lessons of the Rainforest*. San Francisco: Sierra Club Books, 1990.

Huang, Runtian. *Treasured Qigong of Traditional Medical School*. Hong Kong: Hai Feng Pub. Co., 1994.

Jones, Kenneth. *Pau d'Arco: Immune Power from the Rain Forest*. Rochester, VT: Healing Arts Press, 1993.

Jung, C. G., and Meredith Sabini. *The Earth has a Soul: The Nature Writings of C. G. Jung*. Berkeley, CA: North Atlantic Books, 2002.

Kane, Joe. *Savages*. New York: Knopf, 1995.

Keyes, Ken. *The Hundredth Monkey*. St. Mary, KY: Vision Books, 1981.

Kimerling, Judith, and Susan Henriksen. *Amazon Crude*. New York: Natural Resources Defense Council, 1991.

Kutsche, Paul. *Field Ethnography: A Manual for Doing Cultural Anthropology*. Upper Saddle River, NJ: Prentice Hall, 1998.

Labaca Ugarte, Alejandro. *Crónica Huaorani*. Quito, Ecuador: CICAME, Vicariato Apostólico de Aguarico, 1988.

Labate, Beatriz Caiuby, and Wladimir Sena Araújo. *O Uso Ritual da Ayahuasca*. Campinas, São Paulo, Brazil: FAPESP, 2002.

Lamb, F. Bruce, and Manuel Córdova-Rios. *Wizard of the Upper Amazon: The Story of Manuel Córdova-Rios*. Berkeley, CA: North Atlantic Books, 1974.

Lamb, F. Bruce. *Rio Tigre and Beyond: The Amazon Jungle Medicine of Manuel Córdova*. Berkeley, CA: North Atlantic Books, 1985.

Langdon, E. Jean Matteson, and Gerhard Baer. *Portals of Power: Shamanism in South America*. Albuquerque: University of New Mexico Press, 1992.

Langdon, E. Jean Matteson. *The Siona Medical System: Beliefs and Behavior*. Ann Arbor, MI: Xerox Univ. Microfilms, 1974.

Laszlo, Ervin. *The Chaos Point: The World at the Crossroads*. Charlottesville, VA: Hampton Roads Publishing Co., 2006.

Leeming, David Adams. *Mythology: The Voyage of the Hero*. New York: Harper & Row, 1981.

Lévi-Strauss, Claude. *Myth and Meaning: Cracking the Code of Culture*. New York: Schocken Books, 1995.

Lévi-Strauss, Claude. *Tristes Tropiques*. New York: Penguin Books, 1992.

Llosa, Mario. *The Storyteller*. New York: Penguin Books, 1990.

López, Mariana, and Hugo Luzuriaga. *El Hombre que Cura el Cáncer*. Quito, Ecuador: Abya-Yala, 2000.

Losier, Michael J. *Law of Attraction: The Science of Attracting More of What You Want and Less of What You Don't*. Victoria, BC: M. J. Losier, 2006.

Lovelock, James. *Gaia: A New Look at Life on Earth*. Oxford: Oxford University Press, 1987.

Luna, Luis Eduardo, and Pablo Amaringo. *Ayahuasca Visions: The Religious Iconography of a Peruvian Shaman*. Berkeley, CA: North Atlantic Books, 1991.

Luna, Luis Eduardo, and Steven F. White. *Ayahuasca Reader: Encounters with the Amazon's Sacred Vine*. Santa Fe, NM: Synergetic Press, 2000.

McKenna, Terence K. *Food of the Gods: The Search for the Original Tree of Knowledge: A Radical History of Plants, Drugs, and Human Evolution*. New York: Bantam Books, 1992.

McKenna, Terence K., and Dennis J. McKenna. *The Invisible Landscape: Mind, Hallucinogens, and the I Ching*. San Francisco: HarperSanFrancisco, 1993.

McNiff, Shaun. *Art as Medicine: Creating a Therapy of the Imagination*. Boston: Shambhala, 1992.

Metzner, Ralph, and Jace C. Callaway. *Ayahuasca: Hallucinogens, Consciousness, and the Spirit of Nature.* New York: Thunder's Mouth Press, 1999.

Meyers, N. "Threatened Biotas: 'Hotspots' in Tropical Forests," *Environmentalist* 8 (1988): 187–208.

Milagros, Israel. "Una Ventana al Yaje," *Ecuador Terra Incognita*, No. 7 (2000): 4–9.

Miller, Jonathon. "El Jardin del Aguarico," *Ecuador Terra Incognita*, No. 11 (2001): 16–18.

Miller, Jonathon. "Napo-Galeras: Entre la Neblina y el Misterio," *Ecuador Terra Incognita*, No. 20 (2002).

Miller Weisberger, Jonathon. "Granite Spheres of Caño Island," *Bulletin of Primitive Technology*, No. 38 (2009).

Miller Weisberger, Jonathon. *Criterios Técnicos y Científicos para la ampliación del Parque Nacional Sumaco Napo Galeras y Diseños para el Desarrollo local Sostenible en sus Zonas Periféricas,* "Technical and Scientific Criteria for the Enlargement of the Sumaco Napo-Galeras National Park and Designs for Local Sustainable Development in its Periphery Zones." Quito, Ecuador, Fundación OSA (2010).

Miller Weisberger, Jonathon. *Reserva de Biosfera Sumaco: Iniciativas a Favor de la Biodiversidad y sus Habitantes Locales. Un Informe Educativo y Llamado a la acción,* "Sumaco Biosphere Reserve: Initiatives in Favor of Biodiversity and its Local Inhabitants." Quito, Ecuador: Fundación OSA (2010).

Mindell, Arnold. *The Shaman's Body: A New Shamanism for Transforming Health, Relationships, and Community.* San Francisco: HarperSanFrancisco, 1993.

Mitchell, Andrew W. *The Enchanted Canopy: Secrets from the Rainforest Roof.* London: Collins, 1986.

Moritz, Andreas. *The Amazing Liver Cleanse.* Bloomington, IN: 1st Books Library, 1998.

Moritz, Andreas. *The Key to Health and Rejuvenation: Breakthrough Medicine for the 21st Century!* Bloomington, IN: 1st Books Library, 2000.

Moya, Ruth. *Requiem por los Espejos y los Tigres: Una Aproximación a la Literatura y Lengua Secoyas.* Quito, Ecuador: Oficina Regional de Cultura para América Latina y el Caribe, 1992.

Muratorio, Blanca. *The Life and Times of Grandfather Alonso: Culture and History in the Upper Amazon.* New Brunswick, NJ: Rutgers University Press, 1991.

Naranjo, Plutarco. *Ayahuasca: Etnomedicina y Mitología*. Quito, Ecuador: Ediciones Libri Mundi, 1983.

Narby, Jeremy. *The Cosmic Serpent: DNA and the Origins of Knowledge*. New York: Jeremy P. Tarcher/Putnam, 1998.

Neihardt, John Gneisenau. *When the Tree Flowered: An Authentic Tale of the Old Sioux World*. New York: Pocket Books, 1973.

Ni, Hua Ching. *Attaining Unlimited Life: The Teachings of Chuang Tzu*. Los Angeles: Shrine of the Eternal Breath of Tao, College of Tao and Traditional Chinese Healing, 1989.

Ni, Hua Ching. *The Book of Changes and the Unchanging Truth*. Malibu, CA: Shrine of the Eternal Breath of Tao, 1983.

Ni, Hua Ching. *Heavenly Way: The Union of Tao and Universe*. Los Angeles: Shrine of the Eternal Breath of Tao, 1981.

Ni, Hua Ching. *Tao: The Subtle Universal Law and the Integral Way of Life*. Santa Monica, CA: SevenStar Communications Group, 1993.

Ni, Hua Ching. *The Complete Works of Lao Tzu: Tao Teh Ching and Hua Hu Ching*. Santa Monica, CA: SevenStar Communications Group, 1993.

Ni, Hua Ching. *The Power of Natural Healing*. Los Angeles: Shrine of the Eternal Breath of Tao, College of Tao and Traditional Chinese Healing, 1990.

Ni, Hua Ching. *Workbook for Spiritual Development of All People*. Rev. ed. Malibu, CA: Shrine of the Eternal Breath of Tao, 1992.

Ni, Hua, and Maoshing Ni. *Evolve Heaven on Earth: Foundation of a New Spiritual Life*. Los Angeles: Tao of Wellness Press, 2012.

Ni, Maoshing. *Secrets of Self-Healing: Harness Nature's Power to Heal Common Ailments, Boost your Vitality, and Achieve Optimum Wellness*. New York: Avery, 2008.

Nielsen, Arya. *Gua Sha: Traditional Technique for Modern Practice*. Edinburgh, Scotland: Churchill Livingstone, 1995.

Nietzsche, Friedrich Wilhelm, and Duncan Large. *Twilight of the Idols, or, How to Philosophize with a Hammer*. Oxford World's Classics. Oxford: Oxford University Press, 2008.

Ott, Jonathan. *Pharmacotheon: Entheogenic Drugs, Their Plant Sources and History*. Kennewick, WA: Natural Products Co., 1993.

Ott, Jonathan. *The Cacahuatl Eater: Ruminations of an Unabashed Chocolate Addict, Replete with Divers Historical and Scientific Discursions of both an Entertaining and Informative Nature*. Vashon, WA: Natural Products Co., 1985.

Paracelsus, Theophrastus. *The Doctrine of Signatures.* Whitefish, MT: Kessinger Publishing, 2010.

Payaguaje, Fernando, and Miguel Angel Cabodevilla. *The Yage Drinker.* Quito, Ecuador: CICAME, 2008.

Payaguaje, Matilde, and Jorge León. *Ñumine'eo—Mito y Cosmovisión Secoya.* Quito, Ecuador: PETROECUADOR, Gerencia de Protección Ambiental, 2002.

Payne, Buryl. *Magnetic Healing: Advanced Techniques for the Application of Magnetic Forces.* Twin Lakes, WI: Lotus Light Pub., 1997.

Pedersen, H., and H. Balslev. *Ecuadorian Palms for Agroforestry.* Aarhus, Denmark: Aarhus University Botanical Institute, 1990.

Pendell, Dale. *Pharmako/Poeia: Plant Powers, Poisons, and Herbcraft.* Berkeley, CA: North Atlantic Books, 2009.

Pinchbeck, Daniel. *Breaking Open the Head: A Psychedelic Journey into the Heart of Contemporary Shamanism.* New York: Broadway Books, 2002.

Plotkin, Mark J. *Tales of a Shaman's Apprentice: An Ethnobotanist Searches for New Medicines in the Amazon Rain Forest.* New York: Penguin Books, 1994.

Polari de Alverga, Alex. *Forest of Visions: Ayahuasca, Amazonian Spirituality, and the Santo Daime Tradition.* Rochester, VT: Park Street Press, 1999.

Pollan, Michael. *The Botany of Desire: A Plant's Eye View of the World.* New York: Random House, 2001.

Rätsch, Christian. *The Encyclopedia of Psychoactive Plants: Ethnopharmacology and Its Applications.* Rochester, VT: Park Street Press, 2005.

Reichel-Dolmatoff, Gerardo. *The Forest Within: The World-View of the Tukano Amazonian Indians.* Totnes, England: Themis, 1996.

Reichel-Dolmatoff, Gerardo. *The Shaman and the Jaguar: A Study of Narcotic Drugs Among the Indians of Colombia.* Philadelphia: Temple University Press, 1975.

Reps, Paul. *Zen Flesh, Zen Bones: A Collection of Zen & Pre-Zen Writings.* Garden City, NY: Anchor Books/Doubleday, 1961.

Rios, Marlene. *Visionary Vine: Hallucinogenic Healing in the Peruvian Amazon.* Prospect Heights, IL: Waveland Press, 1984.

Rival, Laura M. *Hijos del Sol, Padres del Jaguar: Los Huaorani de Ayer y Hoy.* Quito, Ecuador: Ediciones Abya-Yala, 1996.

Rival, Laura M. *Trekking Through History: The Huaorani of Amazonian Ecuador.* New York: Columbia University Press, 2002.

Rosenberg, Marshall. *Nonviolent Communication: A Language of Life.* Encinitas, CA: PuddleDancer Press, 2003.

Sarkís, Alia, and Víctor Manuel Campos. *Curanderismo Tradicional del Costarricense: Curación con Plantas y Remedios Caseros*. San José, Costa Rica: Lehmann Editores, 1985.

Savinelli, Alfred. *Plants of Power: Native American Ceremony and the Use of Sacred Plants*. Summertown, TN: Native Voices, 2002.

Schultes, Richard Evans, Albert Hofmann, and Christian Rätsch. *Plants of the Gods: Their Sacred, Healing, and Hallucinogenic Powers*. Rochester, VT: Healing Arts Press, 2001.

Schultes, Richard Evans, and Robert F. Raffauf. *The Healing Forest: Medicinal and Toxic Plants of Northwest Amazonia*. Portland, OR: Dioscorides Press, 1990.

Schultes, Richard Evans, and Robert F. Raffauf. *Vine of the Soul: Medicine Men, their Plants and Rituals in the Colombian Amazon*. Santa Fe, NM: Synergetic Press, 2004.

Schultes, Richard Evans. *Where the Gods Reign: Plants and Peoples of the Colombian Amazon*. Oracle, AZ: Synergetic Press, 1988.

Seaborg, David. *Honor Thy Sow Bug*. Berkeley, CA: Beatitude Press, 2008.

Seed, John. *Thinking Like a Mountain: Towards a Council of All Beings*. Philadelphia: New Society Publishers, 1988.

Serrano P., Vladimir (compilador). *Ciencia Andina*, Quito, Ecuador: Ediciones Abya-Yala, 1997.

Siy, Alexandra. *The Waorani: People of the Ecuadorian Rain Forest*. New York: Dillon Press, 1993.

Solís, Misael. *Vademecum de Plantas Medicinales del Ecuador*. Quito, Ecuador: FESO, Ediciones Abya-Yala, 1992.

Stamets, Paul, and C. Dusty Wu Yao. *MycoMedicinals: An Informational Treatise on Mushrooms*. Olympia, WA: MycoMedia, 2002.

Talbot, Michael. *The Holographic Universe*. New York: HarperCollins Publishers, 1991.

Tasorinki, Yanaanka. *Chamanismo Andino-Amazónico: Maestros y Plantas Maestras de Poder, Coca, Ayahuasca, San Pedro, Tabaco, Toe*. Cusco, Perú: Editorial Piki, 2009.

Taussig, Michael. *Shamanism, Colonialism, and the Wild Man: A Study in Terror and Healing*. Chicago: University of Chicago Press, 1987.

Thompson, Lucy. *To the American Indian: Reminiscences of a Yurok Woman*. Berkeley, CA: Heyday Books in conjunction with P. E. Palmquist, 1991.

Tierra, Michael, and David Frawley. *Planetary Herbology: An Integration of Western Herbs into the Traditional Chinese and Ayurvedic Systems*. Twin Lakes, WI: Lotus Press, 1988.

Torre, Stella de la. *Primates de La Amazonía del Ecuador.* Quito, Ecuador: SIMBIOE, 2000.

Towler, Solala. *A Gathering of Cranes: Bringing the Tao to the West.* Eugene, OR: Abode of the Eternal Tao, 1996.

Turolla, Pino. *Beyond the Andes: My Search for the Origins of Pre-Inca Civilization.* New York: Harper & Row, 1980.

Uzendoski, Michael, and Edith Felicia Tapuy. *The Ecology of the Spoken Word: Amazonian Storytelling and Shamanism among the Napo Runa.* Urbana, IL: University of Illinois Press, 2012.

Uzendoski, Michael. *The Napo Runa of Amazonian Ecuador.* Urbana, IL: University of Illinois Press, 2005.

Weil, Andrew. *Natural Health, Natural Medicine: A Comprehensive Manual for Wellness and Self-Care.* Boston: Houghton Mifflin, 1990.

Wesche, Rolf, and Andy Drumm. *Defending Our Rainforest: A Guide to Community-Based Ecotourism in the Ecuadorian Amazon.* Quito, Ecuador: Acción Amazonia, 1999.

Whitten, Norman E. *Sacha Runa: Ethnicity and Adaptation of Ecuadorian Jungle Quichua.* Urbana, IL: University of Illinois Press, 1976.

Whitten, Norman E., and Dorothea S. Whitten. *Puyo Runa: Imagery and Power in Modern Amazonia.* Urbana, IL: University of Illinois Press, 2008.

Wilbert, Johannes. *Tobacco and Shamanism in South America.* New Haven: Yale University Press, 1987.

Willard, Terry. *Reishi Mushroom: Herb of Spiritual Potency and Medical Wonder.* Issaquah, WA: Sylvan Press, 1990.

Wilson, Edward O. *The Diversity of Life.* New York: W. W. Norton, 1993.

Yang, Jwing. *Tai Chi Secrets of the Ancient Masters: Selected Readings with Commentary.* Boston: YMAA Publication Center, 1999.

Yang, Jwing. *The Essence of Tai Chi Chi Kung: Health and Martial Arts.* Jamaica Plain, MA: YMAA Publication Center, 1990.

Yang, Li. *Book of Changes and Traditional Chinese Medicine.* Beijing, China: Beijing Science and Technology Press, 1998.

Yépez, Pablo, S. de la Torre, C. E. Cerón, and W. Palacios. (eds.) *Al Inicio del Sendero: Estudios Etnobotánicos Secoya.* Quito, Ecuador: Ed. Arboleda, 2005.

Yépez, Pablo, Stella de la Torre, Hernán Payaguaje, Alfredo Payaguaje (editores). *Al final del sendero? Aportes la conservación del medio ambiente y la cultura Secoya.* Quito, Ecuador: Fundación VIHOMA, 2010.

INDEX

ACKNOWLEDGMENTS

Thank you to all the people mentioned in this book, to my friends, wisdom teachers, and elders who took the time and confided in me their insights and experiences. I also wish to send special thanks to Don Bright for his help with the color plates and Keith Hinman for his photos—and plenty of technical support. Thank you Murray Cooper for the great photos. Thank you James Ficklin, Bruce Harlow, Matthew Legg, and Daniel Pinchbeck. To Dr. Laura Rival for reviewing Chapter 7 and the Waorani information presented here, thank you. Thank you to all the staff at North Atlantic Books and designer Suzanne Albertson. The biggest heartfelt thanks beyond words to Thomas Wang, Nathan Horowitz, and Kathy Glass: your support and encouragement all through this project have made *Rainforest Medicine* possible.

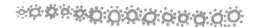

Resources for Getting Involved

Guaria de Osa Ecolodge on Costa Rica's mega-biologically diverse, people-friendly Osa Peninsula wilderness. Visit our calendar of events for upcoming retreats with guest cultural masters: www.guariadeosa .com

To strengthen the bridge between rainforest conservation and good health, drink guayusa tea. To order: www.guayusateahouse.com

Rainforest and wildlife conservation initiatives, cultural revalidation efforts, volunteer opportunities, and the Octo Blog: www.4biodiversity .org

ABOUT THE AUTHOR AND CONTRIBUTORS

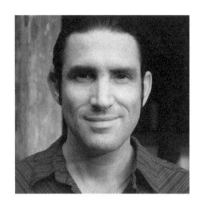

Jonathon Miller Weisberger

Raised to age fifteen in Ecuador and then working there as a young man between 1990 and 2000, Jonathon Miller Weisberger, a.k.a. "Sparrow," lived and worked among five indigenous peoples' communities in the upper Amazon. During those years he was influential in the creation of Napo-Galeras National Park in Ecuador. He participated in the demarcation of Waorani territory and in groundwork that helped the Secoya people retain a significant tract of their ancestral homelands. With a Kichwa-speaking family near Puyo, he collaborated to create a biological reserve bordering Sangay National Park, and in western Ecuador he volunteered in the collaborative establishment of Los Cedros, a biological reserve that protects rare coastal cloud forests rich in endemic species. During this time he delved deeply into the region's mythology while also documenting plant lore, pressing and drying herbarium specimens, discovering five new species (including a new palm from Napo-Galeras), and interviewing traditional elders (accumulating hundred of hours of audio recordings in the process). One of these recordings was edited into an album, released by England's Tumi Music Co., called *Waorani Waponi, Acapelo Chanting in the Amazon*. Today he stewards his family business, Guaria de Osa Ecolodge (www.guariadeosa.com), a rainforest/ocean discovery center located on Costa Rica's Osa peninsula. He continues to guide annual tours into the Ecuadorian Amazon and to collaborate on various conservation projects. His website and blog can be found at www.4biodiversity.org.

Editors

The editors collaborated extensively with the author on a volunteer basis to promote the message of cultural revalidation and rainforest conservation.

Based in the redwood bioregion of northern California, **Kathy Glass** is a writer, editor, traveler, and life-long environmental activist with a passion for the last great forests on Earth. She has worked with North Atlantic Books for more than twenty years, including helping to edit Pablo Amaringo's *Ayahuasca Visions* in 1991, when she first read about rainforest medicine and met Pablo in California. Thanks to friend of the forest James Ficklin for connecting Kathy and Jonathon in 2010; as a result, this book has become a reality.

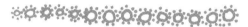

Originally from the USA, **Nathan Horowitz** lived for four years in Latin America before settling in Vienna, Austria, in 2000. He teaches English at universities and proofreads. Translator of *The Yage Drinker* to English from Spanish, Horowitz brought his knowledge of the Secoya culture to his editing of this manuscript. He and the author are old friends, having met in the Amazon in 1995.

Illustrators

Thomas Wang

Black-and-white illustrations of myths and legends

An instructor in the environmental horticulture department at City College of San Francisco, Thomas Wang focuses on the cultivation of gardens and gardeners, and the communion with plants and animals. He says about his volunteer artistic contributions to *Rainforest Medicine*: "I see these drawings as a mix of science and mythology, which is rare in botanical literature, and I'm thankful for the stories as well as the opportunity to illustrate them for a large audience. They are strong legends that pull hard, like power and light together, and in articulating the Amazonian universe I can see the practical pathways these people used to access the energetic realms." More of Thomas Wang's art and stories can be found at www.missionblueproject.com.

Pablo Amaringo

Cover art and color reproductions of oil paintings

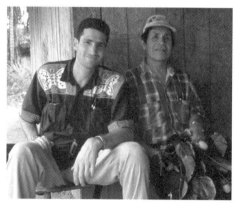

The author (L) and Pablo Amaringo, 1994

Pablo Amaringo (1943–2009) was a Peruvian artist and retired ayahuasquero (in his later years), immortalized through his visionary and landscape art and in the memories of those touched by his far-reaching spirit. The founder of the Neo-Amazonico style of painting and personal friend of the author, Pablo Amaringo is described and referenced throughout this book. (For example, see Chapter 2, endnote 3.) Pablo granted permission to the author to sell reproductions of some of his visionary art, and high-quality prints of the artwork reproduced here and dozens more are available at www.guariadeosa.com, with 100% of sales channeled to charity organizations for rainforest conservation and cultural heritage revalidation projects.

Paintings featured in this book

See the copyright page for details about the book's cover art.

Cascada del Bosque, *"Rainforest Waterfall,"* 2000

One can almost see the water flowing and hear the colorful tanagers in the foreground filling the forest with song as they hop from branch to branch in joy and glee. This painting was created with acrylic paints and a fine brush, bringing the subtle purity found in nature to art.

Poderes del Sumiruna, *"Powers of the Sumiruna,"* **2002**
A sumiruna is an advanced spiritual master, a shaman, who has obtained the ability to enter the dimensions of the water. Here he is seen summoning his spirit allies to effect a complex cure, concentrating on the places where he has accomplished his dietas, the process on behalf of which he has obtained his spiritual powers and authority. The animals, medicinal plants, and symbols represent energetic emanations and astrological phenomena, as well as artifacts of the culture. The powerful and healing energies that he summons make others in the ceremony rise in ecstatic dance. The ayahuasca vine is seen on the right and chagropanga on the left. Purple, the color of the sumiruna, represents deep and far-reaching spiritual merits.

Cosmología Espiritual, *"Spiritual Cosmology,"* **2002**
In this illustration of the three powers of the Peruvian mestizo ayahuasca-drinking tradition, we see three giant "designs serpents." The Wairamama's scintillating energetic aura emanates from the ayahuasca vine, depicted here in full flower, at left. The Yakumama comes from the water and the Sachamama from the forest, all joining together to form a sacred seal of protection around the drinkers, seen as the rainbow aura. The blackcoiled serpent is the Yana-yakumama, the "Black water mother," with the Supai Lancha cruising on its back. Angelic beings descend upon the scene, as do sirenas (mermaids) and many other powerful beings such as ancestors, mythic immortals, and spirits revealed by the sacramental plant medicine, ayahuasca. As in the majority of don Pablo's visionary artworks, we see someone being healed, and someone else purging negativities and toxins. Pablo would relate the name of each entity with precision, and could speak for hours about each of his paintings.

Chirapa Callu, *"Rainbow Tongue,"* **gouache on Arches paper, 2001**
Surrounding a group of mestizo healers are spirits transcendent of time and space whose rainbow tongues indicate that profound spiritual wisdom is being transmitted to the drinkers like information on scrolls pouring from the mouths of divine beings. The drinkers are

being allowed to understand the deeper truths of life that can only be represented symbolically. The orchid, a symbol of the newness of nature, also represents the knowledge that is related to renewal and the ability to transform heavy and brute energy into sublime energies, a necessity in the process of learning to heal. Messenger birds such as the paradise tanager (lower right) carry the supplications of the healers through song to the celestial beings.

Agustin Payaguaje

Sketches and symbols

Known also as "Tintin," traditional Secoya elder **Agustin Rafael Payaguaje** contributed sketches that appear throughout the book, such as those on xxiii (Man Reaching Toward Knowledge) and on all the chapter heads. He is discussed in this book on pages 97 and 145, with a color photo in the center section.

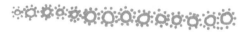

The author (JMW) provided illustrations of petroglyphs from the Misahualli River valley in Napo Province, Ecuador, and of Secoya designs (page 184). Color photography is credited on the color plates and when not specifically credited is by the author, JMW. All guest images courtesy of the artists and photographers. Thank you!